ub.com and http://connect.springerpub.com/

ces Private Ltd.

ng Company, LLC.

print of Springer Publishing Company, LLC.

ce. Research and clinical experience are continually
icular our understanding of proper treatment and
, and publisher have made every effort to ensure
in accordance with the state of knowledge at the
evertheless, the authors, editors, and publisher are
ssions or for any consequences from application of
ake no warranty, expressed or implied, with respect
. Every reader should examine carefully the pack-
rug and should carefully check whether the dosage
e contraindications stated by the manufacturer dif-
his book. Such examination is particularly important
sed or have been newly released on the market.

-Publication Data

editor. | Miller-Chism, Courtney, editor. |

ology / editors, Martha Pritchett Mims,
omina Sosa.
Medical Publishing, [2020] | Includes
index.
int) | LCCN 2019043406 (ebook) | ISBN
SBN 9780826149879 (ebook)
iseases
) | LCC RC636 (ebook) | NLM WH 120 | DDC

n.loc.gov/2019043405
ps://lccn.loc.gov/2019043406

ceive discount rates on bulk purchases.
stomize our books to meet your needs.
n please contact: sales@springerpub.com

d products purchased from third-party sellers are not
icity, or access to any included digital components.

America.

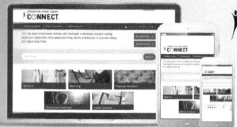

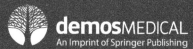

Visit our website at www.Springer[...]
home

ISBN: 978-0-8261-4986-2
ebook ISBN: 978-0-8261-4987-9
DOI: 10.1891/9780826149879

Acquisitions Editor: David D'Addon[...]
Compositor: Exeter Premedia Servi[...]

Copyright © 2020 Springer Publish[...]

Demos Medical Publishing is an im[...]

Library of Congress Cataloging-i[...]

Names: Mims, Martha Pritchett, e[...]
Sosa, Iberia Romina, editor.
Title: Handbook of benign hema[...]
Courtney Miller-Chism, Iberia R[...]
Description: New York : Demos M[...]
bibliographical references and [...]
Identifiers: LCCN 2019043405 (p[...]
9780826149862 (paperback) | I[...]
Subjects: MESH: Hematologic D[...]
Classification: LCC RC636 (prin[...]
616.1/5—dc23
LC record available at https://lc[...]
LC ebook record available at ht[...]

Contact us to re[...]
We can also cu[...]
For more informati[...]

Publisher's Note: New and use[...]
guaranteed for quality, authen[...]

Printed in the United States of [...]
19 20 21 22 / 5 4 3 2 1

Har[...]
Ben[...]

Edito[...]

Martha[...]
Dan L. [...]
Chief, S[...]
Associa[...]
Dan L. [...]
Baylor [...]
Houstor[...]

Courtne[...]
Assistan[...]
Departm[...]
Baylor C[...]
Houston,[...]

Iberia Ro[...]
Assistant[...]
Departme[...]
Baylor Co[...]
Houston, [...]

Contents

v

Contributors

Samer Al-Hadidi, MD, Fellow, Section of Hematology and Oncology, Department of Medicine, Baylor College of Medicine, Houston, Texas

Nicole Canon, MD, PGY3 Resident, Internal Medicine Resident, Baylor College of Medicine, Houston, Texas

Elaine Chang, MD, Medical Officer, Food and Drug Adminstration, Silver Spring, Maryland

Clay T. Cohen, MD, Instructor, Department of Pediatrics, Section of Hematology and Oncology, Texas Children's Cancer and Hematology Centers, Baylor College of Medicine, Houston, Texas

Rosa Díaz, MD, Assistant Professor, Department of Pediatrics, Section of Hematology and Oncology, Texas Children's Cancer and Hematology Centers, Baylor College of Medicine, Houston, Texas

Mahmoud Gaballa, MD, Fellow, Section of Hematology and Oncology, Department of Medicine, Baylor College of Medicine, Houston, Texas

Hatice Gur, MD, Physician, Department of Pathology and Laboratory Medicine, Division of Hematopathology, Northwell Health, Lake Success, New York

Hussein Hamad, MD, Fellow, Section of Hematology and Oncology, Baylor College of Medicine, Houston, Texas

Hyojeong Han, MD, Clinical Postdoctoral Fellow, Department of Pediatrics, Section of Hematology and Oncology, Texas Children's Hospital/Baylor College of Medicine, Houston, Texas

Elizabeth A. Hartwell, MD, Associate Professor, Department of Pathology and Immunology, Baylor College of Medicine, Houston, Texas

Stephanie Holdener, MD, Resident, Department of Pathology and Immunology, Baylor College of Medicine, Houston, Texas

Quillan Huang, MD, Assistant Professor of Medicine, Section of Hematology and Oncology, Baylor College of Medicine, Houston, Texas

Safiya Joseph, BS, Research Assistant, Department of Medicine, Baylor College of Medicine, Houston, Texas

Rosetta Lee, PharmD, Clinical Pharmacy Specialist, Department of Pharmacy, Houston Methodist Hospital, Houston, Texas

Young-na Lee-Kim, MD, Assistant Professor, Department of Pediatrics, Section of Hematology and Oncology, Baylor College of Medicine, Houston, Texas

Premal Lulla, MD, Assistant Professor of Medicine, Center for Cell and Gene Therapy, Section of Hematology and Oncology, Baylor College of Medicine, Houston, Texas

Harish Madala, MD, Physician, Hematology and Oncology, Southwest Virginia Cancer Center, Norton, Virginia

Matthew Miller, MD, Instructor, Department of Pediatrics, Section of Hematology and Oncology, Texas Children's Cancer and Hematology Centers, Baylor College of Medicine, Houston, Texas

Courtney Miller-Chism, MD, Assistant Professor, Department of Medicine, Section of Hematology and Oncology, Baylor College of Medicine, Houston, Texas

Martha Pritchett Mims, MD, PhD, Dan L. Duncan Professor and Chief, Section of Hematology and Oncology; Associate Director for Clinical Research, Dan L. Duncan Cancer Center, Baylor College of Medicine, Houston, Texas

Kirtan D. Nautiyal, MD, Physician, Methodist Hospital, Sugar Land, Texas

Patrick E. Prath, MD, Fellow, Department of Medicine, Section of Hematology and Oncology, Baylor College of Medicine, Houston, Texas

Srijana Rai, MD, Fellow, Department of Medicine, Section of Hematology and Oncology, Baylor College of Medicine, Houston, Texas

Carlos A. Ramos, MD, Associate Professor, Department of Medicine, Section of Hematology and Oncology, Baylor College of Medicine, Houston, Texas

Meredith Reyes, MD, Clinical Assistant Professor, Department of Pathology and Immunology, Baylor College of Medicine, Houston, Texas

Gustavo Rivero, MD, Assistant Professor, Department of Medicine, Section of Hematology and Oncology, Baylor College of Medicine, Houston, Texas

Sarah E. Sartain, MD, Assistant Professor, Department of Pediatrics, Section of Hematology and Oncology, Texas Children's Hospital/Baylor College of Medicine, Houston, Texas

Sumaira Shafi, MD, Physician, Hematology/Oncology, Camden Clark Medical Center, Parkersburg, West Virginia

Iberia Romina Sosa, MD, PhD, Assistant Professor, Department of Medicine, Section of Hematology and Oncology, Baylor College of Medicine, Houston, Texas

Samer A. Srour, MBCHB, Assistant Professor, Stem Cell Transplantation, The University of Texas MD Anderson Cancer Center, Houston, Texas

Robert Streck, **MD**, Medicine Resident, Department of Medicine, Baylor College of Medicine, Houston, Texas

Sravanti Teegavarapu, MD, Assistant Professor, Department of Medicine, Section of Hematology and Oncology, Baylor College of Medicine, Houston, Texas

Mark Udden, MD, Professor, Department of Medicine, Section of Hematology and Oncology, Baylor College of Medicine, Houston, Texas

Anthony Wiseman, MD, Clinical Fellow, Department of Medicine, Section of Hematology and Oncology, Baylor College of Medicine, Houston, Texas

Sarvari Yellapragada, MD, Associate Professor, Department of Medicine, Section of Hematology and Oncology, Baylor College of Medicine, Houston, Texas

.

Preface

As hematologists, we would not describe nonmalignant hematology as benign, but the name is well accepted and well understood to represent all those disorders that one would not characterize as cancer. The notion to create this book came from experiences with our fellows who complained of not having a succinct source to refer to on rounds. Our discussions identified not only a need but also an opportunity to assemble a resource that would be useful to hematology fellows and practicing hematologists and oncologists who are often pressed into service when no hematologist is available. The case-based approach we settled on synthesizes our experiences with difficult clinical problems with a brief background, a carefully assembled case, and a step-by-step approach to diagnosis and treatment. We have tried to identify pitfalls in diagnosis and treatment along with sections on prognosis and future directions. Key points are summarized at the end of each section to reinforce the important issues. Where useful we have included photos of peripheral smears, marrow aspirates, lymph node biopsies, and radiographic images. High-yield tables are included in all chapters for easy reference. Our fellows were incorporated into the writing of this handbook not only as an academic experience for them but also to ensure that the book addresses those points that are critical or difficult for clinicians. We sincerely hope you find value in this work.

As with any large project, we hit barriers and overcame them and learned in the process. We acknowledge the tremendous work of our fellows and faculty colleagues in the writing and rewriting of the chapters that make up this book. A special word of thanks goes to our partners, Jonathan Chism, PhD, Daniel Cohen, MD, PhD, and Don Mims, who supported us through the process of assembling this book.

1 Overview of Normal Hematopoiesis

Mahmoud Gaballa and Carlos A. Ramos

INTRODUCTION

The formed elements of blood include various types of cells or cell fragments, each with different morphology and function. These elements are produced via a process known as hematopoiesis, during which hematopoietic stem cells (HSCs) proliferate and undergo self-renewal or differentiation into lineage-committed progenitors, which continue to differentiate into mature blood cells. This ability to self-renew and the ability to differentiate are two key characteristics of HSCs necessary for normal hematopoiesis (1,2). Self-renewal is the process by which stem cells enter the cell cycle to divide and give rise to more stem cells, thus preserving the stem cell pool. On the other hand, differentiation allows HSCs to develop into more mature cells with progressive lineage commitment. In general, the ability to self-renew diminishes as maturation and lineage commitment progresses.

The capacity of HSCs to differentiate into multiple cell lines is termed multipotency. The hematopoietic hierarchy is a well-orchestrated process that starts with HSCs developing into myeloid and lymphoid progenitor cells. Myeloid progenitor cells continue to develop into erythrocytes, platelets (through fragmentation of megakaryocytes), neutrophils, monocytes, basophils, and eosinophils. In contrast, lymphoid progenitor cells give rise to B lymphocytes, T lymphocytes, natural killer (NK) cells, and a population of dendritic cells (Figure 1.1). Thus, a very complex process in the bone marrow gives rise to at least 10 cellular elements on a daily basis. Blood cell numbers are sustained within relatively narrow ranges through this process, with the ability to boost production if needed in states of increased demand. In this chapter, we illustrate our current understanding of hematopoiesis, its stages, the cellular and non-cellular elements involved, and its regulation.

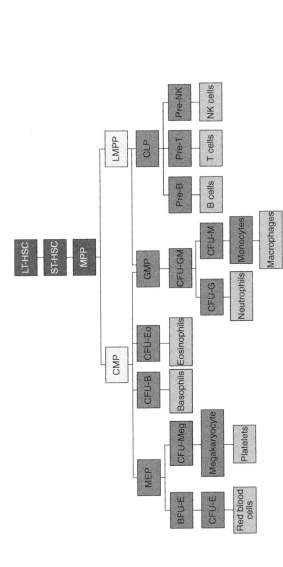

Figure 1.1 Hierarchy of hematopoiesis.

BFU-E, burst-forming unit-erythroid; CFU-B, colony-forming unit-basophil; CFU-E, colony-forming unit-erythrocyte; CFU-Eo, colony-forming unit-eosinophil; CFU-G, colony-forming unit-granulocyte; CFU-GM, colony-forming unit-granulocyte monocyte; CFU-M, colony-forming unit-monocyte; CFU-Meg, colony-forming unit-megakaryocyte; CLP, common lymphoid progenitor; CMP, common myeloid progenitor; GMP, granulocyte–macrophage progenitor; LMPP, lymphoid primed multipotent progenitor; LT-HSC, long-term hematopoietic progenitor; MEP, megakaryocyte–erythrocyte progenitor; MPP, hematopoietic multipotent progenitor; NK, natural killer; pre-NK, pre-natural killer; ST-HSC, short-term hematopoietic stem cell.

STAGES AND SITES OF HEMATOPOIESIS

Hematopoiesis starts during embryonic life and continues through fetal, neonatal, and adult life. Embryonic hematopoiesis comprises two waves of events. The first wave, often referred to as primitive hematopoiesis, takes place specifically in the extraembryonic yolk sac, where nucleated primitive erythrocytes are produced. This is a critical step for the development and survival of the embryo since those primitive erythrocytes are the first elements to facilitate oxygen transportation. In addition, myeloid cells produced in the yolk sac subsequently relocate to the central nervous system and skin to develop into microglia and Langerhans cells, respectively (3). In humans, primitive hematopoiesis lasts from day 19 until week 8 postconception. The second wave, characterized by intraembryonic hematopoiesis, takes place initially in the dorsal aorta (aorta–gonad–mesonephros or AGM region), where hematopoietic progenitors are produced from mesoderm derivatives (4). This process happens once in a lifetime and those cells later continue to develop to form adult HSCs, with the expression of major histocompatibility complex (MHC) class II and cluster of differentiation (CD)45.

In the fetus, hematopoiesis transitions first from the embryonic sites to the liver. At approximately 5 gestational weeks, the HSCs and progenitors travel from the yolk sac or AGM to the liver to establish hematopoiesis (5). At this stage of life, the liver serves as a vital hematopoietic organ where differentiation and expansion of HSCs take place, a process commonly referred to as definitive erythropoiesis (5). In addition, the placenta also becomes a major contributor to hematopoiesis, starting in fetal life and continuing until birth. Furthermore, some HSCs and progenitor cells leave the liver during fetal life and migrate to the spleen, where further differentiation into myeloid and lymphoid lineages occurs transiently (3).

At 4 to 5 months of gestation, hematopoiesis begins to occur in the bone marrow, a process termed medullary hematopoiesis, which continues after birth and throughout postnatal life. As we advance into adulthood, hematopoiesis slowly becomes confined to the skull, pelvic bones, vertebrae, and the metaphyseal region of long bones, with the diaphysis of long bones being gradually replaced with adipose tissue. Thus, the active bone marrow of children is proportionally much larger than that of adults, which is thought to occur due to the higher demand for red cells in neonatal and childhood life compared to adulthood. Importantly, in states of medullary insufficiency, as in patients with thalassemia and myelofibrosis, hematopoiesis can revert to its original sites, including the liver and spleen. This is termed extramedullary hematopoiesis. Figure 1.2 illustrates the sites of hematopoiesis in different stages of life.

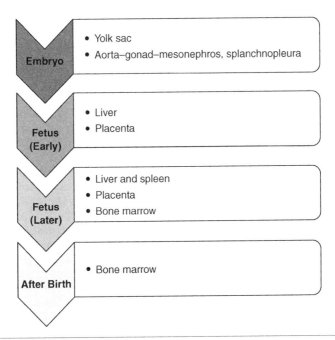

Figure 1.2 Sites of hematopoiesis in different stages of life.

HSCs AND THE HEMATOPOIETIC HIERARCHY

The hematopoietic differentiation cascade is akin to an inverted tree, starting with a small pool of HSCs that develop into a larger pool of progenitors, which then further differentiate into many intermediates and finally develop into different mature blood cells. As the cells travel down their hierarchy, they lose the ability to differentiate into other cell lines and progressively become committed to one lineage, that is, lineage-committed progenitors.

HSCs choose early whether to self-renew or to differentiate into more mature cells, with two models proposed to describe this choice, the stochastic (supportive) and the instructive. In the stochastic model, the choice of self-renewal versus differentiation is random. In contrast, in the instructive model, certain microenvironment factors and cytokines directly influence this decision. Notably, cytokines have critical but different roles in both models. In the instructive model, cytokines actively influence the decision, while in the stochastic model, cytokines do not influence the decision but support the survival and proliferation of progenitor cells that eventually differentiate into mature cells (6). This issue remains controversial with conflicting data supporting both models.

HSCs are further subclassified as long term (LT-HSCs) and short term (ST-HSCs). The main role of LT-HSCs is self-renewal, and most of their progeny will follow this pathway, while lesser numbers become ST-HSCs (1). ST-HSCs have lower self-renewal potential and their predominant fate is to differentiate into multipotent progenitors (MPPs). These, in turn, give rise to common myeloid progenitors (CMPs) and lymphoid primed multipotent progenitors (LMPPs). CMPs and LMPPs then continue their differentiation into lineage-committed progenitors, ending with the different mature blood cells (1).

Hematopoietic progenitors can be classified into multilineage progenitors and single-lineage progenitors according to their differentiation potential. As illustrated in Figure 1.1, there are two main multilineage progenitors recognized, namely, the CMP and the common lymphoid progenitor (CLP; the immediate progeny of LMPPs). The CMPs give rise to erythrocytes, platelets (via megakaryocytes), basophils, eosinophils, neutrophils, and macrophages after a series of intermediate forms, which are generally named burst-forming units (BFUs) or colony-forming units (CFUs) (7). This nomenclature is derived from in vitro assays performed by culturing cells on methylcellulose, a semi-solid medium, mixed with different cytokines intended to induce differentiation into various lineages (8). The timing of appearance, the morphology, the cellular components, and the cytokine requirements of the colonies arising in these assays define each of the intermediate forms, with the convention that a cell population identified by a particular assay is referred to by the assay name. CLPs ultimately differentiate into B, T, and NK cells. While myeloid and lymphoid lineages are thought to arise independently, some studies have suggested that the granulocyte–macrophage progenitor (GMP) can also be derived from LMP.

Whereas many of the intermediates are not morphologically distinguishable, the majority of the final differentiation steps toward individual lineages can be identified by conventional histochemistry, where a blast form gives rise to more mature forms that progressively resemble the fully differentiated elements. Table 1.1 describes the nomenclature of the different processes leading to production of mature blood cells. In addition, Table 1.2 lists the different types of mature blood cells as well as their morphologic characteristics and function.

CLUSTERS OF DIFFERENTIATION

As HSCs and progenitors differentiate, they acquire distinct cell surface antigen markers, also known as CDs, while losing the antigens associated with more primitive cells. CDs can be used

Table 1.1 Hematopoietic Processes

Process	Progenitor	Outcome

Myelopoiesis	CMP	Production of myeloid cells, which can be granulocytic and non-granulocytic
		
		• Granulocytic
		  • Neutrophils
		  • Eosinophils
		  • Basophils
		• Non-granulocytic
		  • Monocytes and macrophages

Lymphopoiesis	CLP	Production of B and T lymphocytes
Erythropoiesis	MEP	Production of red blood cells
Thrombopoiesis	MEP	Production of platelets

CLP, common lymphoid progenitor; CMP, common myeloid progenitor; MEP, megakaryocyte–erythrocyte progenitor.

to identify stem cells and diverse types of progenitors, intermediates, and mature blood cells of different lineages, even at stages when morphology alone would not be enough for cell identification. Identifying cell subpopulations via CDs is often done through monoclonal antibodies and flow cytometry, with marker panels being readily available commercially. The number of described CDs continues to grow and has exceeded 370 to date. Utilization of CDs in the clinical arena has revolutionized the way we understand, diagnose, classify, and treat hematologic diseases, and is now the standard of care to be incorporated in their diagnostic workup.

CDs are considered differentiation antigens, some of which are summarized in Table 1.3 (9), with many being membrane proteins that play an important role in hematopoiesis. These proteins often act as receptors or ligands with subsequently activated signal transduction pathways regulating the behavior of the cells expressing them. Other CDs are not involved in signal transduction, but have other functions such as mediating cell adhesion. Figure 1.3 illustrates selected examples of markers that are associated with different lineages.

CD34 and CD117 (c-KIT) are markers expressed by HSCs from the fetal stages of hematopoiesis through adult life. Importantly, HSCs and primitive progenitors lack CD38 (10). HSCs are rare, and thus, techniques that enhance their enrichment often rely on the identification of those surface markers and exclusion of antigens that define downstream lineages (so-called lineage negativity, Lin⁻) (11). One important clinical example is the use of CD34 to enrich hematopoietic grafts for HSCs.

Table 1.2 Morphology and Function of Blood Elements

Blood cell	Progenitor	Morphology	Main function
Red blood cells	MEP	Biconcave, discoid, and lacking nucleus. Contain hemoglobin	Transport of respiratory gases (oxygen and carbon dioxide) via hemoglobin
Platelets	MEP	Small and lacking nucleus. Develop from fragments of megakaryocytic cytoplasm	Essential for hemostasis via secretion of clotting cofactors, as well as adhesion, aggregation, and provision of a platform for coagulation reactions
Neutrophils	CMP	Multilobed nucleus (two to five lobes). Contain azurophilic cytoplasmic granules Selected CD markers: CD13, CD15, CD16, CD33, CD63, CD66, CD68, and CD141	Members of the innate immune system, especially important against bacterial infections
Eosinophils	CMP	Contain acidophilic cytoplasmic granules Selected CD markers: CD9, CD15, CD16b, CD23, CD49d, CD116, CD193, and CD294	Immunity against parasites and play a role in allergy
Basophils	CMP	Contain basophilic cytoplasmic granules Selected CD markers: CD9, CD49d, CD68, CD123, CD194, and CD294	Role in inflammatory reactions and allergy
Monocytes	GMP	Large, with blue-gray cytoplasm and fine lilac granules (ground-glass appearance) Selected CD markers: CD2, CD11b, CD14, CD16, CD31, CD56, CD62L, CD115, and CD192	Can differentiate into macrophages or dendritic cells. Involved in innate immunity

(continued)

Table 1.2 Morphology and Function of Blood Elements (continued)

Blood cell	Progenitor	Morphology	Main function
Macrophages	GMP	Thought to derive from tissue-resident monocytes. Large cells with abundant clear and vacuolated cytoplasm Selected CD markers: CD11b, CD14, CD16, CD40, CD64, CD68, and CD71	Phagocytosis and antigen presentation. Wound healing and iron hemostasis
T lymphocytes	CLP	Contain scant cytoplasm, dense chromatin in a round nucleus Selected CD markers: CD3, CD4, and CD8	Cell-mediated immunity. Critical role in cancer immunity and viral infections
B lymphocytes	CLP	Contain scant cytoplasm, dense chromatin in a round nucleus Selected CD markers: CD19, CD20, CD22, CD24, CD34, CD38, and CD45R	Humoral immunity via production of antibodies after differentiation into plasma cells, as well as antigen presentation
NK cells	CLP	Large granular lymphocytes Selected CD markers: CD16 and CD56	Innate immune system. Play a role in immunity against viruses and malignant cells

CD, cluster of differentiation; CLP, common lymphoid progenitor; CMP, common myeloid progenitor; GMP, granulocyte–macrophage progenitor; MEP, megakaryocyte–erythrocyte progenitor; NK, natural killer.

Table 1.3 Selected Clusters of Differentiation and Their Function

Cluster of Differentiation	Function
CD2	Involved in T-cell adhesion
CD4	Expressed on the surface of T helper cells. Acts as a co-receptor for Class II MHC
CD8	Expressed on the surface of T cytotoxic cells. Acts as a co-receptor for Class I MHC
CD11	Promotes leukocyte adhesion
CD 19, 20, and 21	B-cell surface antigens necessary for B-cell signal transduction and function
CD28	A co-stimulatory molecule present on the T-cell surface necessary for its immune function
CD34	Thought to promote cell adhesion and/or cell cycle arrest. It is often used as a marker for identifying and selecting hematopoietic stem cells
CD40	A ligand for B cells and involved in immunoglobulin class switching
CD 44, 54, 58, and CD62L	Function as adhesion molecules
CD 80 and 86	Act as co-stimulatory receptors necessary for the function of antigen-presenting cells
CD90	Enhances adhesion of T cells to stromal cells
CD95	Triggers apoptosis
CD110	Receptor for thrombopoietin, the major regulator for formation of megakaryocytes and platelets
CD117 (c-KIT receptor)	Proliferation and survival of HSCs. It is often used as a marker to identify HSCs
CD150	Lymphocyte proliferation
CD154	B-cell receptor that promotes proliferation and is also involved in immunoglobulin class switching
CD164	Involved in blood cell homing and suppressing the proliferation of CD34+/CD38– cells

CD, cluster of differentiation; HSC, hematopoietic stem cell; MHC, major histocompatibility complex.

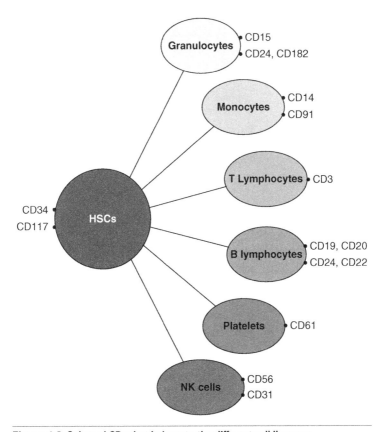

Figure 1.3 Selected CDs that belong to the different cell lineages.

CD, cluster of differentiation; HSC, hematopoietic stem cell; NK, natural killer.

BONE MARROW MICROENVIRONMENT

Bone Marrow Niches

The bone marrow stroma comprises the non-hematopoietic components of bone marrow that provide various growth factors needed to sustain hematopoietic hemostasis and guide trafficking of hematopoietic cells. Many of these components are necessary for the HSCs and progenitors to proliferate and differentiate into various cell lineages. Among the key components are the bone marrow niches. A niche is defined as a local tissue microenvironment involved in maintaining and regulating a specific kind of stem or progenitor cell (12). Importantly, HSCs are thought to colonize two specific niches: the endosteal niche and the vascular niche. The endosteal niche is located between the endocortical surface and the trabecular surface of the bone (2). On the other hand, the vascular niche is located close to sinusoidal endothelial cells and bone marrow stromal cells (2). Current evidence indicates that these two niches, among other factors, play a key role in regulating the function of HSCs, including fate determination, although the relative importance of each of these niches is debated.

In the endosteal niche, a specific type of osteoblast is thought to play a role in HSC maturation, as it expresses N-cadherin, which facilitates the interaction and binding to HSCs also expressing N-cadherin (2). The role of N-cadherin is, however, controversial, with some studies showing that it is not required for the maintenance of HSCs (13). Another protein, angiopoietin receptor-2 (Tie2), on the surface of HSCs, interacts with angiopoietin-1 (Ang-1) expressed on the surface of the lining osteoblasts in the endosteal niche (see Figure 1.4), which leads to enhanced survival of HSCs. In addition, other factors in the endosteal niche have been shown to influence survival and function of HSCs in animal studies (2). In the vascular niche, on the other hand, HSCs lie in close proximity to sinusoidal endothelial cells and stromal cells that seem to be critical for their maturation, with hematopoiesis being thought to take place in the extravascular area between the sinuses (2). Figure 1.4 illustrates both types of niches and the supporting cells involved. In mouse models, evidence suggests that fibroblast growth factor-1 (FGF-1) plays a role in mediating the crosstalk between the two niches to regulate hematopoiesis (14).

Homing is the process that enables circulating HSCs and progenitors to find their way to the bone marrow stroma and selectively reside there. This process is enabled by specific stromal cells and matrix proteins, and is crucial for the maintenance of long-term hematopoiesis. In addition, this property of HSCs is key to the success of stem cell transplantation. HSCs and progenitors interact with endothelial cells and the bone marrow microenvironment via selectins (e.g., cytoadhesion molecules E, P, and L), integrins (discussed in a separate section), and chemokines (e.g., CXCR4 binding to CXCL12) (7).

Drugs that inhibit the interaction of CXCR4 in HSCs and CXCL12 in stromal cells, such as plerixafor, can disrupt the homing steady state and allow mobilization of HSCs into peripheral blood. These drugs can be used to facilitate collection of HSCs from peripheral blood. Nonetheless, the first agent to be used specifically for this purpose was granulocyte colony-stimulating factor (G-CSF) or filgrastim. Apart from its major role in the differentiation and maturation of neutrophils, G-CSF leads to decreased production or increased degradation of stem cell retention factors, including CXCL12, Ang-1, Kit ligand, and vascular adhesion molecule-1 (VCAM-1) (7). The full

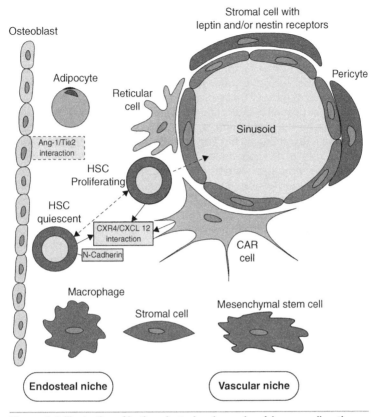

Figure 1.4 **Illustration of both endosteal and vascular niches as well as the supporting cells involved**.

Ang-1, angiopoietin-1; HSC, hematopoietic stem cell.

effects of G-CSF on HSCs are not entirely known, however. Recent animal studies show that G-CSF promotes HSCs' expansion and quiescence, while reducing their repopulating activity. This effect on hematopoietic cell activity occurs at least in part through activation of Toll-like receptor signaling (15). Furthermore, studies in mice indicate that bone marrow macrophages produce factors promoting osteoblast lineage maintenance and subsequently retention of stem cells. G-CSF inhibits the production of these factors, leading to stem cell mobilization (16). Notably, before filgrastim and plerixafor were available, HSC mobilization into peripheral blood was achieved with chemotherapeutic agents, such as cyclophosphamide, which kill rapidly dividing progenitors and thus trigger a burst of hematopoietic repopulation and HSC proliferation.

SUPPORTING CELLS

The bone marrow microenvironment includes a multitude of supporting cells that provide the optimal soil for normal hematopoiesis. These include stromal cells, osteoblasts, osteocytes, osteoclasts, vascular endothelial cells, macrophages, and others (17). Several stromal cell types, such as reticular cells and mesenchymal stromal cells, have been described by different authors. Whether they represent completely distinct cellular entities or a spectrum of a single population is unclear. For instance, a population of reticular cells has long cytoplasmic processes that mesh together to form a lattice along the vascular sinuses, and evidence suggests that it has a role in sustaining HSCs in a proliferative and undifferentiated condition (18). This framework may be further enhanced by other stromal cells that support developing blood cells via cell-to-cell support (being an important element of niches) as well as by producing key hematopoietic growth factors. For example, mesenchymal stem cells (MSCs) can differentiate into osteolineage cells, chondrocytes, adipocytes, and mature stromal cells, all of which help support hematopoiesis. Mature T lymphocytes are also thought to provide adhesion molecules, growth factors, and cytokines that enhance the longevity, maturation, and differentiation of the hematopoietic hierarchy. Table 1.4 lists the different cells in the bone marrow microenvironment and their postulated role in maintaining normal hematopoiesis (19–21).

Regulation and Control

HSCs' self-renewal and lineage fate determination is a complex process controlled via various mechanisms working in harmony to ensure the HSC population is maintained while sustaining the production of different lineages. In addition, hematopoiesis has the capacity to ramp up production to meet excess demand in certain situations. This process is highly regulated but incompletely understood. In general, it is believed that there is a network of intercellular signals triggered by direct cell-to-cell interactions, cell-to-matrix interactions, or in response to cytokines and growth factors. Other factors involved include intracellular transcription factors, cell cycle regulators, and cell adhesion molecules, all subject to genetic as well as epigenetic regulation.

Hematopoietic Growth Factors

Growth factors are secreted molecules that influence cell growth and proliferation through interaction with target receptors on the cell surface and subsequent activation of intracellular signaling cascades and the effects thereof. Prominent hematopoietic growth

Table 1.4 Cell Constituents of the Bone Marrow Niches and Their Role in Supporting Hematopoiesis

Cell		Role in Hematopoiesis
Resident macrophages (osteomacs)		Together with endothelial cells, stromal cells, and osteolineage cells, macrophages form a crisscross 3D scaffolding that harbors different blood-forming cells. In addition, they express COX-2 and produce PGE2, which aids in HSC regulation
Osteolineage cells (including osteoblasts)		Critical niche constituent that supports HSCs' expansion. In some models, loss of osteolineage cells disrupts hematopoiesis. In addition, these cells produce many factors necessary for normal hematopoiesis
Stromal cell populations	**CAR cells**	A population of stromal cells, also known as reticular cells, which are abundant in CXCL12. They have a periendothelial location in the vascular niche. CXCL12 expression is critical for HSCs' retention in bone marrow
	Leptin- and nestin-positive stromal cells	Stromal cells that are located perivascularly and help regulate HSCs. Nestin was recently shown to be involved in HSC maintenance, homeostasis, and mobilization. These cells also produce multiple critical cytokines including SCF and c-KIT ligand. Leptin is known to regulate hematopoiesis, and a synthetic fragment of leptin was found to increase HSC population and increase engraftment capacity. It is not entirely clear if this cell population is distinct from CAR cells
	Mesenchymal stem cells	Multipotent stromal cells that have the ability to differentiate into various connective tissue cells, such as osteoblasts, chondrocytes, and adipocytes, all of which are essential constituents of the bone marrow microenvironment
Vascular endothelial cells		HSCs tend to gather around endothelial vascular cells. Endothelial cells are required for mobilization of HSCs from the marrow to the bloodstream. In addition, the endothelial cells secrete factors that support HSC proliferation and maintenance and help with recovery after myeloablation

CAR, CXCL12-abundant reticular; HSCs, hematopoietic stem cells; SCF, stem cell factor.

factors include stem cell factor (SCF, also known as c-KIT ligand), cytokines such as interleukin (IL)-3 and IL-6, erythropoietin (EPO), thrombopoietin (TPO), granulocyte–macrophage colony-stimulating factor (GM-CSF), G-CSF, and macrophage colony-stimulating factor (M-CSF). Importantly, some of these growth factors are made by the stromal cells in the bone marrow niches.

Regulatory factors may be loosely divided into those that affect the hematopoietic process as a whole (via modulation of early progenitors) and those that act exclusively on specific lineages. General factors that affect overall hematopoiesis especially during its early stages include SCF, IL-3, GM-CSF, IL-11, IL-6, and IL-1. On the other hand, lineage-specific growth factors, including EPO, TPO, G-CSF, M-CSF, and IL-5, are necessary for the production of red blood cells (RBCs), platelets, neutrophils, monocytes, and eosinophils, respectively. Table 1.5 and Figure 1.5 outline the main cytokines and growth factors that regulate the production and differentiation across the hematopoietic hierarchy (9). In addition, Figure 1.6 illustrates the main hematopoietic growth factors that act on specific progenitors.

While numerous growth factors affect hematopoiesis, some are thought to have a key role driving each of the major cell lines. For RBCs, the critical growth factor is EPO. EPO targets committed erythroid progenitors and leads to further differentiation and RBC production. It is also involved in keeping the RBC number within physiologic range via modulation of apoptosis of erythroid progenitors. EPO is synthesized and its levels regulated primarily via specialized cells in the renal cortex that sense blood oxygenation levels. Transcription of the *EPO* gene in these cells is regulated by hypoxia-inducible factor (HIF). EPO binds to EPO receptors on erythroid progenitors with subsequent signal transduction via the JAK2/STAT5 pathway (22) and promotion of erythropoiesis (7). Constitutive, unregulated JAK2 activation is one of the underlying genetic mechanisms for polycythemia vera, a disorder that manifests with excess RBC numbers (23). Interestingly, primitive erythrocytes need much less EPO to develop in contrast to definitive erythrocytes that arise later in life (24). Recombinant forms of EPO are used therapeutically in a number of diseases that are associated with primary anemia. Major indications include anemia related to renal failure, myelodysplastic syndrome (MDS), cancer-related anemia, and situations where patients refuse blood transfusions (e.g., due to certain beliefs). However, the use of recombinant EPO is governed by strict guidelines with the aim to limit the risk of side effects, namely, thromboembolic complications.

Development and production of platelets is chiefly regulated by TPO, largely produced by hepatocytes. TPO functions via activation

Table 1.5 Selected Key Cytokines and Growth Factors Involved in Hematopoiesis

Cytokine	Target	Effect
IL-5	Eosinophils B cells	• Eosinophils: Differentiation, maturation, and survival. It is also a mediator for eosinophil activation • B cells: Promotes B-cell growth and immunoglobulin secretion
IL-7	Early lymphocytes	• Growth regulator of lymphocytes. It is secreted by the stromal cells. It is also important for T-cell memory function, survival, and homeostasis
IL-2	T cells	• Important factor for the differentiation, growth, and function of T cells. It was initially known as T-cell growth factor. It is important to maintain Tregs and for the differentiation of CD4+ T cells into T-cell subsets following antigen presentation and activation. Also promotes differentiation into memory cells
IL-4	B cells and T cells	• B cells: Promotes the growth, helps in activation, and modulates immunoglobulin class switching. IL-4 is sometimes referred to as B-cell growth factor • T cells: Induces differentiation and proliferation
IL-15	T cells, NK cells	• T cells: Regulates T-cell activity and homeostasis. It works with other factors including IL-2 and IL-7 to maintain both naïve and memory T cells. It also enhances the survival of antigen-specific CD8+ T cells • NK cells: Proliferation and activation (through interacting with the components of IL-2 receptor)
SCF	Primitive HSCs and progenitors	• General hematopoietic growth factor that acts to promote growth and development of HSCs, progenitors, and across all downstream lineages
EPO	Erythroid progenitors	• Promotes survival and proliferation of red blood cell progenitors as well as their differentiation into mature red blood cells
TPO	Megakaryocyte progenitors	• Controls the proliferation and maturation of megakaryocytic progenitors

(*continued*)

Table 1.5 Selected Key Cytokines and Growth Factors Involved in Hematopoiesis (*continued*)

Cytokine	Target	Effect
M-CSF	Monocyte progenitors	• Proliferation, differentiation, and survival of monocytic progenitors to sustain macrophage homeostasis
G-CSF	Neutrophil progenitors	• A key stimulant of neutrophil production. Has numerous clinical applications such as stem cell mobilization for stem cell transplantation and in treating neutropenia

EPO, erythropoietin; G-CSF, granulocyte colony-stimulating factor; HSCs, hematopoietic stem cells; IL, interleukin; M-CSF, macrophage colony-stimulating factor; NK, natural killer; SCF, stem cell factor; TPO, thrombopoietin; Tregs, regulatory T cells.

of a cytokine receptor known as MPL present on bone marrow megakaryocytes and their precursors. The ultimate effect of TPO is to raise platelet numbers via initiation of signaling cascades leading to proliferation and differentiation of megakaryocytes from progenitor cells. TPO level is negatively regulated by platelet number, with increased platelets leading to downregulation of TPO mRNA (7). However, the mechanism is not fully understood. Although recombinant TPO has been used clinically to increase the platelet levels, its use was complicated by the development of TPO-neutralizing antibodies and consequent thrombocytopenia in several subjects (25). Thus, its use was abandoned. More recently, TPO receptor agonists (such as eltrombopag and romiplostim) have become available, and are not known to be associated with antibody formation. These drugs can be used to treat chronic immune thrombocytopenic purpura (ITP), aplastic anemia, and chronic hepatitis C–associated thrombocytopenia.

The chief regulatory growth factors driving the granulocytic pathway are GM-CSF and G-CSF. Both GM-CSF and G-CSF activate specific receptors on myeloid precursors, with G-CSF acting on more mature progenitors, leading to subsequent activation of signaling pathways enhancing cell proliferation, survival, and activation of myeloid cells (26). G-CSF production is promoted by several factors including IL-1β, tumor necrosis factor-alpha (TNF-α), and lipopolysaccharide (LPS), all of which are usually elevated during infections or other stress. Therefore, G-CSF plays a critical role in mediating a granulopoietic stress response (15). Both recombinant GM-CSF (sargramostim) and G-CSF (filgrastim) are approved for the treatment of neutropenia (acquired and congenital) as well as

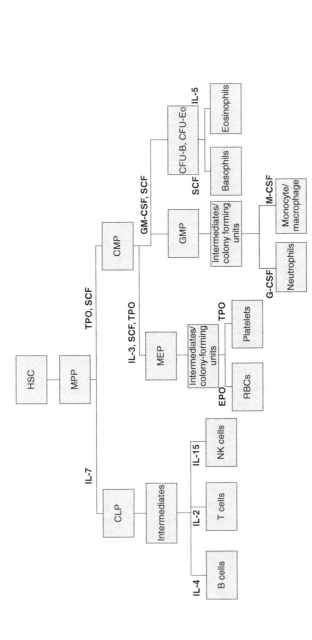

Figure 1.5 Simplified diagram illustrating the key growth factors and cytokines at different stages of the hematopoietic hierarchy.

CFU-B, colony-forming unit-basophil; CFU-Eo, colony-forming unit-eosinophil; CLP, common lymphoid progenitor; CMP, common myeloid progenitor; EPO, erythropoietin; G-CSF, granulocyte colony-stimulating factor; GM-CSF, granulocyte-macrophage colony-stimulating factor; GMP, granulocyte–macrophage progenitor; HSC, hematopoietic stem cell; IL, interleukin; M-CSF, macrophage colony-stimulating factor; MPP, multipotent progenitor; NK, natural killer; RBC, red blood cell; SCF, stem cell factor; TPO, thrombopoietin.

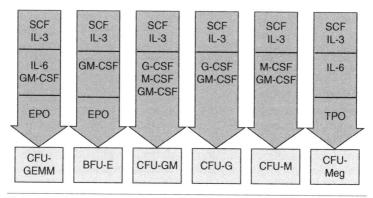

Figure 1.6 Hematopoietic growth factors that target specific progenitors.
BFU-E, burst-forming unit-erythroid; CFU-G, colony-forming unit-granulocyte; CFU-GEMM, colony-forming unit-granulocyte, erythrocyte, megakaryocyte, macrophage; CFU-GM, colony-forming unit-granulocyte monocyte; CFU-M, colony-forming unit-monocyte; CFU-Meg, colony-forming unit-megakaryocyte; EPO, erythropoietin; G-CSF, granulocyte colony-stimulating factor; GM-CSF, granulocyte–macrophage colony-stimulating factor; IL, interleukin; M-CSF, macrophage colony-stimulating factor; SCF, stem cell factor; TPO, thrombopoietin.

for mobilization of HSCs to peripheral blood prior to stem cell harvest. The mechanisms by which G-CSF mobilizes HSCs into peripheral blood are discussed under the section "Bone Marrow Niches." A pegylated form of G-CSF (pegfilgrastim) has the advantage of having sustained action (up to 2 weeks), eliminating the need for daily injections, and is also approved for treatment of chemotherapy-induced neutropenia. Currently, there are only limited data comparing G-CSF and GM-CSF and the results are conflicting.

Integrins

Integrins are transmembrane proteins that facilitate communication between the cell and its extracellular surrounding. They are composed of alpha and beta subunits, both having extracellular and intracellular domains. Ligand binding to the integrin surface domain leads to signal transduction with diverse outcomes, including cell cycle modulation among many other effects. Integrins also have an important role in homing of HSCs to bone marrow stroma and its microenvironment.

HSCs and primitive hematopoietic cells harbor many integrins. Among these is $\alpha_4\beta_1$ integrin, which binds to VCAM-1 or fibronectin and promotes progenitor cell adhesion (27). Other integrins involved in hematopoiesis include $\alpha_4\beta_7$ and $\alpha_5\beta_1$ integrins (7). Of note, the avidity of progenitor cell integrins can be influenced by cytokines and growth factors including SCF, TPO, and CXL12.

VCAM-1, fibronectin, as well as many other integrin ligands are highly expressed in the bone marrow microenvironment. Interactions of these molecules with integrins are thought to contribute to the retention of HSCs in the bone marrow (9).

Intracellular Factors

Transcription factors and other elements such as microRNAs and epigenetic regulators play a unique role in controlling gene transcription. These factors seem to define a road map to guide the hematopoietic process in terms of lineage and differentiation. Similar to growth factors, hematopoietic transcription factors may be divided into those that affect HSCs and early progenitors, and those that are lineage specific. Transcription factors have an important role in regulating HSC expansion as well as in guiding differentiation toward lymphoid and myeloid fates. Important examples are GATA-1, GATA-2, and PU.1. GATA-1 is critical for the differentiation of mature erythrocytes and megakaryocytes. GATA-2 seems to have a role in the final stages of megakaryocyte–erythrocyte progenitor (MEP) differentiation (9). PU.1, on the other hand, has an important role in the development of B cells and macrophages (7). Interestingly, lineage-specific transcription factors promote the expression of lineage-specific genes and work to counteract transcription factors that promote alternative lineages steering the hematopoietic machinery toward a certain lineage when needed (7). In addition, many lineage-specific transcription factors have a positive feedback effect and stimulate their own genes (autoregulation). Of relevance, transcription factors belonging to the HOX family are involved in influencing cell decisions including self-renewal (9).

The specific transcription factors active in a particular cell ultimately influence its gene expression profile, which in turn guides the fate of HSCs and other hematopoietic cells. At each step in the hierarchy, the genes linked to the committed lineage either remain expressed or even become upregulated, while the genes related to the other lineages become silenced. This expression pattern was suggested by studies showing that primitive HSCs express the genes affiliated with multiple lineages, but downstream lineage-committed progenitors express only the genes specific to that lineage (28,29). Mouse studies demonstrate that genes enriched in HSCs include developmental genes, some of which are associated with self-renewal. On the other hand, genes enriched in lineage-committed progenitor cells are linked to differentiation and regulation of immune responses. As HSCs develop into committed progenitors, there is downregulation of "stemness" genes and upregulation of lineage-specific genes (30).

Apart from transcription factors, more recently recognized mechanisms of translational control have also been shown to play an important role in the overall hematopoietic process. MicroRNAs are small, noncoding RNAs that regulate the gene expression by silencing and degrading mRNA, with subsequent inefficient translation. In hematopoiesis, they function to regulate responses to cytokines and transcription factors, and thus have a key role in guiding differentiation and progenitor lineage commitment. Examples include miR-181, which has a role in B-cell differentiation (at least in animal models); miR-155, which inhibits erythropoiesis and megakaryopoiesis; and miR-520h, which is upregulated in primitive stem cells, suggesting a role in stem cell maintenance (9).

KEY POINTS

- Hematopoiesis is a highly regulated process with the end products being 10 formed elements: erythrocytes, platelets, neutrophils, monocytes, basophils, eosinophils, B lymphocytes, T lymphocytes, NK cells, and dendritic cells.
- Sites of hematopoiesis change during development.
- In the embryo, hematopoiesis occurs in the yolk sac. In the fetus, it occurs in the liver, spleen, placenta, and bone marrow. After birth, hematopoiesis occurs solely in the bone marrow, except in states of inefficient hematopoiesis. In such states, hematopoiesis may revert to its fetal sites (liver and spleen).
- Self-renewal and differentiation are the key characteristics of HSCs, which are essential for hematopoiesis.
- The main steps of hematopoiesis include self-renewal of HSCs, HSCs' differentiation, commitment to specific lineages, and finally, maturation and development of lineage-committed progenitors into terminally mature cells.
- As HSCs differentiate into different lineages, their CD expression changes. CDs are thus used to identify the different cells in the hierarchy and have numerous clinical and research applications.
- The bone marrow microenvironment is essential for normal hematopoiesis. The endosteal and vascular niches are thought to play an important role in its preservation and regulation.
- Regulatory factors of hematopoiesis can be classified as external growth factors (such as EPO, TPO, and G-CSF), integrins, and intracellular factors (such as transcription factors, microRNAs, and others).
- Many of the external regulatory factors are produced by the supporting cells in the bone marrow niches.

REFERENCES

1. Aqmasheh S, Shamsasanjan K, Akbarzadehlaleh P, et al. Effects of mesenchymal stem cell derivatives on hematopoiesis and hematopoietic stem cells. *Adv Pharm Bull.* 2017;7(2):165–177. doi:10.15171/apb.2017.021

2. Tamma R, Ribatti D. Bone niches, hematopoietic stem cells, and vessel formation. *Int J Mol Sci.* 2017;18(1):151. doi:10.3390/ijms18010151

3. Golub R, Cumano A. Embryonic hematopoiesis. *Blood Cells Mol Dis.* 2013;51(4):226–231. doi:10.1016/j.bcmd.2013.08.004

4. Chen T, Wang F, Wu M, Wang ZZ. Development of hematopoietic stem and progenitor cells from human pluripotent stem cells. *J Cell Biochem.* 2015;116(7):1179–1189. doi:10.1002/jcb.25097

5. Tavian M, Peault B. Embryonic development of the human hematopoietic system. *Int J Dev Biol.* 2005;49(2–3):243–250. doi:10.1387/ijdb.041957mt

6. Wagers AJ, Christensen JL, Weissman LL. Cell fate determination from stem cells. *Gene Ther.* 2002;9(10):606–612. doi:10.1038/sj.gt.3301717

7. Greer JP, Arber DA, Glader, B, et al. *Wintrobe's Clinical Hematology.* 13th ed. Philadelphia, PA: Wolters Kluwer Health | Lippincott Williams & Wilkins; 2014.

8. Frisch BJ, Calvi LM. Hematopoietic stem cell cultures and assays. *Methods Mol Biol.* 2014;1130:315–324. doi:10.1007/978-1-62703-989-5_24

9. Kaushansky K. Hematopoietic stem cells, progenitors, and cytokines. In: Kaushansky K, Lichtman M, Beutler E, et al., eds. *Williams Hematology.* New York, NY: McGraw-Hill Education; 2015.

10. Terstappen LW, Huang S, Safford M, et al. Sequential generations of hematopoietic colonies derived from single nonlineage-committed CD34+CD38- progenitor cells. *Blood.* 1991;77(6):1218–1227.

11. Takahashi M, Matsuoka Y, Sumide K, et al. CD133 is a positive marker for a distinct class of primitive human cord blood-derived CD34-negative hematopoietic stem cells. *Leukemia.* 2014;28(6):1308–1315. doi:10.1038/leu.2013.326

12. Morrison SJ, Scadden DT. The bone marrow niche for haematopoietic stem cells. *Nature.* 2014;505(7483):327–334. doi:10.1038/nature12984

13. Greenbaum AM, Revollo LD, Woloszynek JR, et al. N-cadherin in osteolineage cells is not required for maintenance of hematopoietic stem cells. *Blood.* 2012;120(2):295–302. doi:10.1182/blood-2011-09-377457

14. de Haan G, Weersing E, Dontje B, et al. In vitro generation of long-term repopulating hematopoietic stem cells by fibroblast growth factor-1. *Dev Cell*. 2003;4(2):241–251. doi:10.1016/S1534-5807(03)00018-2

15. Schuettpelz LG, Borgerding JN, Christopher MJ, et al. G-CSF regulates hematopoietic stem cell activity, in part, through activation of Toll-like receptor signaling. *Leukemia*. 2014;28(9):1851–1860. doi:10.1038/leu.2014.68

16. Christopher MJ, Rao M, Liu F, et al. Expression of the G-CSF receptor in monocytic cells is sufficient to mediate hematopoietic progenitor mobilization by G-CSF in mice. *J Exp Med*. 2011;208(2):251–260. doi:10.1084/jem.20101700

17. Anthony BA, Link DC. Regulation of hematopoietic stem cells by bone marrow stromal cells. *Trends Immunol*. 2014;35(1):32–37. doi:10.1016/j.it.2013.10.002

18. Nagasawa T, Omatsu Y, Sugiyama T. Control of hematopoietic stem cells by the bone marrow stromal niche: the role of reticular cells. *Trends Immunol*. 2011;32(7):315–320. doi:10.1016/j.it.2011.03.009

19. Calvi LM, Link DC. Cellular complexity of the bone marrow hematopoietic stem cell niche. *Calcif Tissue Int*. 2014;94(1):112–124. doi:10.1007/s00223-013-9805-8

20. Xie L, Zeng X, Hu J, Chen Q. Characterization of Nestin, a selective marker for bone marrow derived mesenchymal stem cells. *Stem Cells Int*. 2015;2015:762098. doi:10.1155/2015/762098

21. Dias CC, Nogueira-Pedro A, Tokuyama PY, et al. A synthetic fragment of leptin increase hematopoietic stem cell population and improve its engraftment ability. *J Cell Biochem*. 2015;116(7):1334–1340. doi:10.1002/jcb.25090

22. Kuhrt D, Wojchowski DM. Emerging EPO and EPO receptor regulators and signal transducers. *Blood*. 2015;125(23):3536–3541. doi:10.1182/blood-2014-11-575357

23. Jamieson CHM, Gotlib J, Durocher JA, et al. The JAK2 V617F mutation occurs in hematopoietic stem cells in polycythemia vera and predisposes toward erythroid differentiation. *Proc Natl Acad Sci*. 2006;103(16):6224–6229. doi:10.1073/pnas.0601462103

24. Palis J, Yoder MC. Yolk-sac hematopoiesis: the first blood cells of mouse and man. *Exp Hematol*. 2001;29(8):927–936. doi:10.1016/S0301-472X(01)00669-5

25. Li J, Yang C, Xia Y, et al. Thrombocytopenia caused by the development of antibodies to thrombopoietin. *Blood*. 2001;98(12):3241–3248. doi:10.1182/blood.V98.12.3241

26. Panopoulos AD, Watowich SS. Granulocyte colony-stimulating factor: molecular mechanisms of action during steady state and 'emergency' hematopoiesis. *Cytokine*. 2008;42(3):277–288. doi:10.1016/j.cyto.2008.03.002

27. Vanderslice P, Biediger RJ, Woodside DG, et al. Small molecule agonist of very late antigen-4 (VLA-4) integrin induces progenitor cell adhesion. *J Biol Chem*. 2013;288(27):19414–19428. doi:10.1074/jbc.M113.479634

28. Miyamoto T, Iwasaki H, Reizis B, et al. Myeloid or lymphoid promiscuity as a critical step in hematopoietic lineage commitment. *Dev Cell*. 2002;3(1):137–147. doi:10.1016/S1534-5807(02)00201-0

29. Kiel MJ, Yilmaz OH, Iwashita T, et al. SLAM family receptors distinguish hematopoietic stem and progenitor cells and reveal endothelial niches for stem cells. *Cell*. 2005;121(7):1109–1121. doi:10.1016/j.cell.2005.05.026

30. Terskikh AV, Miyamoto T, Chang C, et al. Gene expression analysis of purified hematopoietic stem cells and committed progenitors. *Blood*. 2003;102(1):94–101. doi:10.1182/blood-2002-08-2509

2 Neutrophil Disorders

Premal Lulla and Srijana Rai

INTRODUCTION

Neutrophils are typically the "first responders" to an invasive bacterial or fungal infection. While they primarily exert their immune effects through phagocytosis, defects in specific genes have uncovered a spectrum of diverse functions of neutrophils. At any given time, only about 2% to 20% of the existing neutrophil pool is circulating in peripheral blood, while the rest are present within the bone marrow and tissue spaces, ready to respond to inflammatory stimuli. Thus, even slight abnormalities in neutrophil numbers measured on a peripheral blood count can indicate a major shift in total body neutrophil quantities. Moreover, alterations in normal functions of neutrophils can result in severe vulnerabilities to bacterial and fungal infections, often without altering the total number of neutrophils. This review highlights the pathophysiology and management of common congenital and acquired defects in neutrophil numbers and functions.

NEUTROPENIA

Clinical Case 2.1

A 66-year-old man was hospitalized with fever and noted to have an absolute neutrophil count (ANC) of 200/mm³. Two weeks earlier, he had received his first cycle of chemotherapy with rituximab, cyclophosphamide, vincristine, adriamycin, and prednisone (R-CHOP) for diffuse large B-cell lymphoma (DLBCL) involving the bone marrow. His current medications included acyclovir and multivitamins. He did not receive granulocyte colony-stimulating factor (G-CSF) after cycle 1.

Introduction

Neutropenia is an absolute reduction in the number of circulating neutrophils. However, ethnicity and age can alter normal neutrophil counts. This is best demonstrated by significantly lower normal neutrophil counts in patients of African descent as compared with Caucasians. A study using U.S. National Health and Nutrition Examination Survey (NHANES) found the normal range of neutrophils to be from 1,300 to 6,600/mm^3 in adult non-Hispanic African American males (1). Furthermore, infants have lower neutrophil counts that gradually increase with age (normal range for infants: 1,200–8,500/mm^3 and for adults: 1,800–8,000/mm^3).

Diagnosis

Neutropenia can be classified as mild (ANC of 1,000–1,500/mm^3), moderate (ANC of 500–1,000/mm^3), and severe (ANC of ≤500/mm^3). In the nonurgent ambulatory setting, a complete blood count with differential repeated two to three times a week for 6 consecutive weeks helps to establish cyclical changes and any relationship with symptoms, if present. Review of a peripheral blood smear should also be done.

Neutropenia can arise from bone marrow failure (or suppression), can be congenital, or can be immune mediated or idiopathic. These entities can be subclassified as congenital and acquired etiologies (Table 2.1). Thus, a diagnostic workup of neutropenia should consider, at a minimum, chronicity, degree of the abnormality, duration of neutropenia, associated symptoms, comorbidity, and other associated hematological abnormalities (isolated neutropenia vs. multilineage cytopenias). A special emphasis on the patient's ethnic background, family, and dietary and medication history can often uncover the common culprits of neutropenia such as benign ethnic neutropenia and drug adverse effects. Laboratory tests beyond a complete blood count and peripheral smear are often needed to narrow the differential diagnosis. For example, a positive ANA or rheumatoid factor could indicate an underlying autoimmune disease.

Key Diagnostic Dilemmas

Observation versus a more aggressive approach to neutropenia may be appropriate in the setting of mild chronic neutropenia. If no cause is identified for isolated severe neutropenia or neutropenia associated with additional hematopoietic cell lineage abnormalities, a bone marrow examination is essential to make the diagnosis. The following tests could be diagnostic in the right context on a suitable bone marrow sample: flow cytometry analysis for hematological malignancies such as leukemias, of which large granular lymphocyte (LGL) leukemia has predominant neutropenia, cytogenetic analysis, chromosome instability tests, whole exome sequencing, or targeted polymerase chain reaction (PCR) assays

Table 2.1 Congenital and Acquired Causes of Neutropenia

Congenital	Presentation	Course	G-CSF?
Severe congenital neutropenia	Infancy	Chronic, severe	Very useful
Benign ethnic neutropenia	Adolescence	Chronic, benign	Not needed
Benign familial neutropenia	Adolescence	Chronic, benign	Not needed
Cyclic neutropenia	Childhood	Chronic, moderate	Useful if repeated infections
Congenital syndromes associated with neutropenia	Infancy	Chronic, variable	Useful depending on the cause
Acquired			
Infections	Any age	Acute, reversible	Not needed
Drugs	Within 7 days of drug administration	Acute, reversible	Useful if it is chemotherapy induced
Autoimmune	Adulthood	Chronic, variable	Useful if repeated infections
Malignancy	Any age	Chronic, variable	Useful if it is chemotherapy induced
Dietary	Any age	Chronic, reversible	Not needed
Chronic idiopathic	Adulthood	Chronic, benign	Not needed

G-CSF, granulocyte colony-stimulating factor.

for known bone marrow failure syndrome mutations, such as testing for *ELANE* mutations in congenital or cyclical neutropenia and so forth.

Management and Prognosis

Identification of the cause of neutropenia is paramount for ascertaining prognosis and guiding treatment. Acutely ill patients without a history of neutropenia are evaluated as a medical emergency as they are most vulnerable to life-threatening infections. Those with an ANC <500/mm^3 present the greatest risk, and patients who have a concomitant fever (>100.4°F) should be hospitalized immediately to administer IV antibiotics with empiric coverage for *Pseudomonas aeruginosa*. Beyond antibiotics, colony-stimulating factors are often used to rapidly correct chemotherapy-related neutropenia.

G-CSF and related granulocyte/macrophage stimulating factors (GM-CSF) are the endogenous cytokines responsible for stimulating and maintaining normal myeloid lineage hematopoiesis. They are normally produced by monocytes, fibroblasts, and endothelial cells, and exogenous supplementation induces myeloid stem cell proliferation and differentiation. Administration of recombinant G-CSF shortens the duration of chemotherapy-related neutropenia and is now U.S. Food and Drug Administration (FDA) approved for the management of chemotherapy-induced febrile neutropenia. The Infectious Diseases Society of America (IDSA) recommends that all patients treated with chemotherapy regimens with >20% risk of febrile neutropenia should receive prophylactic G-CSF after each cycle. Among the formulations of myeloid growth factors available in the United States, filgrastim and pegfilgrastim are the commonest forms of G-CSF, with the latter pegylated version having a longer half-life (up to 7 days vs. 4 hours). Sargramostim is the available formulation of GM-CSF and is reserved for use in allogeneic stem cell transplant recipients who have inadequate engraftment of donor stem cells.

Specific neutropenia syndromes have unique presentations, diagnostic workups, and management, which are discussed subsequently.

1. **Congenital neutropenias:** These can be divided into pure neutropenic syndromes and congenital syndromes that include neutropenia as a component of their phenotypes. For example, neutropenia also occurs as part of the spectrum of a number of congenital syndromes, including Shwachman–Diamond syndrome, Fanconi anemia, dyskeratosis congenita, Chediak–Higashi syndrome, myelokathexis, Griscelli syndrome II, and cartilage–hair hypoplasia, which are discussed in conjunction with qualitative neutrophil defects. Pure neutropenic syndromes are discussed in the following text.

    (a) **Benign ethnic neutropenia:** From 25% to 40% of healthy African Americans harbor lower than expected neutrophil counts, a normal variant known as benign ethnic neutropenia. This condition is characterized by mild, chronic neutropenia in the absence of recurrent infections. It is more common in patients of Mediterranean or African descent. Recent work has uncovered a recurrent single-nucleotide polymorphism (rs2814778) within the Duffy antigen/

receptor chemokine gene (*DARC*) as being highly associated with this condition (2). Furthermore, these patients carry the Duffy minor blood group negative (Fya-b–) phenotype. This is clinically relevant for patients who require treatment with myelotoxic therapies. A recent clinical study in patients with breast cancer noted that African American women were less likely to complete all cycles of adjuvant chemotherapy with frequent delays because of lower baseline neutrophil counts likely due to benign ethnic neutropenia. The authors hypothesize that since these patients may have an otherwise normal pool of neutrophils, they should also have lower ANC thresholds for chemotherapy administration, thereby allowing them to complete curative chemotherapy treatments on schedule. Extensive workup in an otherwise healthy individual of such ethnic background is uninformative and unnecessary (3).

(b) **Benign familial neutropenia**: Benign familial neutropenia has a nearly identical course to that of patients with benign ethnic neutropenia. However, it is not related to a particular ethnic group. Many genes and chromosome locations have been implicated and tend to vary across the families affected. No specific therapies are indicated.

(c) **Severe congenital neutropenia (SCN)**: SCN is a heterogeneous group of inherited disorders, all of which are rare (<500 cases/year in the United States), characterized by agranulocytosis and recurrent infections that begin in infancy. Several genes have been established as pathogenic in recent years:

(i) An autosomal dominant mutation of the neutrophil elastase gene, *ELANE*

(ii) An autosomal recessive mutation of *HAX1* (HS-1–associated protein X)

It is important to perform genetic testing for the commonly implicated genes early, as treatment with G-CSF can be lifesaving as in the case of patients with *ELANE* mutation. A workup should include a bone marrow examination to document maturation arrest and rule out transformation to acute myeloid leukemia (AML), which may develop in 10% to 30% of cases. The frontline therapy for patients with *ELANE* or *HAX-1* mutation in childhood is periodic G-CSF therapy. However, a potentially curative allogeneic hematopoietic stem cell transplantation (HSCT) for those who have a poor response to G-CSF may be required if a suitable donor is available.

(d) **Cyclical neutropenia (CN)**: CN is a rare congenital, autosomal dominant syndrome characterized by episodes of mild neutropenia recurring every 2 to 5 weeks. The length of the cycle may vary, but is consistent for each affected individual. CN can be a diagnostic dilemma because patients can have periods of normal blood counts. To differentiate CN from other neutropenic syndromes, blood counts should be assessed two to three times per week for up to 2 months. The syndrome is usually self-limited, although infections or oral ulcers may affect some patients during their neutrophil nadir. Similar to one of the SCN subtypes, it is also a result of mutation in the *ELANE* gene, though it is unclear why this syndrome presents with a different phenotype. Subcutaneous G-CSF use has been shown to reduce the incidence of neutropenic sepsis and should be used in patients who have CN and gingival complications. In contrast to chemotherapy-induced neutropenia, G-CSF is administered at a lower dose to patients with CN to target an ANC of >500/mm^3. Long-term use of G-CSF has been monitored in the Severe Chronic Neutropenia International Registry (SCNIR), where it has shown an acceptable safety profile in these patients (4).

2. **Acquired neutropenia**: Acquired causes for neutropenia are far more common than congenital causes. Several exogenous and endogenous factors can result in neutropenia as discussed in the following text.

(a) **Infections**: The most common pathogen responsible for neutropenia as opposed to neutrophilia is a recent viral infection, commonly influenza in adults and measles, mumps, or varicella in children. In most cases, postinfectious neutropenia is self-limited. Rarely, pathological activation of the immune system by potent stimulators of toll-like receptors (e.g., lipopolysaccharide [LPS] from bacterial infections) can result in severe sepsis and profound refractory neutropenia. This is more commonly seen in infancy and in the elderly.

(b) **Drugs**: Out of all the acquired causes for neutropenia, drugs are the commonest cause. Although almost any drug can cause neutropenia, either by myelosuppression or antibody-mediated destruction, the usual suspects include chemotherapeutic agents, antipsychotics (clozapine), antithyroid agents (methimazole, propylthiouracil), phenothiazine (chlorpromazine), and anti-inflammatory agents (sulfasalazine, nonsteroidal anti-inflammatory drugs [NSAIDs]). There is usually a temporal relationship between the start of the offending agent and the onset of neutropenia. With regard to non-chemotherapeutic drug-induced neutropenia, the management typically involves a careful medication history and discontinuation of the suspects. Since the life span of a circulating neutrophil is 6 to 8 hours, drug-induced neutropenia can occur within 1 to 7 days after exposure. Conversely, neutrophil recovery can take up to 7 days after discontinuation of the offending agent. G-CSF could be used to manage non-chemotherapeutic drug-induced neutropenia in particularly severe and prolonged cases, although its benefits are unproven in this indication.

(c) **Autoimmune**: Autoantibodies against neutrophil antigens can cause neutropenia. Autoimmune neutropenia may be **primary**, usually seen during the first year of life, or **secondary**, which is primarily seen in adults. Primary autoimmune neutropenia may be moderate or severe and usually remits by 2 years of age. Secondary autoimmune neutropenia occurs in association with systemic autoimmune diseases, such as rheumatoid arthritis (RA) and systemic lupus erythematosus (SLE), is usually mild, and rarely needs treatment. However, if infections develop in the setting of severe neutropenia, treatment with either steroids or IV immunoglobulin may be indicated.

Felty syndrome is a triad of RA, splenomegaly, and neutropenia. The incidence is rare because of widespread use of effective RA disease-modifying agents. Typically, Felty syndrome occurs in patients with long-standing (>10 years) uncontrolled RA. Treatment of the underlying RA with methotrexate, corticosteroids, and/or tumor necrosis factor-alpha (TNF-α)-blocking antibodies can mitigate the neutropenia seen in Felty, resulting in recovery of neutrophils in 1 to 2 weeks. Anecdotal evidence supports the use of G-CSF in prevention of life-threatening sepsis, which is the commonest cause of death in patients with Felty syndrome. Cases of exacerbation of RA and splenic rupture have been reported with G-CSF use in patients with Felty syndrome; thus, careful monitoring must be exercised following G-CSF administration.

LGL leukemia–associated neutropenia is similar to Felty syndrome. Unlike the latter, where the lymphocytes are oligoclonal or polyclonal, LGL-associated neutropenia occurs in the context of a monoclonal population of LGLs again as a result of long-standing autoimmune disease. Neutropenia is often severe and usually requires therapies directed toward the LGLs, such as methotrexate, cyclosporine, or cyclophosphamide.

(d) **Dietary**: Severe caloric malnutrition, resulting in conditions such as anorexia nervosa and folate and vitamin B12 deficiency can cause mild leukopenia. However, neutropenia from malnutrition is often associated with anemia and/or thrombocytopenia.

(e) **Chronic idiopathic neutropenia**: Chronic idiopathic neutropenia is a diagnosis of exclusion and is defined as an ANC lower than $1.5 \times 10^3/mm^3$ for >3 months. This disorder is more common in women. Bone marrow findings usually demonstrate a subtle reduction in neutrophil precursors. Patients with this condition typically are asymptomatic and rarely develop frequent infections. G-CSF is reserved for those who have more frequent severe infections.

(f) **Hypersplenism**: The spleen is an integral part of the reticuloendothelial system. Thus, normal splenic function entails harboring monocytes, macrophages, and neutrophils within the "white pulp." Portal hypertension could induce congestive hypersplenism, which results in increased sequestration of circulating blood cells in sinusoids. Thus, patients with advanced portal hypertension are frequently pancytopenic. Hypersplenism resulting from tropical splenomegaly or Felty syndrome could induce mild to moderate neutropenia. Treatment of the underlying cause of hypersplenism is often indicated to resolve the pancytopenia. For example, a transjugular intrahepatic portosystemic shunt (TIPS) or an orthotopic liver transplant in carefully selected patients with cirrhosis could address the neutropenia from portal hypertension–related hypersplenism. G-CSF use with hypersplenism is risky and relatively contraindicated, given cases of splenic rupture in hematopoietic stem cell donors with underlying hypersplenism during G-CSF stem cell mobilization.

Key Points

- Absolute neutropenia is defined as a neutrophil count <1,500/mm^3, though neutropenia is not considered severe until the count is <500/mm^3.
- Congenital causes of neutropenia can be mild or severe with more severe cases presenting in childhood and requiring genetic evaluation for proper classification and treatment.
- Acquired causes of neutropenia are many and include medications, infections, dietary deficiencies, immune causes, and hypersplenism.

NEUTROPHILIA

Clinical Case 2.2

A 32-year-old man was referred to urgent care for evaluation of an elevated neutrophil count noted in the postoperative clinic (ANC = 12,000/mm³). Ten days ago, he underwent a splenectomy for glucocorticoid-refractory immune thrombocytopenic purpura. He reported to urgent care with a temperature of 99°F, normal hemoglobin, and a platelet count of 461,000/mm³. He had pain at the incision site and mild fatigue. His exam was otherwise unremarkable. He was taking prednisone 20 mg/d on a tapering schedule as well as lithium for stable bipolar disorder.

Introduction

Neutrophilia is a laboratory abnormality that is secondary to an underlying disorder. It results from increased production of neutrophils in the bone marrow or reduced tissue demargination.

Diagnosis

Normal circulating neutrophil counts vary between 2 and 7×10^9/L. Neutrophilia is defined as an ANC >7,700/mm³. While diagnosis of neutrophilia can be made with a simple peripheral blood count assessment, the underlying cause requires a careful clinical history and physical examination. Physiological causes such as pregnancy, medications such as corticosteroids and lithium, cigarette smoking, extreme exercise, and asplenia can all be identified through a systematic history without extensive laboratory testing (Table 2.2).

Table 2.2 Causes of Neutrophilia

Autonomous:	
Hematological	Leukemias (acute and chronic myeloid)
Non-hematological	Solid cancers that produce G-CSF
Genetic/inherited	Trisomy 18, 21 (transient myeloproliferation)
Reactive:	
Infection	Bacterial, fungal, parasitic (commonest)
Inflammation	Vasculitis, IBD, autoimmune
Drugs	G-CSF, glucocorticoids, epinephrine, lithium
Exposures/iatrogenic	Smoking, exercise, asplenia
Endocrine	DKA, pheochromocytoma, Cushing's syndrome

DKA, diabetic ketoacidosis; G-CSF, granulocyte colony-stimulating factor; IBD, inflammatory bowel disease.

Rarely, complementary laboratory testing can help resolve diagnostic dilemmas.

Key Diagnostic Dilemma

Subtle neutrophilia in otherwise healthy individuals is a common outpatient hematology consult. In the majority of cases, a diagnosis is made during history taking or physical examination. If a diagnosis remains elusive, for asymptomatic patients, trending neutrophil levels over a 2 to 3 month period is often helpful to determine the chronicity and possible variations. This strategy can uncover cyclical changes in hormone levels, as well as periods of physical or emotional stress or subclinical inflammation after which patients should have normal neutrophil counts. For patients who do not demonstrate normalization of neutrophil counts despite observation and a thorough search for an underlying myeloproliferative disorder, systemic inflammation secondary to metabolic syndrome should be considered in the appropriate clinical context. In a minority of cases, a definite cause of subtle neutrophilia cannot be determined. While they could represent natural variations among subjects, monitoring periodic neutrophil counts as well as a yearly clinical evaluation are recommended.

When approaching a patient with marked leukocytosis (white blood cells [WBCs] >50,000/mm^3), it is important to differentiate a clonal proliferation from reactive neutrophilia. Patients with reactive causes for marked neutrophilia present with acute illness secondary to sepsis or acute exacerbation of autoimmune diseases such as ulcerative colitis. In contrast, patients with myeloproliferative neoplasms such as chronic myeloid leukemia (CML) usually present with marked neutrophilia with no symptoms or, in advanced cases, with symptoms related to "hypermetabolism" (weight loss, sweats, and fevers). Examination of a peripheral blood smear can often differentiate reactive from malignant causes of neutrophilia. For example, patients with CML often have absolute basophilia and eosinophilia in the presence of immature myeloid cells including myeloblasts, while patients with underlying sepsis commonly have eosinopenia and only rarely have circulating myeloblasts.

Additional laboratory testing is often necessary to confirm a diagnosis of a myeloproliferative disease. For instance, prior to the advent of cytogenetics and molecular testing, a leukocyte alkaline phosphatase (LAP) score, typically low with CML and high with leukemoid reaction, was used to differentiate between the two diagnoses. Currently, more sensitive and specific tests for CML are available, such as testing for Philadelphia chromosome or reverse transcriptase PCR assays for *BCR-ABL* transcripts.

Differential Diagnoses

Aside from the use of corticosteroids or from specific congenital disorders that limit neutrophil demargination, the most common culprit is increased production of neutrophils by the bone marrow driven by proinflammatory cytokines such as G-CSF, GM-CSF, TNF, interleukin (IL)-1, IL-6, IL-8, and so forth. Thus, various causes of neutrophilia overlap considerably with the causes of tissue inflammation.

1. **Infection:** Neutrophilia is a classical manifestation of bacterial infections and is a necessary physiological response to cytokines such as IL-6, TNF, and G-CSF. All types of organisms, bacterial, fungal, viral, and parasitic—can elicit neutrophilia. Infectious causes that may induce marked leukocytosis or a "leukemoid reaction" include staphylococcal bacteremia, *Clostridium difficile* colitis, miliary tuberculosis, acute pertussis, and, in tropical countries, visceral larva migrans. Some features of neutrophils when viewed on a peripheral blood smear can indicate an ongoing infection or inflammation, such as prominent neutrophil vacuolization and Dohle bodies. In addition to significant neutrophilia, patients typically present with an acute illness and even septic shock that requires emergent intervention with appropriate anti-infectives.

2. **Autoimmune disease:** Neutrophilia commonly accompanies autoimmune disorders such as lupus vasculitis, inflammatory bowel disease (IBD), adult Still's disease, and RA. In rare cases, neutrophilia might precede clinical symptoms or signs of the underlying disorder. Autoimmune-related neutrophilia can be chronic. An erythrocyte sedimentation rate (ESR) or a C-reactive protein (CRP) measurement can serve as a marker of ongoing disease. Successful management of the underlying autoimmune disorder with immunosuppressive therapies should resolve the neutrophilia.

3. **Physiological stressors:** Several physiological stressors have been implicated as causes for transient neutrophilia. Intensive exercise, pregnancy and childbirth, acute pain, major hemorrhage, and heat stroke result in the activation of stress hormones such as catecholamines and glucocorticoids which induce neutrophilia. Acute injuries such as myocardial infarction, fractures, pain crises secondary to sickle cell anemia, and a stroke result in both physiological elevation of stress hormones as well as tissue inflammation that can induce neutrophilia. In most cases related to a stressor, the neutrophilia is acute, temporally related to the stressor, and resolves over time with alleviation of the acute stressor.

4. **Drugs:** Medications are commonly implicated as causes for neutrophilia. Cytokines such as G-CSF and GM-CSF directly stimulate proliferation of neutrophils and precursors. Medications such as lithium or catecholamines have subtle effects on proinflammatory cytokines, resulting in low-grade neutrophilia. On the other hand, systemic glucocorticoids interfere with adhesion of neutrophils to the capillary wall and decrease their turnover. As with most medication-related side effects, withdrawal of the offending agent often reverses the neutrophilia.

5. **Asplenia:** Neutrophilia is usually observed early after splenectomy, although mild chronic neutrophilia may also be seen. Presence of Howell–Jolly bodies within red blood cells on a peripheral blood smear is a classic sign of functional asplenia. The neutrophilia does not require treatment; however, asplenic patients are at risk for sepsis from encapsulated organisms which would abruptly increase circulating neutrophil counts. Appropriate prophylactic measures such as vaccination and penicillin prophylaxis in children are the standard practice for patients with asplenia.

6. **Smoking:** Cigarette, cigar, and pipe smoking are associated with mild neutrophilia and may be related to a chronic underlying inflammatory state that is well described in chronic smokers even in the absence of obstructive lung disease. WBC counts can increase by 25% and remain chronically elevated in response to continuous smoking. This may persist up to 5 years after smoking cessation (5).

7. **Endocrine disorders:** Elevation in the serum levels of corticosteroids, catecholamines, progesterone, and human chorionic gonadotropin hormone is associated with increased neutrophil count. Disorders with excess hormones, such as pheochromocytoma and Cushing's syndrome, and even physiological elevations in these hormones, such as during pregnancy, can result in mild to moderate neutrophilia. Furthermore, acute endocrine stresses, such as thyrotoxicosis and diabetic ketoacidosis, even in the absence of an infection, may be associated with neutrophilia.

8. **Non-hematological malignancy:** Solid tumors can cause leukocytosis without direct bone marrow involvement. This is often secondary to tissue inflammation. However, some tumors (lung adenocarcinoma and neuroendocrine tumors) secrete cytokines like GM-CSF which result in neutrophilia.

9. **Hereditary chronic idiopathic neutrophilia** is a rare disorder where an autosomal mutation in the *CSF3R* gene constitutively activates the G-CSF receptor, promoting granulocyte

proliferation and differentiation, leading to a chronic neutrophilia. Various mutations in the *CSF3R* gene have now been identified and they result in several phenotypes of neutrophil disorders. Rare activating mutations can result in persistent congenital neutrophilia and a loss-of-function mutation may result in neutropenia and other qualitative defects (6).

Management and Prognosis

Neutrophilia is most often secondary to an underlying cause. Treatment and prognosis for patients with acquired neutrophilia depend on accurate identification and management of the underlying etiology.

Key Points

- Neutrophilia is defined as an ANC of >7,700/mm^3 and it results from increased production of neutrophils in the bone marrow or reduced tissue demargination.
- The commonest cause of neutrophilia is increased marrow production driven by inflammatory cytokines in infections and immune disorders.
- A variety of circumstances can cause mild neutrophilia, including smoking, endocrine disorders, physiological stress, and drugs such as catecholamines, lithium, and glucocorticoids.

QUALITATIVE NEUTROPHIL DEFECTS

Clinical Case 2.3

A 5-month-old boy was hospitalized for the second time with a staphylococcal pneumonia. Two months before, he had completed a prolonged course of penicillin for an umbilical site cellulitis. He was ill appearing, with a respiratory rate of 52/minute, temperature of 101°F, and bibasilar crackles on lung exam. Labs demonstrated the following: WBC: 8.8 K/µL, Hb: 10.1 g/dL, and platelets: 118 K/µL.

Introduction

Qualitative neutrophil defects are rare inherited diseases. In normal physiology, chemotactic substances such as IL-8 and monocyte chemotactic factor (MCF) produced by tissue-resident phagocytes stimulate the migration of circulating neutrophils to the sites of inflammation. As the neutrophil approaches the diseased sites, it slows down and rolls over the vascular endothelium mediated by selectin and firmly attaches itself to the endothelium surface mediated by integrin family molecules. After attaching to the endothelial surface, the neutrophil migrates to the extravascular space using either a paracellular or transcellular route. Once in the extravascular space, the neutrophils have an array of surface receptors that enable them to bind to and ingest foreign particles and microbes by a process known as phagocytosis. Phagocytosis is followed by neutrophil activation, degranulation, and respiratory burst activity leading to death of the target. The respiratory burst is an oxygen-dependent pathway for microbial killing which involves the generation of superoxide, hydrogen peroxide, hydroxyl radical, and subsequently hypochlorous acid and chloramine. Degranulation, on the other hand, is an oxygen-independent pathway involving release of the contents of the cell granules aiding bactericidal activity. Thus, disorders that result in a loss or gain of function in any one of the above essential neutrophil functions can result in specific qualitative defects (7).

Diagnosis

Qualitative neutrophil disorders are rare and typically diagnosed within the first year of life. Neutrophil defects often accompany congenital syndromes that impact several organ systems. Each disorder has a distinct clinical presentation that prompts specific workup testing and/or molecular analysis. Molecular techniques such as whole exome sequencing have emerged as a mainstream strategy to diagnose congenital neutrophil disorders. Thus, the workup and diagnosis of specific neutrophil disorders are discussed individually subsequently.

Key Diagnostic Dilemma

Affected patients present with a common theme of recurrent bacterial or fungal infections soon after birth. Since there is no newborn screening performed for these disorders, patients come to attention at the time of diagnosis of opportunistic or recurrent infections. In some cases, a bacterial infection of the umbilical stump soon after birth may be the first sign of a qualitative neutrophil defect. The diagnosis of the specific cause of recurrent infections in the newborn can be challenging because several individual neutrophil defects can lead to a similar phenotype. In this regard, our approach is to first perform a thorough physical examination and basic laboratory testing which could uncover phenotypic clues such as albinism associated with Chediak–Higashi syndrome and elevated IgE levels associated with hyper-IgE syndrome (HIES). Subsequently, we proceed with functional testing of neutrophils, such as the nitroblue tetrazolium (NBT), which evaluates the respiratory burst in neutrophils, and platelet aggregation testing to assess the function of integrins in patients with suspected leukocyte adhesion defects (LADs). Finally, targeted gene mutation testing is performed by PCR for confirmation. If a diagnosis cannot be reached despite the systematic approach, most centers in the current era refer patients and first-degree family members for whole exome sequencing (8).

Differential Diagnosis

Defects in the function of neutrophils are congenital disorders and can be classified as defects in (a) chemotaxis/adhesion, (b) neutrophil activation and degranulation, (c) the respiratory burst, and (d) other disorders of intracellular killing. These are individually discussed subsequently.

Disorders of Chemotaxis/Adhesion

LAD: Neutrophils migration to the target organs is mediated by various adhesion molecules like integrins and selectins and their ligands. Each integrin molecule is a heterodimer consisting of an alpha and a beta chain and is essential for firm adhesion of the leukocyte to the endothelium and subsequent transendothelial migration. Selectins, on the other hand, are another family of adhesion molecules that are responsible for the "rolling" interaction between leukocytes and the endothelium. Defects in any of these adhesion molecules can, therefore, adversely impact neutrophil migration and would not be corrected by G-CSF administration. Thus, patients who have genetic mutations involving these proteins are susceptible to a wide variety of invasive organisms, depending on the defect, as discussed subsequently.

LAD I: LAD I is an autosomal recessive defect in beta-2 integrins (*ITGB2* defect). As a result, neutrophils are unable to tightly adhere and migrate, but rolling over the endothelium remains intact. As with most migration defects, the first clinical presentation is usually an infection invading the skin or mucous membrane surface. The infected sites undergo necrosis, but fail to develop pus, even though patients are capable of mounting a robust peripheral neutrophilia (neutrophil counts can reach as high as 100,000/mm^3 during an infection). Infections left untreated can result in sepsis and eventual death. Indeed, >75% of all children with the severe form of this defect die from an infection before the age of 5 years without a curative allogeneic HSCT. One of the earliest clinical presentations of this syndrome is delayed cord detachment with marked peripheral neutrophilia soon after birth. A diagnosis requires demonstration of mutations within the leukocyte integrin beta-2 (CD18), but flow cytometry analysis of blood from the newborn may demonstrate reduced expression of CD11 or CD18 (additional beta integrins). Furthermore, severity of the defect is directly related to the amount of CD18 expression (severe for <2% expression and mild to moderate for >2%). Families known to harbor *LAD-1* mutations should undergo genetic counseling, and mutation analysis during gestation is highly recommended.

LAD II: This is a rare disorder (approximately 10 patients and associated families have been described) in which defect in the fucose transferase enzyme (gene: *SLC35C1*) leads to inappropriate glycosylation of the selectin molecule, Lewis-X (CD15s), in addition to several other molecules that are necessary for homeostasis. Although the defect involves abnormal "rolling" or binding with P-selectin or E-selectin, patients can still have emigration of neutrophils and mount an immune response. Most patients have neutrophilia (10–40,000/mm^3) and less-severe sinopulmonary, skin, and mucous membrane infections as in LAD I. Thus, most cases are apparent later in life when anatomical defects that accompany LAD II become apparent, such as short stature, abnormal facies, periodontitis, severe cognitive impairment, and frequent mild to moderate sinopulmonary infections. This disorder is closely associated with the "Bombay" blood group (*hh* phenotype) or an absence of the usual A, B, and H antigens, which can sometimes be the first sign of glycosylation defects. Sometimes, when enzyme activity is still present at low levels, as was the case in one patient studied extensively, high-dose fucose (substrate: up to 492 mg/kg five times a day) supplementation could reverse the defects and be therapeutic when instituted early in infancy.

LAD III: LAD III is a variant of LAD I, wherein the genetic defect lies within the kindlin-3 (gene: *FMTR3*) protein that is essential for inside-out signaling of all beta integrins (1, 2, and 3) within the body. Thus, in addition to the defects seen with LAD I, patients present with a Glanzmann's thrombasthenia type of bleeding from birth because of ineffective beta-3 integrin signaling (*ITGB3*). Thus, assessment of platelet aggregation in addition to measurement of CD18 levels in a newborn suspected of having LAD could distinguish between types I and III. This can impact treatment as bleeding in these neonates may require platelet transfusions. Assessment for deleterious mutations within the kindlin-3 gene may confirm this diagnosis. As with LAD I, an allogeneic HSCT is the only curative therapy.

HIES or Job's syndrome: HIES is a rare primary immunodeficiency state and usually presents in infancy with recurrent staphylococcal skin and lung infections. Two forms have been described, autosomal dominant (AD-HIES, type 1 or Job's syndrome) and autosomal recessive (AR-HIES, type 2) forms. Type 1, which is the most common, is associated with heterozygous mutations in the transcription factor *STAT3*, which promotes inflammatory responses by individual immune cells in response to cytokine (such as IL-6, IL10, IL-12, etc.) signaling. The dominant negative mutation prevents dimerization with the normal *STAT3* produced from the unaffected allele, thereby inhibiting its function and presenting as an autosomal dominant disease. In addition to causing severe defects in neutrophil trafficking and emigration in response to cytokine signals, *STAT3* defects have other multiple phenotypic presentations such as skeletal and dermatological disorders.

Type 2 (autosomal recessive form) is extremely rare and is limited to specific families commonly where consanguinity rates are high. The pathogenic mutations again impact normal *STAT3* functions, such as defects in dedicator of cytokinesis 8 gene (*DOCK8*), tyrosine kinase 2 (*TYK-2*) gene, and phosphoglucomutase 3 gene (*PGM3*). In general, patients with HIES are diagnosed in early childhood (rarely diagnosed in infancy) and they present with a spectrum of findings such as eczema, recurrent skin abscesses, and sinopulmonary infection. Severe recurrent viral infections with herpes simplex virus and herpes zoster are more indicative of type 2 due to T-cell dysfunction and more commonly have autoimmune manifestations. Type 1 individuals have more connective tissue and skeletal abnormalities such as osteoporosis, two rows of teeth, scoliosis, and fractures. Increased IgE levels and peripheral eosinophilia are common in both forms. Serum IgG, IgA, and IgM are typically normal in type 1, whereas IgM and T-cell counts are low in type 2. Definitive diagnosis can be established with genetic analysis of the *STAT3* and/or *DOCK8/TYK-2* or *PGM3* genes, but a clinical diagnosis can be made if a score of 30 or higher is made based on the National Institutes of Health (NIH) clinical scale which incorporates the following findings: IgE >1,000 IU/mL, typical facies, internal organ abscesses, severe infections, pneumatoceles, nail candidiasis, fractures, and scoliosis.

While an allogeneic hematopoietic stem cell transplant has been shown to cure the hematological and immunological defects of HIES, it is not effective in reversing non-hematological organ damage. Thus, the management is usually supportive with the goal of preventing long-term pulmonary complications from recurrent infections. These patients receive prophylactic antimicrobials, intravenous immunoglobulin (IVIG), and daily chlorhexidine washes to prevent infections. In those who develop severe autoimmune or allergic manifestations, systemic steroids and other T-cell immunosuppressants such as cyclosporine have been used.

Disorder of Degranulation

Neutrophil granules contain toxic proteins for the purpose of killing phagocytosed and neighboring microbes. Defects in granule production and/or degranulation can present with low normal neutrophil counts in the setting of normal chemotaxis, but inability to clear acute bacterial infections. The most common disorders of degranulation are Chediak–Higashi syndrome and specific granule deficiency.

Chediak–Higashi syndrome: Chediak–Higashi syndrome is an autosomal recessive disorder caused by mutations in the lysosomal trafficking regulator gene, *LYST*. There is uncontrolled granule fusion leading to large defective granules in granule-containing cells such as Schwann cells, melanosomes, and neutrophils. These large lysosomal vacuoles can be visualized within granulocytes on a peripheral blood smear or within the bone marrow on biopsy. Children often present with neutropenia and are associated with defects in other cells like lymphocytes, natural killer (NK) cells, and platelets. They have hypopigmented patches of hair, eye (iris), and skin (albinism), along with recurrent infections. Beyond childhood, severe neurological defects may begin to manifest because of dysfunctional Schwann cells. There are two known clinical phases of the disease: (a) stable phase and (b) accelerated phase. The stable phase is usually managed by routine measure to prevent and treat any antecedent infections. The accelerated phase, on the other hand, is thought to be triggered by a viral infection like Epstein–Barr virus (EBV) and causes uncontrollable proliferation of neutrophils which infiltrate the vital organs leading to organ failure. This is treated with steroids and chemotherapeutic agents, but is often fatal. Thus, most patients who present while in stable phase should be referred for a potentially curative allogeneic HSCT.

Specific granule deficiency: This is an extremely rare autosomal recessive disorder characterized by absence of granules in neutrophils. Most of the patients have a mutation in the *CEBPE* gene, which inhibits neutrophil maturation beyond the promyelocyte stage in the bone marrow. Patients present early in life with repeated pyogenic infections, with atypical infections being the key manifestation. Patients are primarily managed with prophylactic antibiotics and aggressive treatment of infections.

Disorder of Respiratory Burst

Chronic granulomatous disease (CGD): CGD usually presents early in life and is characterized by recurrent, life-threatening bacterial or fungal infections. It is caused by defects in the phagocyte nicotinamide adenine dinucleotide phosphate (NADPH) oxidase, which is responsible for the generation of microbicidal reactive oxygen species (ROS). The common sites of infections are the lungs, liver, lymph nodes, and skin. The diagnosis is commonly made by the age of 5 years, although a growing number of patients are now diagnosed during adulthood. Males are primarily affected as most of the mutations are X-linked. Carriers of CGD are asymptomatic. Patients with CGD usually present with recurrent infections by catalase-positive organisms (most bacterial and all fungal pathogens), which cause, on the descending order of frequency, pneumonia, abscesses, suppurative adenitis, osteomyelitis, bacteremia/fungemia, and superficial skin infections. Physical examination may reveal hepatosplenomegaly and lymphadenopathy. Patients may have hypergammaglobulinemia, elevated erythrocyte sedimentation rate (ESR), hypoalbuminemia, and anemia of chronic disease. One of the hallmarks of this disease is presence of granulomas caused by chronic inflammatory reaction to the pathogen. Functional assessment of neutrophils is performed by the NBT test which evaluates the ability of immune cells to convert colorless NBT to deep blue color. In this assay, neutrophils are exposed to phorbol myristate acetate (PMA) and incubated with NBT. One hundred neutrophils are stained and counted. More than 95% of neutrophils from healthy individuals stain positive as opposed to <5% of neutrophils in CGD. Females with the X-linked CGD show 30% to 70% positive neutrophils. However, false-positive or false-negative tests can occur, especially with mild diseases and variants of CGD. Similarly, a diagnosis can be made by assessing the number of dihydrorhodamine (DHR)-positive neutrophils after PMA stimulation in a DHR flow cytometry assay. The DHR test is now considered more accurate than the NBT, and the number of positive DHR cells after stimulation can indicate the genotype as well (carrier vs. homozygote). Further mutation analysis by PCR-based whole exome or next-generation sequencing can not only confirm the diagnosis, but also identify carrier states with abnormal respiratory burst.

Management of patients with CGD relies on prevention, rapid diagnosis, and aggressive treatment of the underlying infection. All yearly vaccinations are strongly recommended, except for Bacillus Calmette–Guérin (BCG).

Lifelong prophylaxis with antibiotics (trimethoprim/sulfamethoxazole, dicloxacillin, or levofloxacin) is the standard practice to avoid recurrent infections, although there is weaker evidence supporting the use of fungal prophylaxis. Itraconazole, however, is used for patients who have had recurrent episodes of fungal infections. As with most neutrophil defects, an allogeneic HSCT is curative, but carries significant treatment-related toxicities for patients with CGD. Therefore, gene therapy trials are ongoing for X-linked CGD, wherein patients are transplanted with genetically modified autologous hematopoietic stem cells.

Other Disorders of Intracellular Killing

Myeloperoxidase (MPO) deficiency: MPO is an enzyme required for the formation of hydrochlorous acid, which is an end product that kills the infective organism. The *MPO* gene is located on chromosome 17. Generally, quantitative or qualitative defect of MPO does not lead to severe manifestations of immunodeficiency, but often these individuals are susceptible to candidal infections and tend to have diabetes mellitus. Patients present later in life, sometimes in adolescence. Diagnosis can be challenging, since this disorder is rare and the phenotype is not severe. So, once suspected, a diagnosis can be confirmed by immunohistochemical staining for MPO on myeloid lineage cells in the blood or marrow. Since the antibody for MPO can cross-react with another peroxidase found in eosinophils, it is important to assess the levels of MPO within neutrophils or monocytes.

Generally, prophylactic antibiotics are not recommended for these patients; however, those who have underlying diabetes should be vigilant for signs and symptoms of early infections. Environmental mold exposures and use of prolonged antibacterial agents greatly increase the risk of fungal infections, which may be life-threatening for this patient population, and thus should be avoided.

Glutathione synthetase deficiency: Glutathione is a potent antioxidant that prevents cell damage by neutralizing harmful oxidative molecules generated during energy production. The deficiency may be categorized into mild, moderate, and severe. Patients who have severe deficiencies of this enzyme (<20% functioning) are susceptible to opportunistic infections because of the failure of neutrophils to mount a respiratory burst. Specifically, ingestion of foreign particles or bacteria results in an oxidative stress to the neutrophil membranes. In the absence of sufficient glutathione synthetase, the neutrophils die before initiating the respiratory burst cascade. In select individuals who have been closely studied, bouts of infection are accompanied with episodes of severe neutropenia and high neutrophil turnover. Mild and moderate forms of this disease usually present with hemolytic anemias without phenotypic defects in neutrophil function. A severe form of this disease has been isolated in select families and is not a common disorder. Diagnosis is first suspected when patients experience hemolytic anemia and can be confirmed by demonstrating low levels of this enzyme in red blood cells. Conversely, high levels of 5-oxoproline, a metabolite of oxidative stress, can be detected in the urine by gas chromatography–mass spectrometry. The mainstay of treatment is avoidance of medications or substances that can increase oxidative stress. In severe cases, an allogeneic HSCT should be considered.

Severe glucose-6-phosphate dehydrogenase (G6PD) deficiency: G6PD is an enzyme necessary for ensuring adequate availability of NADPH during respiratory burst. Individuals with G6PD deficiency present with hemolytic anemia and jaundice after exposure to an oxidative stress. This disorder is more common and has a similar pathogenesis to glutathione synthetase deficiency. In severe cases, neutrophils fail to mount a sufficient respiratory burst because of inadequate available NADPH. Although the hemolytic anemia after oxidative stress exposure leads to the initial diagnosis, the specific neutrophil defects in severe cases can be uncovered by NBT dye reduction in neutrophils and are confirmed by undetectable G6PD in red cells and leukocytes. Since the red cell and neutrophil defects manifest in the presence of an oxidative stress, the mainstay of management is avoidance of substances such as dapsone or fava beans which have the potential to induce hemolysis and neutrophil defects (see Table 2.3).

Table 2.3 Common Inherited Neutrophil Defects and Their Pathogenesis

Function	Disease	Pathogenesis
Chemotaxis/ adhesion	1. Leukocyte adhesion deficiency	Defects in integrin and selectin molecules leading to defective adherence, and rolling and migration of neutrophils
	2. Hyper-IgE syndrome	Mutation in transcription factor STAT3 causes defect in neutrophil trafficking and emigration
Neutrophil activation	1. Chediak–Higashi syndrome	Mutation in lysosomal trafficking regulator gene LYST causes formation of large defective neutrophilic granules
	2. Specific granule deficiency	Mutation in CEBPE gene inhibits neutrophil maturation
Disorder of respiratory burst	Chronic granulomatous disease	Defect in NADPH oxidase causes ineffective microbial killing
Other mechanisms of intracellular killing	1. Myeloperoxidase deficiency	Several known mutations

(continued)

Table 2.3 Common Inherited Neutrophil Defects and Their Pathogenesis (*continued*)

Function	Disease	Pathogenesis
	2. Glutathione synthetase deficiency	
	3. Severe G6PD deficiency	

G6PD, glucose-6-phosphate dehydrogenase; NADPH, nicotinamide adenine dinucleotide phosphate.

Management and Prognosis

While the mainstay of treatment for severe congenital neutrophil defects involves allogeneic HSCT (9,10), supportive care, management of less-severe phenotypes, and prognosis of these disorders have been individually discussed in the text.

Key Points

- Qualitative neutrophil defects are rare inherited diseases typically diagnosed in the first year of life.
- Affected patients present with recurrent bacterial or fungal infections soon after birth.
- Qualitative neutrophil defects can be classified as defects in (a) chemotaxis/adhesion, (b) neutrophil activation and degranulation, (c) the respiratory burst, and (d) other disorders of intracellular killing.
- Initial evaluation should begin with a thorough history and physical exam which may replace clues to the diagnosis. If the diagnosis is unclear, then NBT testing of neutrophils should be performed to examine the respiratory burst, followed by platelet aggregation testing to assess the function of integrins.

REFERENCES

1. Lim E-M, Cembrowski G, Cembrowski M, Clarke G. Race-specific WBC and neutrophil count reference intervals. *Int J Lab Hematol.* 2010;32(6 pt 2):590–597. doi:10.1111/j.1751-553X.2010.01223.x
2. Charles BA, Hsieh MM, Adeyemo AA, et al. Analyses of genome wide associated data, cytokines and gene expression in African-Americans with benign ethnic neutropenia. *PLoS One.* 2018;13(3):e0194400. doi:10.1371/journal.pone.0194400

3. Gibson C, Berliner N. How we evaluate and treat neutropenia in adults. *Blood.* 2014;124(8):1251–1258. doi:10.1182/blood-2014-02-482612

4. Dale DC, Bolyard A, Marrero T, et al. Long-term effects of G-CSF therapy in cyclic neutropenia. *N Engl J Med.* 2017;377(23):2290. doi:10.1056/NEJMc1709258

5. Stemmelin GR, Doti C, Shanley CM, et al. Smoking as a cause for mild chronic neutrophilia. *Blood.* 2004;104(11):3796.

6. Triot A, Järvinen PM, Arostegui JI, et al. Inherited biallelic CSF3R mutations in severe congenital neutropenia. *Blood.* 2014;123(24):3811–3817. doi:10.1182/blood-2013-11-535419

7. Dinauer MC. Primary immune deficiencies with defects in neutrophil function. *Hematology Am Soc Hematol Educ Program.* 2016;2016(1):43–50. doi:10.1182/asheducation-2016.1.43

8. Rabbani B, Tekin M, Mahdieh N. The promise of whole-exome sequencing in medical genetics. *J Human Genet.* 2014;59:5–15. doi:10.1038/jhg.2013.114

9. Connelly JA, Choi SW, Levine JE. Hematopoietic stem cell transplantation for severe congenital neutropenia. *Curr Opin Hematol.* 2012;19(1):44–51. doi:10.1097/MOH.0b013e32834da96e

10. Elhasid R, Rowe, JM. Hematopoetic stem cell transplantation in neutrophil disorders: severe congenital neutropenia, leukocyte adhesion deficiency and chronic granulomatous disease. *Clinic Rev Allerg Immunol.* 2010;38:61. doi:10.1007/s12016-009-8129-y

3 Myeloid Disorders

Quillan Huang, Nicole Canon, Sravanti Teegavarapu,
and Sarvari Yellapragada

SYSTEMIC MASTOCYTOSIS

Clinical Case 3.1

A 79-year-old man with a history of definitively treated prostate and renal cell carcinoma was referred to hematology for workup of a moderate macrocytic anemia which developed over a period of several years. At presentation, his hemoglobin was 9.4 g/dL and mean cell volume (MCV) was 102.6 fL. Routine anemia workup including vitamin levels was negative, but his serum erythropoietin was elevated to 32 mU/mL. Bone marrow biopsy showed trilineage dysplasia and 2% bone marrow blasts. Cytogenetic and fluorescence in-situ hybridization (FISH) analyses were notable for trisomy 8. He was diagnosed with myelodysplastic syndrome (MDS) with trilineage dysplasia, intermediate risk by Revised International Prognostic Scoring System (IPSS-R). He was followed for his asymptomatic MDS and a year later was found to have lytic and sclerotic lesions throughout the thoracolumbar spine and pelvic bones. At this time, he had no evidence of recurrence of his prostate or renal cell carcinoma. A bone biopsy showed a dense infiltrate of cells expressing CD117 and tryptase. A repeat bone marrow biopsy demonstrated 90% cellularity with 5% blasts, trilineage dysplasia, as well as 15% mature mast cells. Polymerase chain reaction (PCR) was positive for the KIT D816V mutation, and serum tryptase levels were above 200 ng/mL. The World Health Organization (WHO) diagnostic criteria for aggressive systemic mastocytosis with associated hematologic neoplasm (ASM–AHN) were met. His MDS progressed, and azacitidine was initiated with a plan to consider adding midostaurin, but azacitidine was tolerated poorly. The patient decided to pursue best supportive care.

Introduction

Mastocytosis is a spectrum of disorders characterized by accumulation of neoplastic mast cells in tissues. Mastocytic disorders are classified into cutaneous mastocytosis (CM), systemic mastocytosis (SM), and localized mast cell tumors based on the site of involvement. Although the majority of childhood cases of masto-cytosis are limited to the skin, most adults are diagnosed with sys-temic disease. This section primarily focuses on SM.

SM is a myeloid neoplasm in which abnormal mast cells accu-mulate in the skin, bone marrow, and visceral organs, most notably the liver and spleen. A driver mutation, *KIT* D816V, is present in over 90% of cases and leads to a constitutively active tyrosine kinase (1). Symptoms stem from the systemic secretion of mast cell–derived vasoactive mediators as well as direct organ infiltration of mast cells. Thus, clinical presentations may include anaphylaxis, diar-rhea, flushing, and neuropsychiatric symptoms. Moreover, mani-festations of direct organ infiltration (termed "C-findings") include hepatosplenomegaly, malabsorption, and lytic or sclerotic bone lesions, with or without pathologic fractures.

The clinical spectrum of SM ranges from indolent and smol-dering forms characterized by a lack of direct organ infiltration to more aggressive forms characterized by a higher mast cell burden with C-findings. Anaphylaxis occurs more frequently with indo-lent forms of SM, though it can occur in all subtypes, with 50% of patients experiencing at least one episode. Though associated with fewer mast cell mediator–derived symptoms, advanced SM has a very poor prognosis.

Diagnosis

The initial evaluation of a patient suspected to have SM should include the following:

- Complete blood count and differential with smear review and serum chemistries, including serum tryptase level (which is invariably high in SM) and IgE levels
- Peripheral blood PCR for *KIT* D816V, which can be detected in up to 70% of SM, making it a potentially useful screen in cases of suspected SM
- Bone marrow aspiration and biopsy, including immunohisto-chemistry and/or flow cytometry analyses for CD2, CD25, CD117 (*KIT*), and mast cell tryptase. Coexisting hematologic diseases and alternative causes of mastocytosis such as hypereosinophilic syndromes should also be assessed (Figures 3.2, 3.3, and 3.4)
- Imaging in patients with bone pain to evaluate for osteolytic lesions. Dual-energy x-ray absorptiometry (DEXA) scanning may be performed to evaluate for secondary osteoporosis
- Abdominal imaging to assess for hepatosplenomegaly and/or lymphadenopathy

The primary distinction between CM and SM is infiltrating mast cells in the bone marrow or visceral organs. A diagnosis of SM is

Table 3.1 2016 WHO Classification and Diagnostic Criteria for Mastocytosis

CM: Skin lesions demonstrating the typical clinical findings of urticaria pigmentosa/maculopapular CM, diffuse CM, or solitary mastocytoma, and typical histologic infiltrates of mast cells in a multifocal or diffuse pattern in an adequate skin biopsy. Diagnostic criteria for SM cannot be met

SM: Either one major criterion and one minor criterion, or three minor criteria

Major criterion

Multifocal, dense infiltrates of mast cells detected in sections of bone marrow and/or other extracutaneous organs (≥15 mast cells in aggregates)

Minor criteria

1. In biopsy sections of bone marrow or other extracutaneous organs, >25% of the mast cells in the infiltrate are spindle shaped or have atypical morphology or, of all mast cells in the bone marrow aspirate smears, >25% are immature or atypical (Figure 3.1)
2. Detection of an activating point mutation at codon 816 of *KIT* in bone marrow, blood, or another extracutaneous organ
3. Mast cells in bone marrow, blood, or other extracutaneous organs express CD2 and/or CD25 in addition to normal mast cell markers
4. Serum total tryptase persistently exceeds 20 ng/mL (unless there is an associated clonal myeloid disorder, in which case this parameter is not valid)

CM, cutaneous mastocytosis; SM, systemic mastocytosis.

Source: Data from Valent P, Akin C, Metcalfe DD. Mastocytosis: 2016 updated WHO classification and novel emerging treatment concepts. *Blood.* 2017;129(11):1420–1427. doi:10.1182/blood-2016-09-731893

made when the major criterion and one minor criterion, or at least three minor criteria are met (see Table 3.1). Determination of the subtype of SM is made based on the presence of B findings (reflecting mast cell infiltration without organ dysfunction) and C findings (reflecting organ dysfunction resulting from mast cell infiltration). If only B findings are present, the diagnosis is either indolent systemic mastocytosis (ISM) or smoldering systemic mastocytosis (SSM). SM with an associated hematologic neoplasm (SM-AHN), aggressive systemic mastocytosis (ASM), and mast cell leukemia (MCL) are the poorer prognosis variants of SM, and together are considered to be "advanced" SM (Table 3.2). The advanced forms of SM are characterized by either C findings (indicating ASM), >20% mast cells on marrow aspirate (indicating MCL), or the presence of another hematologic neoplasm separately meeting WHO diagnostic criteria (indicating SM-AHN).

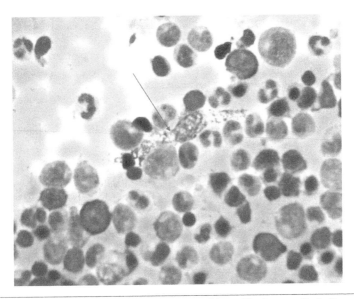

Figure 3.1 Mast cell image from bone marrow biopsy. The image reflects the classic spindle-shaped morphology of the mast cell with evident degranulation within its cytoplasm.

Source: Courtesy of Dr. Mark Udden.

In SM-AHN, the associated hematologic neoplasm is almost always myeloid, with myeloproliferative neoplasms, chronic myelomonocytic leukemia (CMML), and MDS being the most commonly associated diseases. By contrast, acute leukemias or lymphoid diseases such as lymphoma or myeloma are rare.

The *KIT* D816V mutation is detected in over 90% of patients with mastocytosis, including adults with ISM who otherwise have a normal life expectancy. This suggests that *KIT*-independent factors are important for disease progression and prognosis. A number of other somatic mutations have prognostic and predictive value in mastocytosis. Commonly mutated sites include *TET2, SRSF2, ASXL1, CBL,* and *RUNX1.*

Under the revised 2016 WHO classification of hematolymphoid diseases, mastocytosis is no longer classified under "myeloproliferative neoplasms" and now has its own unique major category. There have been some nomenclature changes, with "systemic mastocytosis with an associated hematologic non–mast cell lineage disease (SM-AHNMD)" now renamed as "SM-AHN." There have also been subcategory changes proposed to better risk-stratify patients within existing categories. "Aggressive systemic mastocytosis in transformation (ASM-t)" has been proposed as a

Table 3.2 Classification of Mastocytosis

1. CM

2. SM
   a. ISM—Zero to one B finding, no C findings
   b. SSM—Two to three B findings, no C findings
   c. SM-AHN—Any variant, with AHN found
   d. ASM—C findings present
   e. MCL—20% neoplastic mast cells in bone marrow smears

3. Localized mast cell tumors, including mast cell sarcoma and extracutaneous mastocytoma

"B" findings (high mast cell burden, without evidence of organ damage)	"C" findings (indicative of organ damage caused by mast cell infiltration)
1. Bone marrow biopsy showing >30% infiltration by mast cells (focal, dense aggregates) and/or serum total tryptase >200 mg/mL	1. Bone marrow dysfunction manifested by one or more cytopenias (ANC <1 × 10⁹/L, Hb <10 g/dL, or platelets <100 × 10⁹/L), but no obvious non–mast cell hematopoietic malignancy
2. Signs of dysplasia or myeloproliferation, in non–mast cell lineages, but insufficient criteria for diagnosis of SM-AHN, with normal or only slightly abnormal blood counts	2. Palpable hepatomegaly with impairment of liver function, ascites, and/or portal HTN
3. Hepatomegaly without impairment of liver function, and/or palpable splenomegaly without hypersplenism, and/or lymphadenopathy	3. Skeletal involvement with large osteolytic lesions and/or pathologic fractures (pathologic fractures caused by osteoporosis do not qualify)
	4. Palpable splenomegaly with hypersplenism
	5. Malabsorption with weight loss due to GI mast cell infiltrates

ANC, absolute neutrophil count; ASM, aggressive systemic mastocytosis; CM, cutaneous mastocytosis; GI, gastrointestinal; Hb, hemoglobin; HTN, hypertension; ISM, indolent systemic mastocytosis; MCL, mast cell leukemia; SM, systemic mastocytosis; SM-AHN, systemic mastocytosis with an associated hematologic neoplasm; SSM, smoldering systemic mastocytosis.

Source: Adapted from Arber DA, Orazi A, Hasserjian R, et al. The 2016 revision to the World Health Organization classification of myeloid neoplasms and acute leukemia. *Blood.* 2016;127(20):2391–2405; Valent P, Akin C, Metcalfe DD. Mastocytosis: 2016 updated WHO classification and novel emerging treatment concepts. *Blood.* 2017;129(11):1420–1427. doi:10.1182/blood-2016-09-731893

subcategory defined as ASM with 5% to 19% blast cells in the bone marrow, as these patients have a significantly higher risk of transformation to MCL. It has also been proposed that MCL be further refined to include "acute" versus "chronic" MCL, with acute MCL being defined as MCL with C findings and a worse prognosis.

Diagnostic Dilemmas

Mastocytosis is a difficult diagnosis due to its low incidence and variable clinical presentation. Patients who do not have characteristic skin lesions amenable to biopsy present unique challenges that can result in incorrect and/or delayed diagnosis. More common entities, such as MDS, are often considered in patients with hematologic abnormalities, and the final diagnosis may be delayed until a biopsy of the bone marrow or another involved site is performed. If a patient is diagnosed initially with another hematologic disease such as MDS, one clue to the concomitant presence of SM-AHN would be the incidental finding of a *KIT* mutation which is rarely seen in MDS. Patients presenting with recurrent episodes of flushing or allergic reactions/anaphylaxis may be misdiagnosed with primary allergic diseases or functional neuroendocrine malignancies. Table 3.3 lists a number of alternative diagnoses which may present similarly to SM.

Prognosis

The WHO subclassification of SM is the primary driver of prognosis. Patients with ISM have a low progression rate compared to more advanced forms of SM, with one retrospective study showing a rate of approximately 3% after median follow-up of over 12 years (2). Patients with ASM have a less predictable clinical course, especially in the era of novel therapies (see the section on treatment). However, prognosis is generally much worse in advanced SM, ranging from 3.5 years in patients with ASM to <6 months in those with mast cell leukemia (3). In patients with SM-AHNMD, the prognosis is typically driven by the associated hematologic neoplasm.

The prognostic role of molecular and cytogenetic findings in SM is an area of active investigation. In patients with a *KIT* D816V mutation, the allele burden correlates with survival (4). In this study, patients in whom the *KIT* D816V mutation burden exceeded 2% had a 10-year survival of around 50%, as compared to over 80% in patients with an allele burden <2%. Absence of *KIT* D816V has not clearly correlated with survival, but investigations are limited by the high frequency of D816V as well as the lack of next-generation sequencing in older studies of molecular drivers of SM.

The presence of additional somatic mutations correlates with advanced disease state and shorter overall survival. In the midostaurin era, *SRSF2*, *ASXL1*, and *RUNX1* have predictive value (5). Patients mutated at one of these loci (S/A/R[pos]) have a 39% overall response rate (ORR) when treated with midostaurin, compared to 75% in wild-type patients. Cytogenetics independently affects prognosis, with survival in non-indolent SM strongly correlating with the presence or absence of poor-risk karyotypic features such as complex cytogenetics or a monosomal karyotype (6).

Table 3.3 Differential Diagnosis of Systemic Mastocytosis

Mediator release symptoms	• Secondary mast cell activation disorders (allergic diseases, physical urticaria)
	• Mast cell activation secondary to malignancy
	  ○ Hypereosinophilic syndromes
	  ○ Hodgkin lymphoma
	  ○ Miscellaneous solid tumors
	• Idiopathic mast cell activation syndrome/idiopathic anaphylaxis
	• Functional neuroendocrine tumors
	  ○ Carcinoid syndrome (24-hour urine 5-HIAA, serum chromogranin)
	  ○ Pheochromocytoma (urine and plasma metanephrines)
	  ○ VIPoma (serum VIP)

Organ infiltration	• Metastatic malignancy
	  ○ Hematologic malignancies (lymphoma, myeloma, myeloproliferative neoplasms, histiocytic diseases)
	  ○ Solid tumors
	• Systemic/infiltrative diseases
	  ○ Sarcoidosis
	  ○ Amyloidosis
	  ○ Lysosomal storage diseases
	  ○ Autoimmune diseases

Presence of *KIT* D816V mutation (seen in 90%–95% of SM)	• Present in 20% to 30% of core-binding factor AML (t(8;21), inv(16), t(16;16)), where it confers poorer prognosis • *KIT* mutations (including D816V) have also been described in melanoma and seminoma • The *PDGFRA* D842V mutation seen in gastrointestinal stromal tumors is structurally and functionally analogous to D816V

5-HIAA, 5-hydroxyindoleacetic acid; AML, acute myeloid leukemia; SM, systemic mastocytosis; VIP, vasoactive intestinal peptide.

Management

General Measures

Patients with all subtypes of SM may have symptoms attributable to mast cell–derived mediators which usually respond to a combination of H1/H2 receptor blockers. As anaphylaxis is common in all subtypes of SM (often from a concomitant IgE-mediated allergy), patients should carry epinephrine auto-injectors. Patients should be educated on the potential triggers for anaphylaxis, which may include environmental and emotional stressors, medications, or medical procedures. Prophylactic therapies to consider include corticosteroids, mast cell stabilizers, and leukotriene inhibitors. Osteoporosis is common and treated with calcium/vitamin D supplementation with or without bisphosphonates. Gastrointestinal symptoms can be treated with the addition of proton pump inhibitors to H2 receptor blockers.

Cytoreductive Therapy for Advanced Disease

Midostaurin received U.S. Food and Drug Administration (FDA) approval in 2017 for the treatment of advanced SM (ASM, SM-AHM, and MCL) regardless of *KIT* mutational status, and is a reasonable first-line option for treatment. The standard dose is 100 mg twice daily. Midostaurin inhibits the protein product of *KIT*, including *KIT* with the D816V mutation. A phase 2 trial of 89 patients with advanced SM demonstrated an ORR of 60%, with 45% having a major response defined as complete resolution of at least one type of end-organ damage. In patients with any degree of response, the median duration of response was 24.1 months. Of the 16 patients in the study with MCL, the ORR was 50% with a median overall survival of 9.4 months. Importantly, responses were maintained in those patients without a *KIT* D816V mutation (ORR 44%). Midostaurin was generally well tolerated, with the most common adverse events being low-grade nausea, vomiting, and diarrhea (7).

Prior to the approval of midostaurin, cytoreductive treatment options included cladribine, interferon-alfa, and hydroxyurea. Cladribine is an option for patients with advanced SM who have failed to respond to midostaurin. One study including 32 patients with advanced SM demonstrated an ORR of 50%, with a median duration of response lasting 2.47 years. Clinical improvement in both mediator release and mast cell infiltration–related symptoms was observed (8). Patients with advanced SM that is progressing slowly can be treated with interferon, giving response rates around 20% (9). In patients with advanced SM who are intolerant of more aggressive therapy, hydroxyurea has been an option for palliation.

In addition to midostaurin, several other tyrosine kinase inhibitors have been studied in SM. Imatinib is FDA approved for the treatment of ASM without D816V mutation, which confers imatinib resistance. Since the vast majority of patients with SM carry the D816V mutation, most patients are not imatinib candidates. Dasatinib demonstrated a 33% response rate in a small phase 2 trial, though responses may have been less pronounced in patients carrying the D816V mutation (10). In another phase 2 study of ASM, nilotinib demonstrated a response rate of 22% including patients with D816V mutation (11).

Masitinib is an inhibitor of wild-type (not D816V-mutated) *KIT*, which has been evaluated in a phase 3 trial for symptom control in ISM and SSM (12). The primary endpoint was improvement in any of the following symptoms: pruritus, flushing, depression, or fatigue after a 24-week period. Nineteen percent of the treatment group achieved response as compared to 7% in the placebo arm. This was balanced by an increase in diarrhea, rash, and asthenia. Given that ISM generally has a similar life expectancy compared to the healthy population, symptomatic benefits need to be carefully weighed with side effects.

Treatment of more advanced forms of SM such as MCL remains poorly defined. In young and fit patients, the usual approach is to treat with a combination of cytotoxic agents with or without midostaurin. Consolidative allogeneic hematopoietic stem cell transplantation (HSCT) is the only curative treatment option in SM, albeit with significant treatment-related mortality. Limited data on the outcomes after allogeneic HSCT are available, with one retrospective series of 57 patients reporting a 3-year survival of 43% in ASM and 17% in MCL. Consensus guidelines published in 2016 recommend early consideration for allogeneic transplant in advanced SM patients who achieve at least a partial response to initial therapy and who are otherwise reasonable candidates for transplant (i.e., those with a suitable donor and lack of significant comorbid conditions) (13). Treatment of SM-AHM generally involves concurrent treatment of the associated hematologic malignancy and mastocytosis, with care taken to avoid excessive drug interactions or additive toxicity.

Future Directions

Ongoing areas of active research include the development of novel agents targeting *KIT*, combinations of targeted agents with chemotherapy (especially in the setting of SM-AHN), and better clarifying the role and timing of stem cell transplantation. Avapritinib (formerly BLU-285) is a selective inhibitor of the *KIT* D816V mutation which is in phase 1 clinical trials for the treatment of advanced SM.

Key Points

- SM is characterized by clonal mast cell accumulation in various organs, most notably the skin, bone marrow, and liver/spleen.
- The *KIT* D816V driver mutation is seen in 90% to 95% of cases.
- SM is further subclassified based on the degree of organ involvement, circulating mast cell level, and the presence or absence of additional hematologic neoplasms.
- Midostaurin, a multikinase inhibitor with activity against the *KIT* D816V mutation, is FDA approved for advanced SM.
- Imatinib is ineffective against the D816V mutation.

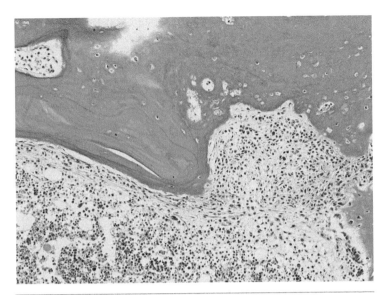

Figure 3.2 Hematoxylin and eosin stain of systemic mastocytosis.
Source: Courtesy of Dr. Perumal Thiagarajan.

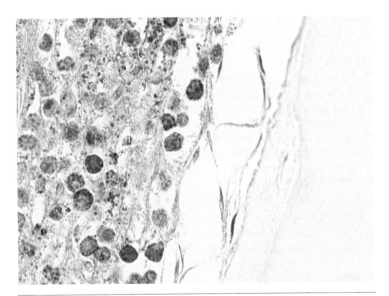

Figure 3.3 CD117 immunohistochemistry of systemic mastocytosis.
Source: Courtesy of Dr. Perumal Thiagarajan.

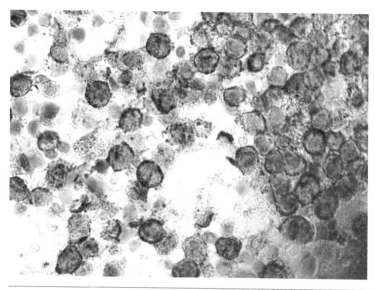

Figure 3.4 Tryptase stain of systemic mastocytosis.
Source: Courtesy of Dr. Perumal Thiagarajan.

LANGERHANS CELL HISTIOCYTOSIS

Clinical Case 3.2

A 32-year-old woman presented with central diabetes insipidus, hypothyroidism, and adrenal insufficiency. She was also noted to have bilateral groin lesions (Figure 3.5). Biopsy revealed Langerhans cell histiocytosis (LCH). MRI of the brain showed a 1.2-cm lesion of the pituitary stalk (Figure 3.6). A BRAF V600E mutation was detected. Her blood counts and routine chemistries were unremarkable. CT of the body revealed nonspecific subcentimeter pulmonary nodules, but was otherwise negative for hepatosplenomegaly or bony disease. Given the presence of multisystem disease involving the skin and central nervous system (CNS) with endocrinopathy, the decision was made to start systemic therapy. She was initiated on cytarabine at a dose of 100 mg/m²/d over 5 days, for four cycles. Although her skin lesions improved, follow-up brain imaging demonstrated an increase in the size of her pituitary stalk lesion. She was then started on vemurafenib. Her skin lesions fully resolved over a few weeks, and subsequent MRI of the brain demonstrated a partial response in her pituitary mass. After 2 years of follow-up, her disease is stable. She continues to have pan-hypopituitarism, and remains on desmopressin, dexamethasone, and levothyroxine.

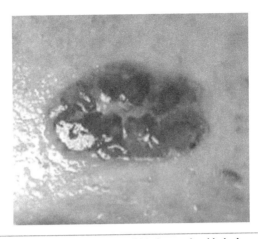

Figure 3.5 Langerhans cell histiocytosis, skin lesion.

Introduction

LCH is a rare dendritic cell disorder characterized by diffuse organ infiltration by pathologic myeloid-derived dendritic cells. Originally, it was thought that the pathologic Langerhans cells arose from inappropriate activation of normal epidermal Langerhans cells, but gene expression profiling now suggests that the pathologic LCH cell is likely an immature dendritic cell of myeloid rather than of epidermal origin (14).

Pathologic activation of the RAS–RAF–MEK–ERK pathway has been found in virtually all LCH patients, with activating *BRAF*V600E mutations occurring in over half of them. In patients without *BRAF* mutations, *MAP2K1* mutations have been found in a significant

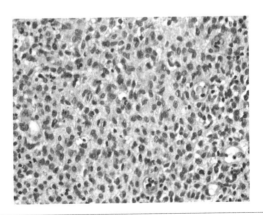

Figure 3.6 Langerhans cell histiocytosis, skin biopsy, high power.

subset. As discussed subsequently, the presence of these mutations has both predictive and prognostic value.

LCH is most commonly seen in children younger than 3 years of age, though it can be seen in all age groups. The incidence in adults is approximately one to two cases per million. Around half of the patients have disease limited to a single organ system (termed single-system LCH [SS-LCH]). Lytic bone lesions are the most common clinical manifestations, with other common sites of involvement being the skin, bone marrow, lymph nodes, liver, spleen, and lung. SS-LCH of the lung is nearly universally associated with smoking, in contrast to other forms of LCH in which cigarette smoking does not play a role. Involvement of the CNS is less common, though LCH has a predilection for hypothalamic–pituitary axis which manifests as endocrinopathies including diabetes insipidus and anterior pituitary hormone deficiency.

LCH is classified as a histiocytic disorder, a group of diseases of abnormal accumulation of dendritic cells, such as in LCH, or macrophages. Other diseases in this grouping include hemophagocytic lymphohistiocytosis (HLH; discussed elsewhere in this chapter), Rosai–Dorfman disease, Erdheim–Chester disease, and juvenile xanthogranuloma. Some pathophysiologic characteristics are shared among this group of disorders; for example, Erdheim–Chester disease is also characterized by a high frequency of *BRAF* V600E mutations (Tables 3.4 and 3.5) (15,16).

Diagnosis

The diagnosis of LCH is made by tissue biopsy showing clusters of abnormal Langerhans cells which express CD1a and CD207

Table 3.4 2016 World Health Organization Classification of Histiocytoses	
Histiocytic and dendritic cell neoplasms	Histiocytic sarcoma
	Langerhans cell histiocytosis
	Langerhans cell sarcoma
	Indeterminate dendritic cell tumor
	Interdigitating dendritic cell sarcoma
	Follicular dendritic cell sarcoma
	Fibroblastic reticular cell tumor
	Disseminated juvenile xanthogranuloma
	Erdheim–Chester disease

Source: From Swerdlow SH, Campo E, Pileri SA, et al. The 2016 revision of the World Health Organization classification of lymphoid neoplasms. *Blood.* 2016;127:2375–2390. doi:10.1182/blood-2016-01-643569

Table 3.5 Histiocyte Society—2016 Proposed Classification

L group	Langerhans cell histiocytosis (including LCH-SS, LCH lung, LCH-MS) Indeterminate cell histiocytosis Erdheim–Chester disease Mixed LCH/ECD
C group	Cutaneous non-LCH, xanthogranuloma family Cutaneous non-LCH, non-xanthogranuloma family Cutaneous non-LCH with a major systemic component
R group	Familial Rosai–Dorfman disease Sporadic RDD, including classical RDD, extranodal RDD, RDD with neoplasia or immune disease, unclassified RDD
M group	Primary malignant histiocytosis Secondary malignant histiocytosis
H group	Primary HLH Secondary HLH HLH of unknown/uncertain origin

ECD, Erdheim–Chester disease; HLH, hemophagocytic lymphohistiocytosis; LCH, Langerhans cell histiocytosis; LCH-MS, multi-system LCH; LCH-SS, single-system LCH; RDD, Rosai–Dorfman disease.

Source: From Emile JF, Abla O, Fraitag S, et al. Revised classification of histiocytoses and neoplasms of the macrophage-dendritic cell lineages. *Blood.* 2016;127:2672–2681. doi:10.1182/blood-2016-01-690636

(langerin). Other features include S100 expression and Birbeck granules, which are induced by langerin. There is typically a characteristic inflammatory infiltrate composed of macrophages, activated lymphocytes, eosinophils, and plasma cells. The tissue sample should be sent for *BRAF* V600E mutation testing, which is present in over 50% of LCH cases.

Once the diagnosis is made, all patients should undergo a pretreatment evaluation aimed at uncovering other sites of disease, especially so-called "high-risk" sites which have prognostic and/or treatment implications. This evaluation consists of complete blood counts and chemistries, coagulation studies, urine specific gravity and osmolality (as screening for diabetes insipidus [DI]), abdominal ultrasound (to evaluate hepatosplenomegaly), chest imaging, and a skeletal survey or low-dose whole-body bone CT. Positron emission tomography (PET) scan is an effective alternative and can be used to follow treatment response. MRI of the brain should be obtained for any suspected CNS involvement. Testing based on suspected specific organ involvement is summarized in Table 3.6.

Table 3.6 Recommended Testing for Langerhans Cell Histiocytosis

Indication	Assessment/Test
Cytopenia(s)	Bone marrow aspiration/biopsy, *BRAF*V600E qPCR, may detect cases of marrow involvement missed by morphologic assessment
Liver dysfunction	Consider additional imaging with MRI or PET/CT. Liver biopsy only recommended if there is clinically significant liver involvement and the result will alter treatment (i.e., to differentiate between active LCH and sclerosing cholangitis)
Lung involvement	High-resolution CT chest. Consider PFTs, bronchoscopy with BAL, lung biopsy
Suspected craniofacial lesions, including visual/aural or neurologic abnormalities	MRI head with contrast, to include brain, hypothalamus–pituitary axis, craniofacial bones. Baseline hearing evaluation if auditory canal or temporal bones are involved
Suspected endocrine abnormality (i.e., short stature, growth failure, polyuria, polydipsia, hypothalamic syndromes, precocious or delayed puberty)	MRI head with contrast, to include brain, hypothalamus–pituitary axis, craniofacial bones. History-directed testing for diabetes insipidus, anterior pituitary deficiencies (GH, FSH/LH, ACTH, TSH, prolactin)
Malabsorption/hypoalbuminemia failure to thrive, chronic diarrhea	Endoscopy

BAL, bronchoalveolar lavage; FSH, follicle stimulating hormone; GH, growth hormone; LCH, Langerhans cell histiocytosis; LH, luteinizing hormone; PET, positron emission tomography; PFT, pulmonary function test; qPCR, quantitative polymerase chain reaction; TSH, thyroid stimulating hormone.

Risk Stratification and Classification

Based on the pretreatment evaluation, LCH is classified as either SS-LCH or multisystem LCH (MS-LCH). Further stratification is performed depending on the specific site(s) of disease involvement.

High-risk disease (RO+): Involvement of the liver, spleen, or bone marrow is classified as "high-risk" disease portending a poorer prognosis (RO+). Traditionally, the lung was classified as a high-risk organ, but newer data in the pediatric population suggest it may not be important as an independent prognosticator. Most experts currently include only the liver, spleen, and hematopoietic system as high-risk organ systems (17).

CNS risk lesions: The separate term "CNS risk lesion" refers to the presence of bony lesions in the skull (including the mastoid, sphenoid, orbit, clivus, and temporal bones) which increase the risk of development of diabetes insipidus (DI) and/or neurodegenerative CNS LCH.

Special site lesions: These include lesions located in functionally critical anatomic sites like the odontoid peg and vertebral lesions with associated intraspinal soft tissue extension.

Key Diagnostic Dilemmas

LCH remains a difficult diagnosis due to its low incidence and its ability to involve multiple organ systems. The key to diagnosis remains clinical suspicion and tissue sampling. Skin and bone lesions are easily accessible for biopsy and can yield the diagnosis even in the absence of a high clinical suspicion. Less commonly, the disease can present with isolated pituitary stalk involvement. The differential diagnosis includes malignancies such as lymphoproliferative disease or germ cell tumors, and due to the difficulties of a pituitary biopsy, it may be reasonable to initiate empiric LCH therapy after excluding other diagnoses (17). In these situations, testing for the *BRAF* V600E mutation in either blood or cerebrospinal fluid (CSF) may also suggest the diagnosis, with the caveat that these mutations can also be seen in other histiocyte disorders. It is important to distinguish between LCH and these other rare systemic histiocytic disorders such as Rosai–Dorfman disease and Erdheim–Chester disease. Similar to LCH, the histiocytes in Erdheim–Chester disease can contain the *BRAF* V600E mutation. Unlike LCH, staining for CD1a or S100 is negative. Rosai–Dorfman can be distinguished histologically based on the presence of emperipolesis (phagocytosed but otherwise normal-appearing lymphocytes within macrophages) which is pathognomonic of the disease.

Prognosis

Prognosis in LCH is primarily associated with the risk classification system based on critical organ involvement. These risk classifications were validated and studied in pediatric populations, thus their significance in adults remains unproven. The long-term survival of low-risk patients (risk organ negative [RO–] patients without high-risk organ involvement) is 90% to 100%. The long-term survival of high-risk patients is somewhat worse, though in pediatric patients treated with modern intensive regimens, the 5-year survival remains over 80% (18). *BRAF* V600E mutation status portends higher rates of relapse after initial treatment, but without a detrimental effect on survival (19).

Management

Systemic therapy is warranted for all patients with multisystem disease (MS-LCH), as well as for those with high-risk single-system disease, including SS-LCH with "CNS-risk" lesions, "special site" lesions, or multifocal bone lesions (more than one bone lesion). If feasible, enrollment in a clinical trial is encouraged for all patients, especially for those with multisystem disease. It is also important to note that treatment recommendations in adults are based primarily on extrapolations from the pediatric population and expert opinion, due to the lower incidence of disease in the adult population.

Single-System Langerhans Cell Histiocytosis

Treatment of SS-LCH varies based on the specific site of involvement. Skin-limited LCH may spontaneously resolve and can be closely observed, though 40% of infants in one cohort were found to have MS-LCH subsequently, and thus, evaluating for multisystemic disease becomes important (20). Numerous topical and systemic therapies are potentially useful in this setting, but some experts recommend oral methotrexate and 6-mercaptopurine (6-MP) as the initial therapy for symptomatic skin-limited SS-LCH (17). Solitary bone lesions in low-CNS risk areas such as lesions not involving the craniofacial region recur in <10% of patients after local treatment with surgical curettage with or without corticosteroids (21). Radiation therapy is another option for local control which produces excellent responses. Isolated pulmonary LCH in adults may resolve with smoking cessation alone.

Patients with bone lesions classified as CNS-risk lesions, "special site" lesions, or multifocal bone disease are typically treated with systemic therapy as described subsequently. Bisphosphonates should be considered for patients with multifocal bone disease. Specific bone lesions at risk for fracture may be treated prophylactically with radiation therapy, though in children, the risk of long-term skeletal morbidity must be considered.

MS-LCH, Regardless of "Risk-Organ" Involvement by Children Versus Adults

MS-LCH in Children

In children, the standard induction regimen for patients who require systemic therapy is a 6-week course of vinblastine and prednisone or prednisolone, as utilized in the LCH-III trial (18). Vinblastine is given at a dose of 6 mg/m^2 weekly, and prednisone is given at a dose of 40 mg/m^2/d for 4 weeks, followed by a 2-week taper. The LCH-II and LCH-III studies have examined the addition of etoposide and methotrexate to the vinblastine/prednisone backbone, respectively, without significant improvements in outcome. Response assessment should be performed after 6 weeks.

Continuation therapy is necessary due to high rates of relapse even in patients who attain a good initial response. If an initial complete response to induction is attained, continuation therapy for a total of 12 months is the current standard of care. This recommendation is based on cross-trial historical comparisons between LCH-III, in which 12 months' continuation was used, versus its predecessor trials LCH-I/-II, in which 6 months' continuation was used. The 5-year survival rate with 12 months of continuation was 84%, compared with 62% to 69% with 6 months of continuation. The rate of reactivation was lower as well (27% with 12 months' continuation, 45% with 6 months' continuation). Continuation therapy consists of vinblastine and prednisone 5-day pulses, given at 3-week intervals, with the addition of daily 6-MP for those patients with risk-organ involvement as used in LCH-III. The LCH-IV study is currently underway and includes an arm extending the continuation therapy to 24 months.

Those patients who attain less than a complete response require further therapy prior to continuation, typically with a reinduction course of 6 weeks of vinblastine and prednisone. However, patients who either progress or show no improvement with induction (especially those with risk-organ involvement) should be considered for immediate second-line therapy rather than retreatment with vinblastine/prednisone.

Salvage treatment for those who are refractory to induction or for those with early relapse remains challenging. The LCH-S-2005 study regimen of cytarabine and cladribine appears to be the most effective published regimen, though with significant associated toxicity (22). In that study, an ORR of 92% was attained in a group of 27 RO+ patients. In the LCH-S-98 study, the single agent cladribine produced responses in 62% of RO– patients, but in only 22% of RO+ patients (23).

There are also limited data supporting the use of lower-dose clofarabine, which appeared well tolerated. Patients who progress on multiple salvage regimens should be referred for allogeneic stem cell transplant (see Table 3.7). Approximate survival at 3 years appears to be between 70% and 80% regardless of the conditioning regimen, though ablative conditioning was associated with lower relapse rates when compared to reduced-intensity regimens (8% vs. 28%) (24).

MS-LCH in Adults

Unlike in children, there have not been prospective trials comparing different regimens. Based on retrospective data, adults

Table 3.7 Selected Pediatric Salvage Regimens

LCH-S-98 (23)	**Two to six** 5-day courses, every 21 days: cladribine 5 mg/m^2/d
LCH-S-2005 (22)	**2+** 5-day courses, 28 days apart: cytarabine 1 g/m^2/d + cladribine 9 mg/m^2/d
Abraham, 2013 (25)	**Six** 5-day courses, every 3–4 weeks: clofarabine 25–30 mg/m^2/d

requiring systemic therapy for LCH may be effectively and safely treated with low-dose cytarabine (100 mg/m^2/d for 5 days, repeated monthly for 12 months) (26). Data to support this come from a retrospective analysis of 58 patients treated at an LCH center. The regimens compared were vinblastine/prednisone as used in pediatric trials, cytarabine, and cladribine. The 1-year failure rate for cytarabine was 21%, compared with 59% with cladribine and 84% with vinblastine/prednisone. Toxicities were also significant in the vinblastine-treated group, with grade 3+ neuropathy developing in 75%. Of note, cytarabine and cladribine have the added benefit of crossing the blood–brain barrier in patients with CNS involvement. Some experts advocate treating CNS disease or CNS-risk lesions with a higher dose of cytarabine (150 mg/m^2 instead of 100 mg/m^2) (17). Some European centers continue to prefer vinblastine/prednisolone as used in the pediatric population, and European treatment guidelines also list etoposide as an active regimen to consider for patients requiring systemic therapy but without risk-organ involvement (27). Intensive combination chemotherapy with methotrexate, doxorubicin, cyclophosphamide, vincristine, prednisone, bleomycin (MACOP-B) has shown promising activity in a single-institution experience of 11 patients, with a complete remission (CR) rate of 73% and 82% overall survival (OS) after median 6.7-year follow-up. Finally, less-intensive regimens for patients without risk-organ involvement include weekly oral methotrexate, oral azathioprine, and thalidomide.

There are even fewer data available on adult salvage therapy options. One published study of cladribine in a heavily pretreated population showed an ORR of 75% (CR 58%), with median response duration of 33 months; the main toxicity was neutropenia (28). This represents an attractive option, especially in cases of CNS involvement as cladribine crosses the blood–brain barrier. Hydroxyurea has recently been shown to have efficacy in a small combined pediatric and adult cohort which had been refractory to multiple lines of treatment (29). Allogeneic stem cell transplant can be considered for adults with aggressive or refractory disease.

Because the majority of LCH patients harbor the *BRAF* V600E mutation, the use of *BRAF* inhibitors to block MAPK/ERK pathway activation represents a logical targeted approach. One basket trial enrolling patients of all types with *BRAF* V600E-mutant tumors included 18 patients with LCH or Erdheim–Chester. The overall response rate (ORR) in this group was 43% with durable responses, albeit with a median treatment duration of only 5.9 months. The VE-BASKET trial is a phase 2 study using the *BRAF* inhibitor vemurafenib in 26 patients with either LCH or Erdheim–Chester disease and *BRAF*V600 mutations. Although only four patients in this study had LCH, all four had at least partial responses (30). Awada et al. in 2018 reported on the successful combination of *BRAF–MEK* inhibition as used in *BRAF*-mutated melanoma; this report was also unique in its use of *BRAF*V600E ctDNA as a biomarker of response (31).

Future Directions

The multi-stratum trial LCH-IV is currently underway as a follow-up to the established backbone of vinblastine and prednisone studied in LCH-III described earlier. This study includes arms adding intensification with 6-MP and cytarabine, salvage with cladribine/cytarabine, prolongation of continuation therapy from 12 to 24 months, and the addition of indomethacin or 6-MP as part of continuation therapy. The LCH-REASON trial is another multicenter phase 3 trial evaluating the frontline use of cytarabine. Enrollment in both these trials is limited to the pediatric and young adult population. More data are also needed on the use of targeted therapy such as *BRAF* inhibitors, particularly regarding the durability of responses, as well as additional data with combination therapy with *BRAF* and *MEK* pathway inhibition.

Key Points

- LCH is a rare dendritic cell neoplasm with potential multisystem organ involvement.
- Patients are risk-stratified based on involvement of high-risk organs (liver, spleen, bone marrow) as well as involvement of the CNS or "CNS-risk" sites.
- Multisystem involvement, if treated outside the context of a clinical trial, generally warrants intensive therapy.
  - Treatment in children is based on the regimen used in the LCH-III trial, with a 6-week induction course of vinblastine and prednisone followed by 1 year of continuation therapy with vinblastine/prednisone as well as 6-MP for high-risk patients.

- ○ Treatment in adults is less clear; but some experts suggest a 1-year course of low-dose cytarabine.
- *BRAF* V600E mutations are seen in over 50% of cases and are predictive of response to *BRAF* pathway inhibition.

HEMOPHAGOCYTIC LYMPHOHISTIOCYTOSIS

Clinical Case 3.3

A 20-year-old Hispanic man without significant medical or family history presented with 3 weeks of fevers and fatigue. One week earlier, he was diagnosed with infectious mononucleosis based on a positive Monospot test. At his current presentation, he was febrile to 103°F, with a platelet count of 68,000/µL, hemoglobin of 12.3 g/dL, white blood cell (WBC) count of 5.2 × 10⁹/L with normal differential, a bilirubin of 10.7 (direct 8.3), alanine transaminase (ALT) of 366, aspartate transaminase (AST) of 389, and lactate dehydrogenase (LDH) of 1,063 U/L. Cross-sectional imaging demonstrated splenomegaly of 16 cm along with diffuse lymphadenopathy in the abdomen. Further laboratory workup revealed a ferritin of 13,715 ng/mL, fasting triglycerides of 289, positive IgA/IgM antibodies against Epstein–Barr virus (EBV) viral capsid antigen, and an EBV viral load of 1.7 million copies/mL; testing for all other viral infections including hepatitis and HIV was negative. Lymph node biopsy showed plasmablastic lymphoma with a Ki-67 of greater than 90%, and a bone marrow biopsy showed marked hemophagocytosis. He was diagnosed with hemophagocytic lymphohistiocytosis (HLH), likely secondary to EBV infection and EBV-associated aggressive lymphoma. The patient was started within 24 hours of arrival on HLH-directed therapy with dexamethasone and etoposide. However, he had an aggressive clinical course, developing multiorgan failure within several days of presentation, including acute kidney injury requiring hemodialysis, respiratory failure requiring mechanical ventilation, and coagulopathy along with vancomycin-resistant enterococcus. (VRE) bacteremia. Over the following week, he also received treatment with intravenous immunoglobulin (IVIG), followed by EBV-directed therapy with rituximab given his high viral load, along with dose-reduced ifosfamide, carboplatin, and continued etoposide (ICE). Both his ferritin and EBV viral load downtrended, and his counts began to recover after chemotherapy. Unfortunately, he succumbed to hospital-acquired infections and multiple bleeding complications.

Introduction

HLH is a syndrome characterized by excessive and pathologic immune activation, leading to life-threatening multiorgan dysfunction. The hallmark of HLH is supraphysiologic systemic activation of macrophages and lymphocytes with highly elevated levels of proinflammatory cytokines such as interferon-gamma (IFN-γ), tumor necrosis factor-alpha (TNF-α), interleukin (IL)-6, macrophage colony-stimulating factor (M-CSF), and CD25, resulting in cytokine storm and multiorgan dysfunction. The name of the syndrome derives from the ability of activated macrophages to phagocytose blood cells, which can be seen on bone marrow biopsy samples. HLH is often classified as "primary" versus "secondary."

Primary HLH is characterized by inherited immune defects with typical presentations in infancy or early childhood, while secondary HLH classically occurs in adults and has identifiable triggers such as infection or malignancy. In one study, malignancy was associated with 45% of adult HLH cases as compared to only 8% of pediatric cases (32). More recently, it has been recognized that HLH exists on a continuous spectrum of both intrinsic and acquired contributions to immune dysfunction. Within this conceptual framework, patients with some degree of intrinsic genetic susceptibility can develop overt HLH after immune homeostasis is disrupted by an extrinsic trigger such as viral infections (Box 3.1) (35,36).

Of note, the term "macrophage activation syndrome" (MAS) is typically used to describe an inflammatory syndrome similar to HLH, but occurring in the specific setting of an autoimmune disorder such as systemic lupus erythematosus. Although there is significant overlap in both the pathophysiology and the clinical presentation between MAS and HLH, chronic IL-18 elevation has been suggested as a distinguishing factor between MAS and familial HLH.

Clinically, the distinction remains important as the treatment for MAS typically involves pulse-dose corticosteroids without HLH-specific therapy such as etoposide.

Diagnosis

The diagnostic criteria most commonly used in clinical practice are those used as inclusion criteria for the pediatric HLH-2004 trial (see Table 3.8). Of note, these criteria are not fully inclusive of common clinical features seen in HLH. Other common manifestations include progressive liver failure, disseminated intravascular coagulation, elevated LDH, renal insufficiency, and CNS findings such as encephalitis or CSF pleocytosis. Despite the name, the degree of bone marrow hemophagocytosis correlates poorly with the clinical diagnosis of HLH, and the finding of marrow hemophagocytosis is not pathognomonic of HLH. Extremely high ferritin levels appear to correlate well with a diagnosis of HLH in the pediatric population; in one study, a serum ferritin >10,000 ng/mL was reported as being 90% sensitive and 96% specific for HLH (37). However, studies in adult patients have reported lower specificity and sensitivity for extremely high (>10,000 ng/mL) ferritin levels, with multiple differential diagnoses to consider, including iron overload, liver and renal failure, rheumatologic disease, and hematologic malignancy. In an attempt to provide better diagnostic tools to distinguish HLH

Box 3.1 Examples of Hemophagocytic Lymphohistiocytosis Triggers

Intrinsic (genetic)

Lymphocyte cytotoxicity defects:
PRF1, UNC13D, STX11, STXBP2, RAB27A, LYST

Dysregulated inflammasome activity:
NLRC4, XIAP

Mutations affecting T-cell function/viral control:
ITK, CD27, SH2D1A

Immunodeficiency syndromes: Griscelli syndrome type II, Chediak–Higashi, Hermansky–Pudlak type II, X-linked lymphoproliferative disease

Extrinsic (acquired)

Infection—most commonly EBV, but other implicated viral pathogens include HIV, CMV, HSV, VZV, parvovirus, HHV-8. Other organisms include AFB, fungi, and typical bacteria (33)

Malignancy—most commonly hematologic malignancies, including Hodgkin and non-Hodgkin lymphomas, acute leukemia (34)

Autoimmune (termed macrophage activation syndrome)—SLE, juvenile RA

Iatrogenic (termed cytokine release syndrome)—posttransplant, immunotherapy associated (CAR-T, BITE, CTL)

AFB, acid fast bacilli; BITE,bBispecific T-cell engager; CAR-T, chimeric antigen receptor T-cell therapy; CMV, cytomegalovirus; CTL, cytotoxic T-lymphocyte therapy; EBV, Epstein–Barr virus; HHV-8, human herpes virus 8; HSV, herpes simplex virus; RA, rheumatoid arthritis; SLE, systemic lupus erythematosus; VZV, varicella zoster virus.

Source: From Allen CE, McClain KL. Pathophysiology and epidemiology of hemophagocytic lymphohistiocytosis. *Hematology.* 2015;2015:177–182. doi:10.1182/asheducation-2015.1.177; Chinn IK, Eckstein OS, Peckham-Gregory EC, et al. Genetic and mechanistic diversity in pediatric hemophagocytic lymphohistiocytosis. *Blood.* 2018;132:89–100. doi:10.1182/blood-2017-11-814244

---

from these alternative diagnoses in adults, an expert panel consensus was reached on nine criteria felt to be important; these included lab-based criteria (hyperferritinemia, hypertriglyceridemia, transaminase elevation above the upper limit of normal, hypofibrinogenemia, cytopenias), clinical variables (fevers, hepatosplenomegaly, underlying immunosuppression), and one cytologic variable (hemophagocytosis). These variables were combined and validated as the "HScore," with the probability of HLH being <1% for an HScore ≤90 and >99% for an HScore ≥250 (38).

The HScore can be calculated using a free online calculator (available at saintantoine.aphp.fr/score/). Patients (especially pediatric patients) meeting the HLH-2004 criteria should be highly

Table 3.8 Hemophagocytic Lymphohistiocytosis Diagnostic Criteria

The diagnosis of HLH can be established if either one or two of the following are fulfilled

1.	A molecular diagnosis consistent with HLH is made (e.g., familial *HLH* gene mutation)
2. (Five of eight criteria)	Fever Splenomegaly Cytopenias affecting two or more cell lines: • Hemoglobin <9 g/dL • Platelets <100 × 10^9/L • Neutrophils <1 × 10^9/L Hypertriglyceridemia and/or hypofibrinogenemia • Fasting triglycerides ≥265 mg/dL • Fibrinogen ≤1.5 g/L Hemophagocytosis in bone marrow, spleen, or lymph nodes Low or absent NK cell activity* Ferritin ≥500 µg/L Soluble CD25 (IL2r) ≥2,400 U/mL

*Traditionally, a chromium release assay, but may be augmented with perforin and CD107a testing.

HLH, hemophagocytic lymphohistiocytosis; NK, natural killer.

Source: Adapted from HLH-2004 Trial Inclusion Criteria.

considered for additional diagnostic testing for potential primary drivers of HLH, including testing for natural killer (NK) cell function and further genetic testing for known HLH predisposing mutations.

Diagnostic Dilemmas

HLH is often difficult to distinguish in the acute setting from sepsis or other multiorgan dysfunction syndromes. Because the diagnosis is made on clinical criteria rather than pathologic features, a high clinical suspicion is important. Markedly high serum ferritin levels should raise suspicion for HLH and prompt further workup, although the specificity of a very high ferritin level is lower in adults compared to that in children. HLH triggers such as EBV infection or hematologic malignancy should also prompt suspicion for HLH. Importantly, the HLH-2004 criteria (see Table 3.8) do not capture all cases of HLH warranting therapy and should not be used to exclude patients from treatment. Treatment also should not be delayed in patients in whom a high clinical suspicion for HLH exists but for whom specialized testing (genetic testing, NK cell activity, soluble CD25) is pending. Additionally, underlying immunodeficiency syndromes may be the predisposing factor for infections that trigger HLH.

Prognosis

Prognosis of HLH depends on multiple factors, including age, disease severity, underlying predisposing conditions, and treatment. Historically, the mortality rate of untreated HLH was over 90%. By comparison, the mortality rate of HLH treated with HLH-specific therapy is around 50%, based on long-term follow-up of the pediatric HLH-94 study which showed a survival rate of 54% (39). Of note, in HLH-94, mortality was not significantly different between "familial" and non-familial HLH, supporting the notion that all HLH should be treated aggressively regardless of the underlying predisposing factors. In adults, factors that have been associated with worse outcome include lack of aggressive etoposide-based treatment, age, liver function derangements, and underlying hematologic malignancy (40). In a retrospective series of 156 adults in whom the predominant predisposing factor was hematologic malignancy (56%), the 1-month mortality rate was 20% overall and the long-term survival rate was 58%. In children, both ferritin at the time of diagnosis as well as the rate of decline of ferritin after initiation of therapy correlated with outcomes.

Management

Given the natural history of untreated patients, HLH-specific therapy must be considered early in all patients in whom HLH is suspected. HLH-specific treatment is most commonly based on the protocol used in the HLH-94 protocol utilizing induction etoposide and dexamethasone. A lumbar puncture should be performed if clinical status permits, with intrathecal methotrexate and steroids given in patients in whom CSF pleocytosis is found. It is important to note that the original study for this protocol was a pediatric population with a high percentage of hereditary HLH; thus, recommendations based on this protocol in adult patients are derived from expert opinion. Etoposide is a cornerstone of all HLH treatment via its ability to selectively deplete activated T cells. Of note, etoposide may require dose reductions for age as well as hepatic or renal dysfunction, both of which often complicate cases of HLH.

The HLH-2004 study was undertaken in an attempt to improve the HLH-94 regimen by moving cyclosporine into the initial induction portion of therapy and by adding hydrocortisone to intrathecal therapy. Updated results to this trial were published in 2017, demonstrating a nonsignificant reduction in pretransplant mortality when compared to HLH-94 (27% vs. 19%, $p = .06$) (41). Based on these results, cyclosporine is generally not used as part of induction therapy. Furthermore, due to the risk of developing posterior reversible encephalopathy syndrome (PRES), some experts advocate not utilizing this agent at all or reserving it for higher severity cases. Tacrolimus is also sometimes substituted for cyclosporine.

Although HLH-94 serves as a general backbone of therapy regardless of specific secondary etiology, there are some additional considerations for therapy in secondary HLH. Any identified infectious triggers should be treated with the appropriate antimicrobials. EBV-associated HLH should be treated with rituximab with or without IVIG, as EBV replicates predominantly in B lymphocytes. Malignancy-associated HLH requires treatment both with HLH-directed and cancer-directed therapy. If the associated malignancy is a non-Hodgkin lymphoma, then an etoposide-containing regimen should be considered.

Emapalumab, a novel anti-IFN-γ fully human monoclonal antibody that binds and neutralizes IFN-γ, is FDA approved for relapsed or refractory HLH based on a study of 34 pediatric patients with primary HLH, many of whom had failed initial therapy (42).

Unfortunately, relapse rates after initial response to induction therapy are high, especially in young patients with known genetic predisposition. Such patients should be considered for allogeneic stem cell transplantation, typically with reduced intensity regimens. Adults in whom the HLH trigger is suspected to be acquired, either in cases of relapsed/refractory disease or in those in whom the trigger is a hematologic malignancy, may require transplantation as well. Alemtuzumab can be used as a bridge to transplantation in patients who fail initial etoposide/dexamethasone-based treatment.

As mentioned previously, MAS is treated differently from HLH and requires high-dose steroids and disease-specific immunosuppression without HLH-specific therapy or stem cell transplant. Cytokine-release syndrome (CRS) is a similar condition of immune dysregulation and excessive macrophage activation which occurs after cancer immunotherapy, such as with CAR-T or the CD19/CD3 bispecific T-cell engaging antibody blinatumomab. The anti-IL-6 antibody tocilizumab has been shown to be effective in this setting.

Future Directions

One major area of ongoing investigation is the development of novel plasma-based biomarkers for diagnostic and prognostic purposes. Trials are ongoing to evaluate the addition of various immunosuppressants and novel agents to standard induction with etoposide/dexamethasone including anti-thymocyte globulin (ATG), the anti-CD52 monoclonal antibody alemtuzumab, and the anti-IL-6 antibody tocilizumab. The JAK1/2 inhibitor ruxolitinib is being tested in a phase 1 study. There remains a paucity of data regarding treatment of adults with HLH as well as specific subgroups such as malignancy-associated HLH.

Key Points

- Diagnosis of HLH is often made based on the criteria used in the HLH-2004 trial, which identifies a very high-risk cohort of HLH patients. However, other clinical features such as liver function test (LFT) abnormalities can also be seen. Treatment should not be withheld in patients who do not meet the HLH-2004 criteria if there is a high clinical suspicion for HLH.

- HLH-specific therapy should be promptly initiated in patients with a high suspicion for HLH, and consists of an induction course of etoposide with dexamethasone, with intrathecal therapy for patients with CNS involvement.

- In relapsed/refractory HLH, the humanized anti-IFN-γ antibody emapalumab is a newly FDA-approved treatment option.

- Allogeneic stem cell transplantation should be considered in patients with relapsed/refractory HLH.

REFERENCES

1. Garcia-Montero AC, Jara-Acevedo M, Teodosio C, et al. KIT mutation in mast cells and other bone marrow hematopoietic cell lineages in systemic mast cell disorders: a prospective study of the Spanish Network on Mastocytosis (REMA) in a series of 113 patients. *Blood*. 2006;108:2366–2372. doi:10.1182/blood-2006-04-015545

2. Escribano L, Alvarez-Twose I, Sánchez-Muñoz L, et al. Prognosis in adult indolent systemic mastocytosis: a long-term study of the Spanish Network on Mastocytosis in a series of 145 patients. *J Allergy Clin Immunol*. 2009;124:514–521. doi:10.1016/j.jaci.2009.05.003

3. Lim KH, Tefferi A, Lasho TL, et al. Systemic mastocytosis in 342 consecutive adults: survival studies and prognostic factors. *Blood*. 2009;113:5727–5736. doi:10.1182/blood-2009-02-205237

4. Hoermann G, Gleixner KV, Dinu GE, et al. The KIT D816V allele burden predicts survival in patients with mastocytosis and correlates with the WHO type of the disease. *Allergy*. 2014;69:810–813. doi:10.1111/all.12409

5. Jawhar M, Schwaab J, Naumann N, et al. Response and progression on midostaurin in advanced systemic mastocytosis: KIT D816V and other molecular markers. *Blood*. 2017;130:137–145. doi:10.1182/blood-2017-01-764423

6. Naumann N, Jawhar M, Schwaab J, et al. Incidence and prognostic impact of cytogenetic aberrations in patients with systemic mastocytosis. *Gene Chromosome Canc*. 2018;57:252–259. doi:10.1002/gcc.22526

7. Gotlib J, Kluin-Nelemans HC, George TI, et al. Efficacy and safety of midostaurin in advanced systemic mastocytosis. *NEJM*. 2016;374:2530–2541. doi:10.1056/NEJMoa1513098

8. Barete S, Lortholary O, Damaj G, et al. Long-term efficacy and safety of cladribine (2-CdA) in adult patients with mastocytosis. *Blood*. 2015;126:1009–1016. doi:10.1182/blood-2014-12-614743

9. Lim KH, Pardanani A, Butterfield JH, et al. Outcome analysis and response prediction during treatment with interferon-alpha, hydroxyurea, imatinib mesylate or 2-chlorodeoxyadenosine. *Am J Hematol*. 2009;84:790–794. doi:10.1002/ajh.21561

10. Verstovsek S, Tefferi A, Cortes J, et al. Phase II study of dasatinib in Philadelphia chromosome-negative acute and chronic myeloid diseases, including systemic mastocytosis. *Clin Cancer Res*. 2008;14:3906–3915. doi:10.1158/1078-0432.CCR-08-0366

11. Hochhaus A, Baccarani M, Giles FJ, et al. Nilotinib in patients with systemic mastocytosis: analysis of the phase 2, open-label, single-arm nilotinib registration study. *J Cancer Res Clin Oncol*. 2015;141:2047–2060. doi:10.1007/s00432-015-1988-0

12. Lortholary O, Chandesris MO, Bulai Livideanu C, et al. Masitinib for treatment of severely symptomatic indolent systemic mastocytosis: a randomised, placebo-controlled, phase 3 study. *Lancet*. 2017;389:612–620. doi:10.1016/S0140-6736(16)31403-9

13. Ustun C, Gotlib J, Popat U, et al. Consensus opinion on allogeneic hematopoietic cell transplantation in advanced systemic mastocytosis. *Biol Blood Marrow Transplant*. 2016;22:1348–1356. doi:10.1016/j.bbmt.2016.04.018

14. Allen CE, Li L, Peters TL, et al. Cell-specific gene expression in Langerhans cell histiocytosis lesions reveals a distinct profile compared with epidermal Langerhans cells. *J Immunol*. 2010;184:4557–4567. doi:10.4049/jimmunol.0902336

15. Swerdlow SH, Campo E, Pileri SA, et al. The 2016 revision of the World Health Organization classification of lymphoid neoplasms. *Blood*. 2016;127:2375–2390. doi:10.1182/blood-2016-01-643569

16. Emile JF, Abla O, Fraitag S, et al. Revised classification of histiocytoses and neoplasms of the macrophage-dendritic cell lineages. *Blood*. 2016;127:2672–2681. doi:10.1182/blood-2016-01-690636

17. Allen CE, Ladisch S, McClain KL. How I treat Langerhans cell histiocytosis. *Blood*. 2015;126:26–35. doi:10.1182/blood-2014-12-569301

18. Gadner H, Minkov M, Grois N, et al. Improved outcome in multisystem Langerhans cell histiocytosis is associated with therapy intensification. *Blood*. 2013;121:5006–5014. doi:10.1182/blood-2012-09-455774

19. Berres ML, Lim KP, Peters T, et al. BRAF-V600E expression in precursor versus differentiated dendritic cells defines clinically distinct LCH risk groups. *J Exp Med.* 2014;211:669–683. doi:10.1084/jem.20130977

20. Simko SJ, Garmezy B, Abhyankar H, et al. Differentiating skin-limited and multisystem Langerhans cell histiocytosis. *J Pediatr.* 2014;165:990–996. doi:10.1016/j.jpeds.2014.07.063

21. Jubran RF, Marachelian A, Dorey F, Malogolowkin M. Predictors of outcome in children with Langerhans cell histiocytosis. *Pediatr Blood Cancer.* 2005;45:37–42. doi:10.1002/pbc.20364

22. Donadieu J, Bernard F, van Noesel M, et al. Cladribine and cytarabine in refractory multisystem Langerhans cell histiocytosis: results of an international phase 2 study. *Blood.* 2015;126:1415–1423. doi:10.1182/blood-2015-03-635151

23. Weitzman S, Braier J, Donadieu J, et al. 2'-Chlorodeoxyadenosine (2-CdA) as salvage therapy for Langerhans cell histiocytosis (LCH). Results of the LCH-S-98 protocol of the Histiocyte Society. *Pediatr Blood Cancer.* 2009;53:1271–1276. doi:10.1002/pbc.22229

24. Veys PA, Nanduri V, Baker KS, et al. Haematopoietic stem cell transplantation for refractory Langerhans cell histiocytosis: outcome by intensity of conditioning. *Br J Haematol.* 2015;169:711–718. doi:10.1111/bjh.13347

25. Abraham A, Alsultan A, Jeng M, et al. Clofarabine salvage therapy for refractory high-risk Langerhans cell histiocytosis. *Pediatr Blood Cancer.* 2013;60:E19–E22. doi:10.1002/pbc.24436

26. Cantu MA, Lupo PJ, Bilgi M, et al. Optimal therapy for adults with Langerhans cell histiocytosis bone lesions. *PLoS One.* 2012;7:e43257. doi:10.1371/journal.pone.0043257

27. Girschikofsky M, Arico M, Castillo D, et al. Management of adult patients with Langerhans cell histiocytosis: recommendations from an expert panel on behalf of Euro-Histio-Net. *Orphanet J Rare Dis.* 2013;8:72. doi:10.1186/1750-1172-8-72

28. Saven A, Burian C. Cladribine activity in adult Langerhans-cell histiocytosis. *Blood.* 1999;93:4125–4130.

29. Zinn DJ, Grimes AB, Lin H, et al. Hydroxyurea: a new old therapy for Langerhans cell histiocytosis. *Blood.* 2016;128:2462–2465. doi:10.1182/blood-2016-06-721993

30. Diamond EL, Subbiah V, Lockhart AC, et al. Vemurafenib for BRAF V600–mutant Erdheim-Chester disease and Langerhans cell histiocytosis: analysis of data from the histology-independent, phase 2, open-label VE-BASKET study. *JAMA Oncol.* 2018;4:384–388. doi:10.1001/jamaoncol.2017.5029

31. Awada G, Seremet T, Fostier K, et al. Long-term disease control of Langerhans cell histiocytosis using combined BRAF and MEK inhibition. *Blood Adv*. 2018;2:2156–2158. doi:10.1182/bloodadvances.2018021782

32. Lehmberg K, Sprekels B, Nichols KE, et al. Malignancy-associated haemophagocytic lymphohistiocytosis in children and adolescents. *Br J Haematol*. 2015;170:539–549. doi:10.1111/bjh.13462

33. Ramos-Casals M, Brito-Zerón P, López-Guillermo A, et al. Adult haemophagocytic syndrome. *Lancet*. 2014;383(9927):1503–1516.

34. Otrock ZK, Eby CS. Clinical characteristics, prognostic factors, and outcomes of adult patients with hemophagocytic lymphohistiocytosis. *Am J Hematol*. 2015;90(3):220–224.

35. Allen CE, McClain KL. Pathophysiology and epidemiology of hemophagocytic lymphohistiocytosis. *Hematology*. 2015;2015:177–182. doi:10.1182/asheducation-2015.1.177

36. Chinn IK, Eckstein OS, Peckham-Gregory EC, et al. Genetic and mechanistic diversity in pediatric hemophagocytic lymphohistiocytosis. *Blood*. 2018;132:89–100. doi:10.1182/blood-2017-11-814244

37. Allen CE, Yu X, Kozinetz CA, McClain KL. Highly elevated ferritin levels and the diagnosis of hemophagocytic lymphohistiocytosis. *Pediatr Blood Cancer*. 2008;50:1227–1235. doi:10.1002/pbc.21423

38. Fardet L, Galicier L, Lambotte O, et al. Development and validation of the HScore, a score for the diagnosis of reactive hemophagocytic syndrome. *Arthritis Rheumatol*. 2014;66:2613–2620. doi:10.1002/art.38690

39. Trottestam H, Horne A, Aricò M, et al. Chemoimmunotherapy for hemophagocytic lymphohistiocytosis: long-term results of the HLH-94 treatment protocol. *Blood*. 2011;118:4577–4584. doi:10.1182/blood-2011-06-356261

40. Arca M, Fardet L, Galicier L, et al. Prognostic factors of early death in a cohort of 162 adult haemophagocytic syndrome: impact of triggering disease and early treatment with etoposide. *Br J Haematol*. 2015;168:63–68. doi:10.1111/bjh.13102

41. Bergsten E, Horne A, Aricó M, et al. Confirmed efficacy of etoposide and dexamethasone in HLH treatment: long-term results of the cooperative HLH-2004 study. *Blood*. 2017;130:2728–2738. doi:10.1182/blood-2017-06-788349

42. Locatelli F, Jordan MB, Allen CE, et al. Safety and Efficacy of Emapalumab in Pediatric Patients with Primary Hemophagocytic Lymphohistiocytosis. Presented at: 2018 ASH Annual Meeting and Exposition; 2018.

4 Acquired Aplastic Anemia and Inherited Bone Marrow Failure Syndromes

Clay T. Cohen, Matthew Miller, and Rosa Díaz

INTRODUCTION

Bone marrow failure (BMF) refers to the inability of hematopoiesis to meet the physiologic demands for the production of functional blood cells. BMF can be classified into three categories based on the presumed etiology: idiopathic, secondary, and inherited. The first section of this chapter discusses idiopathic and secondary BMF, which is usually called acquired aplastic anemia (AA), and subsequent sections review the most common inherited bone marrow failure syndromes (IBMFSs). The clear differences in clinical management and outcomes in patients with IBMFSs compared to those with acquired AA highlight the need to have a clear understanding of these disorders and how to recognize them.

ACQUIRED APLASTIC ANEMIA

Clinical Case 4.1

A previously healthy 17-year-old male presented to the emergency department after a syncopal episode. The family reported weight loss, increased fatigue, and nosebleeds. Patient denied any recent illness and was taking no medications. A complete blood count (CBC) showed white blood cell (WBC) count of 900 cells/μL, hemoglobin (Hgb) of 4.5 g/dL, mean corpuscular volume (MCV) of 105 FL, platelet count of 1,000 cells/μL, and absolute neutrophil count (ANC) of 190 cells/μL.

Introduction

Acquired AA is a life-threatening form of BMF that refers to pancytopenia in association with bone marrow hypoplasia or aplasia and has diverse underlying causes (Table 4.1). Autoimmune damage to hematopoietic stem cells (HSC), with resultant decrease in mature blood cells, causes or contributes to most cases of acquired AA (1).

Table 4.1 Causes of Acquired Aplastic Anemia

Idiopathic

Secondary*

    Drugs (phenytoin, carbamazepine, sulfonamides, chloramphenicol)

    Radiation

    Toxic chemicals (benzene, solvents)

    Viral infections (EBV, seronegative hepatitis, HIV)

    Immune disorders (SLE)

    Others (paroxysmal nocturnal hemoglobinuria, thymoma, pregnancy)

*Predictable, transient episodes of bone marrow suppression secondary to drug exposure or viral infection are not considered AA.

AA, aplastic anemia; EBV, Epstein–Barr virus; SLE, systemic lupus erythematosus.

Diagnosis

Patients with acquired AA are usually healthy prior to the diagnosis. Common presenting symptoms include easy bruising or bleeding, pallor, and fatigue. Hepatosplenomegaly and/or lymphadenopathy do not usually occur in patients with acquired AA. Features such as poor growth, developmental delay, limb abnormalities, and skin and nail lesions should raise suspicion of an IBMFS.

The CBC reveals pancytopenia with reticulocytopenia. Patients with mild cytopenias and no clinical complications may be monitored over days to a few weeks, particularly if the history reveals a reversible cause of AA (drug, infection). However, if no improvement or worsening is observed or complications of cytopenias arise, the patient should promptly undergo further testing. Patients with critical cytopenias and/or life-threatening complications should undergo immediate assessment including bone marrow aspirate and biopsy. These patients should be evaluated urgently as the interval between diagnosis of AA and treatment is a strong predictor of survival. The diagnostic approach to patients with suspected AA is summarized in Table 4.2, including the tests that can be used to screen for IBMFS (2).

Bone marrow biopsy will identify marrow hypoplasia or aplasia and exclude diagnoses such as leukemia, metastatic cancer, myelodysplastic syndrome (MDS), among others. A bone marrow aspirate is obtained for cytogenetic and/or fluorescent in situ hybridization (FISH) analysis to identify chromosome abnormalities that may coexist with AA. AA is categorized as severe or non-severe based on peripheral blood counts and bone marrow findings (Table 4.3).

Table 4.2 Diagnostic Approach to a Patient With Suspected Aplastic Anemia

General	Complete blood count and reticulocyte*
	Bone marrow aspirate and biopsy
	Bone marrow cytogenetics and/or FISH analysis
r/o Secondary AA	Chemistries, including LDH and uric acid
	Liver function tests
	Viral serologies when indicated (HIV, hepatitis panel, EBV, CMV, parvovirus)
	Serum vitamin B12* and red blood cell folate
	Hemoglobin F*
	Quantitative immunoglobulins
	ANA and anti-dsDNA titers, DAT
	Flow cytometry for PNH†
r/o IBMF	Chromosome breakage analysis‡
	Telomere length testing‡
	Targeted mutation analysis for specific syndromes when suspected

*Elevated MCV, vitamin B12, and hemoglobin F levels suggest IBMFS.

†Recommended for **all** patients.

‡Recommended prompt testing for all as patients may lack the classic features of these syndromes and early detection can impact management decisions.

AA, aplastic anemia; ANA, antinuclear antibody; CMV, cytomegalovirus; DAT, direct antiglobulin test; EBV, Epstein–Barr virus; FISH, fluorescent in situ hybridization; IBMFS, inherited bone marrow failure syndromes; LDH, lactate dehydrogenase; MCV, mean corpuscular volume; PNH, paroxysmal nocturnal hemoglobinuria; r/o, rule out.

Table 4.3 Diagnostic Criteria of AA for the Purposes of Risk Stratification and Selection of Therapy (Must Meet Both Peripheral Blood and Bone Marrow Criteria)

	Peripheral Blood	Bone Marrow
Severe*	At least two of the following: ANC <500/µL, platelet count <20,000/µL, or reticulocyte count <20,000/µL	Cellularity <25% (or 25%–50% if <30% of the residual cells are hematopoietic)
Non-severe	Do not fulfill criteria as described for severe	Hypocellular BM as described for severe

*Very severe AA includes the criteria for SAA and ANC <200/µL.

AA, aplastic anemia; ANC, absolute neutrophil count; BM, bone marrow; SAA, severe AA.

Drug and chemical exposures should be elicited, but these may be hard to evaluate quantitatively and are subject to recall bias. If these are suspected, physicians may monitor after discontinuation of the offending agent. However, this must be weighed against the risk of delaying treatment in the hope of spontaneous recovery, which can result in serious complications before definitive treatment is administered. Exhaustive attempts to identify a trigger in patients with acquired AA can be challenging, and outcomes are not likely to differ from idiopathic disease.

A small paroxysmal nocturnal hemoglobinuria (PNH) clone can be identified in 40% to 60% of patients with newly diagnosed acquired AA. PNH is a rare clonal disorder in which an acquired mutation of the *PIG-A* gene in an HSC can lead to global absence of certain proteins on the surface of blood cells, thereby altering their immune appearance and reducing their ability to resist destruction by complement. The classic presenting features of PNH include hemolytic anemia and atypical thrombosis. However, PNH clones in patients with acquired AA are usually asymptomatic and, in general, do not require PNH-specific therapy. Flow cytometry on at least two cell lineages is the preferred diagnostic test as it will show reduced levels of glycosylphosphatidylinositol-anchored proteins (CD59, CD55) on peripheral blood cells. Whether the presence of a small PNH clone has clinical significance or predicts response to treatment and outcomes is controversial.

Once the diagnosis of AA has been confirmed via peripheral blood and bone marrow studies, human leukocyte antigen (HLA) typing of the patient and first-degree relatives should be completed promptly and prior to initiation of treatment.

Key Diagnostic Dilemma

Hepatosplenomegaly and/or lymphadenopathy do not usually occur in patients with acquired AA or IBMFS, and their presence is most suggestive of malignancy or hemophagocytic lymphohistiocytosis.

The clinical presentation and bone marrow findings in patients with inherited and acquired BMF may be identical. The absence of syndromic features and/or classic family history does not rule out an underlying IBMFS in a patient with newly diagnosed AA. Many publications suggest 40 years as a threshold for performing testing to rule out IBMFS, but testing of older patients should be strongly considered if concerning features are identified on physical exam and/or family history is even minimally suggestive of an IBMFS. Failure to recognize an IBMFS can have devastating consequences. Patients with IBMFS do not respond to immunosuppressive therapy, require dose reductions in transplant conditioning due to high risk for toxicities, and need careful monitoring for a multitude of non-hematologic complications.

Management

Supportive care of patients with AA includes the following (3):

Transfusion therapy is integral to caring for patients with AA. Red blood cells or platelets should be administered for symptomatic/severe anemia or bleeding/severe thrombocytopenia, respectively, and different thresholds have been suggested. Leukoreduced, irradiated products reduce the risk of alloimmunization, febrile nonhemolytic transfusion reactions, cytomegalovirus (CMV) infection, and graft-versus-host disease (GVHD).

Prevention of infections by administering prophylactic antibiotics or antifungal drugs is controversial, but may be considered, particularly in those with prolonged, very severe neutropenia and/or lymphopenia.

Fever in a patient with AA is a medical emergency. Blood cultures should be obtained promptly and broad-spectrum IV antibiotics administered.

AA-specific treatment depends on the underlying cause and severity of the disease as summarized in Table 4.4 (4,5).

Prognosis

The prognosis of patients with severe AA has improved dramatically thanks to improved supportive care, the increasing availability of hematopoietic stem cell transplant (HSCT), and more effective immunosuppressive therapy (IST) with the survival rates being as high as 80% to 90% (3,4). Improved survival is associated with younger age, higher ANC, and use of HSCT as the primary therapy. Relapse occurs in approximately 30% of patients who initially respond to IST. Clonal evolution, MDS, and acute myeloid leukemia (AML) are the possible complications after IST.

Future Directions

Trials using eltrombopag are addressing the optimal timing and dosing of therapy, duration of response, discontinuation of drug, and safety in patients with clonal abnormalities. Other areas of

Table 4.4 Treatment for Acquired Aplastic Anemia

	Treatment
Secondary AA (medication, infection)	If secondary AA is very likely, discontinuation of the offending agent and/or treatment of the underlying disease and an observation period may be appropriate. If treatment is necessary, proceed with a similar approach as described for patients with idiopathic AA

(continued)

Table 4.4 Treatment for Acquired Aplastic Anemia (*continued*)

	Treatment
Idiopathic AA	
Non-severe	Optimal therapy is unknown, but observation may be sufficient, especially if the patient remains transfusion independent
Severe/very severe	Matched related HSCT is the preferred treatment when feasible as it is curative, particularly for patients <40 to 50 years old*

Severe/very severe (continued):

IST is most commonly used as the first therapy as most patients are not candidates for HSCT due to lack of a matched sibling donor, age, comorbidities, or access to transplantation

Standard IST includes the following:

- hATG
  - Dose: 40 mg/kg IV daily for 4 days
  - SE: Serum sickness (fever, rash, malaise) is a significant concern; therefore, steroids are administered concurrently and continued for approximately 2 weeks, followed by a rapid taper and discontinuation. Other SE include rigors, hypotension, hypoxemia, and allergic reactions
- CSA
  - Dose: 10 to 12 mg/kg/d orally divided in two doses, then adjusted to target trough levels of 200 to 400 ng/mL
  - CSA is continued usually for a minimum of 6 to 12 months and then tapered slowly in patients with count recovery
  - SE: hypertension, renal injury, elevations in creatinine, hypomagnesemia, neurotoxicity, tremor, gingival hyperplasia, and hypertrichosis
- Eltrombopag is now being used as the first-line therapy for adults, in combination with IST (6)
  - Dose: 150 mg orally once per day in adults of non-Asian ancestry. Patients of East of Southeast Asian ancestry are given half the normal dose. Dose is reduced/temporarily held for high platelet counts or elevations in liver enzymes
  - SE: elevation in hepatic enzymes, high platelet counts, risk of thrombosis

*Not a strict cutoff, and decision must be based on a case-by-case basis taking into account the patient's clinical status and if they could tolerate HSCT or not. Elderly patients or those with serious comorbidities may not benefit from aggressive interventions if they are stable and quality of life is maintained with regular transfusions.

AA, aplastic anemia; CSA, cyclosporine; hATG, horse antithymocytes globulin; HSCT, hematopoietic stem cell transplant; IST, immunosuppressive therapy; SE, side effects.

interest include optimizing conditioning regimens for patients undergoing HSCT and use of matched unrelated HSCT as the first-line therapy.

Key Points

- AA is a life-threatening condition that refers to pancytopenia with bone marrow hypoplasia or aplasia.
- AA may be idiopathic, secondary, or inherited (IBMFS). The clinical presentation and bone marrow findings may be identical regardless of the underlying etiology; thus, a thorough diagnostic evaluation is critical prior to starting treatment.
- Idiopathic and secondary AA may be treated with HSCT or IST, typically with excellent outcomes.

FANCONI ANEMIA

Clinical Case 4.1 (*continued*)

The father of the 17-year-old patient had history of mild thrombocytopenia. No other blood disorders or cancers were reported in the family. The patient's physical exam demonstrated only pallor and bruising on his extremities. Bone marrow studies showed a markedly hypocellular bone marrow (5%) without evidence of malignancy or dysplasia. Blood chemistries, liver panel, and flow cytometry for PNH were all negative. Results of chromosome breakage analysis and telomere length testing are pending.

Introduction

Fanconi anemia (FA) is an IBMFS characterized by congenital anomalies and a predisposition to malignancies. FA is a clinically heterogeneous disease that can affect almost every organ system. Affected cells have spontaneous chromosomal instability and hypersensitivity to DNA interstrand cross-linking agents. The prevalence of FA is about 2.5 individuals per million, with a male to female ratio of 1.2:1. FA is most commonly autosomal recessive, though may be X-linked rarely. Median age of diagnosis is 7 years, which is typical when BMF develops.

Diagnosis

Diagnosing or ruling out FA is important as FA patients do not respond to immunosuppressive agents used to treat severe AA and are hypersensitive to chemotherapeutic agents and radiation often used in FA-associated malignancies. The Fanconi Anemia Research Fund published detailed guidelines on diagnosis and evaluation of FA (7).

Hematologic abnormalities: BMF often develops between ages 5 and 15, but can develop well into adulthood. BMF is thought to be caused by increasing apoptosis in stem and progenitor cells and affects Hgb, platelets, and leukocytes. Anemia in FA is characterized by macrocytosis, along with an elevated Hgb F level and increased expression of the i antigen on red cells. After developing thrombocytopenia, 50% of patients progress to pancytopenia in 3 to 4 years. Serum alpha-fetoprotein is characteristically elevated in FA. Bone marrow examination often shows hypocellularity for age due to decreased numbers of hematopoietic precursors with normal morphology.

Key diagnostic test: **Chromosome fragility testing**. When exposed to DNA cross-linking agents such as diepoxybutane (DEB) or mitomycin C (MMC), FA leukocytes and fibroblasts have a 3- to 10-fold increase in chromosomal breakage compared to normal controls.

Confirmation of FA can be done by detecting biallelic mutations in one of the 16 identified *FANC* genes associated with FA. *FANC* gene products function in a DNA repair signaling pathway, repairing interstrand cross-links that impede replication and transcription by inhibiting DNA strand separation. The most commonly affected genes are *FANCA* (60%), *FANCC* (15%), and *FANCG* (10%).

Congenital anomalies: Sixty percent of patients have major physical malformations. The most common anomalies are short stature/intrauterine growth retardation (40%), café-au-lait spots or abnormal (either hyper- or hypo-) skin pigmentation (40%), radial ray abnormalities (may have absent or hypoplastic radii with absent thumbs) (35%), microcephaly, micropthalmia, renal anomalies, and hypogonadism (20%–25%). Beyond the most common anomalies, nearly every organ system can be affected in FA. Following diagnosis, important organ evaluations include audiometry, ophthalmic exam, renal ultrasound, and an endocrine assessment.

About 75% of FA patients have at least one endocrinopathy. Commonly affected endocrine organ disorders include short stature, growth hormone insufficiency, hypothyroidism, glucose intolerance, gonadal dysfunction, midbrain abnormalities (hypothalamus–pituitary axis defects), dyslipidemia, metabolic syndrome, and osteopenia.

Prognosis

Median survival is estimated to be 29 years of age. The major causes of death are complications from BMF (including sepsis and hemorrhagic complications), HSCT, and FA-associated malignancies.

Key Diagnostic Dilemma

The combination of congenital anomalies and progressive BMF in FA overlaps with other IBMFSs. Thrombocytopenia absent radius (TAR) syndrome presents early in life with thrombocyto-penia and the absence of radii. Unlike FA, however, the thumbs are always present and unaffected in TAR. Radial ray abnormali-ties can be seen in FA, but are associated with abnormal thumb development.

Predisposition to Malignancy

Leukemia and MDS often develop in FA in adolescence or young adulthood. Acute myeloblastic leukemia (AML) is the most com-mon leukemia seen in FA, though acute lymphoblastic leukemia and chronic myeloid leukemia may occur as well. The risk of AML is 600 times that of the general population in FA, and may occur without a preceding MDS. The initial manifestation of FA may be the development of AML or MDS, though 90% of patients present with BMF. Due to low tolerance for DNA-damaging chemothera-peutic agents, chemotherapy regimens often need to be modified to avoid excessive toxicity. Routine monitoring of peripheral blood counts and bone marrow evaluations are important to monitor for evidence of MDS or AML. Once MDS develops in FA, prognosis is poor with 5-year survival declining to 9%.

Solid tumors often develop in adult patients. The chance of devel-oping a solid tumor is 500 to 700 times that of the general popu-lation, with the median age of presentation being 26 years (with a cumulative incidence of 30% by 40 years of age). Malignancies are often head, neck, esophageal, or gynecologic carcinomas, and commonly, human papilloma virus–associated squamous cell carcinomas. Oral and gynecologic (at menarche) surveillance is important for early diagnosis. FA cells have increased sensitivity to ionizing radiation and oxygen radicals; therefore, it is important for patients to avoid carcinogens including tobacco and radiation when possible. Patients with FA have a more severe phenotype due to mutations in *FANCD1/BRCA2*, with an earlier onset of leuke-mia and solid tumors and a 97% probability of developing malig-nancy by age 5.

Management

Treatment options for patients with FA include HSCT and andro-gens (8,9).

HSCT is the only cure for the hematologic manifestations of FA, though it does not cure other manifestations of the disease. HSCT from an HLA-matched sibling donor can cure the BMF of FA and prevent the progression to MDS and AML. Genetic testing and chromosome breakage studies on immediate family members are important to determine who may be suitable bone marrow donors. The ideal timeline for HSCT in FA is controversial; it is best for patients to receive a transplant prior to developing MDS or AML, and outcomes are better if HSCT is performed before age 10. Conditioning regimens for FA patients limit the amount of radiation and alkylating agents like cyclophosphamide. Often, fludarabine-based regimens are used with T-cell depletion to reduce the increased GVHD seen in FA.

Androgen therapy transiently improves the cytopenias in 50% to 60% of FA patients. Treatment with androgens may delay the need for HSCT for months or years in responsive patients (may be helpful for those without a suitable donor, for those facing lack of access to HSCT facilities, or for those in whom transplant would pose a higher risk of toxicity). Androgens do not prevent progression to MDS or AML, and have significant side effects including virilization, premature closure of epiphyses/short stature, aggressiveness, development of hepatic adenoma or hepatocellular carcinoma, and hypertension. Treatment should be considered when blood counts drop to clinically significant levels, but before the bone marrow becomes devoid of HSC. Commonly used androgens are oxymetholone and danazol; response rates are similar, but liver toxicity appears more common with oxymetholone. Hematologic response is usually seen within 3 months, and then the drug is slowly tapered to an effective dose with minimal side effects.

Future Directions

Future therapies for FA involve the use of gene therapy to correct the genetic defect in the patient's own HSC. The use of metformin to improve hematopoiesis in patients with FA is also being evaluated after a study showed that this drug improved HSC function and reduced cancer risk in a mouse model of FA.

Key Points

- FA is an IBMFS characterized by macrocytic anemia, thrombocytopenia, and neutropenia.
- Congenital anomalies are commonly seen in FA.
- Chromosome fragility testing demonstrates increased chromosomal breakage in FA leukocytes when exposed to DNA cross-linking agents.
- There is a predisposition for FA patients to develop AML/MDS at a young age and solid tumors in adulthood.
- HSCT offers a cure for the hematologic manifestations of FA, though androgen therapy may provide transient improvement of the cytopenias.

DYSKERATOSIS CONGENITA AND OTHER TELOMERE BIOLOGY DISORDERS

Clinical Case 4.1 (*continued*)

While awaiting the test result, the family disclosed that the patient's 12-year-old brother had several birth marks, the paternal grandmother had thrombocytopenia of unclear etiology and expired from cirrhosis in her 50s, and several relatives had lung disease. The patient's father developed gray hair in his early 20s as did other members of his family. Results of telomere length testing became available 2 weeks later and showed very short telomeres in five out of six of the tested WBC types. Chromosome breakage analysis was normal.

Introduction

Dyskeratosis congenita (DC) is a multisystemic IBMFS disorder with marked clinical heterogeneity. Classic DC is characterized by the mucocutaneous triad of abnormal skin pigmentation, nail dystrophy, and leukoplakia, as well as BMF and predisposition to cancer. There is considerable variation among patients with respect to age of onset and severity of disease, even within the same family. The mucocutaneous triad often appears in childhood, followed by BMF frequently by the age of 20. However, some patients present with BMF or an abnormality in another system in the absence of the classic mucocutaneous triad. While the true prevalence of DC and other telomere biology disorders is unknown, it has been estimated to be approximately one in 1 million people in the general population and 2% to 5% of patients with BMF.

Diagnosis

DC is a disorder of telomere dysfunction. Telomeres are the repetitive non-coding DNA at the end of chromosomes consisting of hundreds of repeats of TTAGGG. Specific shelterin proteins bind to the DNA repeats and protect them from being discarded as useless DNA or from accidental DNA breaks during cell replication. Without the protection of these proteins, which coat the chromosomes' ends, they would shorten during cell division and replication. When chromosomes become too short, the cell is no longer able to divide. Mutations in the genes that code for the proteins of the shelterin complex as well as in the genes that encode enzymes and other proteins important for telomere maintenance have been implicated in telomere biology disorders, of which DC is the best known. Approximately 70% of patients have mutations in genes implicated in telomere function that lead to abnormally short

Table 4.5 Genetic Mutations of Dyskeratosis Congenita

X-linked	*DKC1*
Autosomal dominant	*TINF2*
	TERC
	TERT
Autosomal recessive	*NOP10*
	NOLA3
	NHP2
	NOLA2

telomeres; inheritance can be X-linked recessive, autosomal dominant, or autosomal recessive (Table 4.5).

Major Clinical Features of DC—the Mucocutaneous Triad:

Three findings define the mucocutaneous triad which is a hallmark of DC. A patient may not have all three at diagnosis as they can develop as the patient ages. Seventy-five percent of DC patients have at least one finding and 46% have all three features.

- Reticulated skin pigmentation

  Skin changes may occur at any site, but are on the neck, upper chest, proximal portions of the extremities, and hypopigmentation in the groin.

- Nail dystrophy

  Nail findings include ridging, thinning, peeling, or slow growth. Severity ranges widely, and some nails may be more affected than others.

- Oral leukoplakia

  Lesions resemble mucositis on the buccal mucosa or tongue.

A multitude of other clinical features can be seen in patients with DC (Table 4.6).

Two distinct subsets of DC have a more severe phenotype:

- Hoyeraal–Hreidarsson syndrome: DC with cerebellar hypoplasia
- Revesz syndrome: DC with exudative retinopathy

If a patient has the clinical features of DC, then *telomere length testing* in leukocyte subsets by multicolor flow FISH by a validated laboratory is indicated. Very short telomere length in all, or nearly all, the WBCs is highly indicative of DC and further genetic testing can be obtained. Other diagnostic criteria for DC include one of the classic mucocutaneous triad plus a hypoplastic marrow with any two additional physical findings.

Table 4.6 Clinical Features of Dyskeratosis Congenita

Eyes	Lacrimal duct stenosis, blepharitis, exudative retinopathy, epiphora
Hair	Early graying, sparse eyelashes
Gastrointestinal	Esophageal stricture, liver fibrosis, cirrhosis, peptic ulceration, enteropathy
Stature	Short
Dental	Caries, missing teeth, periodontitis, decreased crown/root ratio, taurodontism
Skeletal	Osteoporosis, hip avascular necrosis
Head/neurodevelopmental	Microcephaly, cerebellar hypoplasia (ataxia, spasticity, hypotonia), intracranial calcification
Perinatal	Low birth weight, intrauterine growth retardation
Pulmonary	Fibrosis, AV fistulas
Gonadal	Small testes, undescended testes, phimosis, meatal stenosis, urethral stricture, hypospadias
Neurodevelopmental	Learning disability, developmental delay, intellectual disability, depression, anxiety

AV, arteriovenous.

Key Diagnostic Dilemma

While the presence of the mucocutaneous triad is helpful for iden-tifying patients with cytopenias or BMF secondary to DC, these fea-tures may not be present simultaneously or at all in some cases. Some patients may present with abnormalities in other systems (such as pulmonary or liver fibrosis, or cancer) prior to BMF. A high index of suspicion and serial physical exams are essential, as well as a detailed family history that focuses on questions about early graying of hair, nail abnormalities, cytopenias and BMF, MDS/AML, pulmonary or liver fibrosis, cancer in young relatives, and/or early unexplained deaths due to infections. Disease anticipation, that is, earlier onset and more severe disease in successive generations, is reported in families with DC. For more information about the diagnosis and management of DC and other telomere biology disorders, please refer to "*Dyskeratosis Congenita and Telomere Biology Disorders: Diagnosis and Management Guidelines*" (10).

Prognosis

Eighty percent of patients with classic DC develop BMF by age 30. The severity of hematologic findings can vary significantly, but thrombocytopenia is typically the first cytopenia. The more severe phenotypes, Hoyeraal–Hreidarsson and Revesz syndromes, present earlier in life. DC patients are at increased risk of developing other malignancies, notably head and neck squamous cell cancer and MDS/AML, in addition to progressive pulmonary fibrosis. Ongoing cancer screening is recommended given the increased risk of malignancy, and routine surveillance includes regular dental visits, dermatologic evaluation, routine blood counts, and possibly bone marrow evaluations. Preventive measures include limiting smoking and alcohol consumption and avoiding sun exposure. Overall survival for DC patients based on data from 1910 to 1999 was 34 years; however, in more recent decades, this has increased to 49 years. The most common causes of mortality in DC patients were complications of BMF, HSCT, and other malignancies.

Management

BMF is the main cause of premature mortality in patients with DC. In general, for a patient with normal or mildly low blood counts and no cytogenetic abnormality in the bone marrow, serial follow-up of blood counts and bone marrow studies may be appropriate. Appropriate plans for intervention should be in place in case the patient experiences progressively worsening cytopenias, worsening BMF, clonal progression or evolution, or evidence of leukemia. Treatment options for patients with severe BMF include HSCT or androgens (9,11).

HSCT is the only curative treatment for BMF, MDS, and leukemia in patients with DC. A related donor who is confirmed to not have DC is preferred, though HSCT from an unrelated donor can be considered in patients lacking a matched, related donor. HSCT for patients with DC should be done with reduced intensity conditioning as these patients have high risk of pulmonary toxicity from chemotherapy and irradiation. While HSCT may cure the hematologic manifestations of DC, it does not impact the risk for developing solid cancers (and, in fact, may accelerate the development of such a malignancy) or progression of pulmonary or hepatic fibrosis.

Androgens are a reasonable option in patients who are not candidates for HSCT. Androgens, however, do not cure BMF or prevent the progression to MDS or AML. The literature on androgen use in patients with DC is limited, but as many as 50% to 70% of patients with DC receiving androgens may show a hematopoietic response with improvements in Hgb, platelets, and neutrophil counts. Oxymetholone was the most commonly used androgen, but recently, danazol, a synthetic androgen derivative, has gained popularity given less-severe side effects. The suggested starting dose of danazol is 2.5 to 5 mg/kg/d in children and 100 to 150 mg twice a day in adults. The dose is adjusted based on the hematologic response and side effects. Possible side effects include virilization, mood changes, liver toxicity, alterations in blood lipid profile, growth spurt/premature closure of growth plates in children, liver adenomas, peliosis in spleen or liver, and rarely, hepatocellular carcinomas.

Future Directions

New trials are warranted to better guide clinical choices regarding minimal effective doses of androgens to lessen or avoid androgen-related side effects. An ongoing trial with nandolone decanoate is assessing safety and reduction in telomere attrition rate. HSCT trials in DC patients are focusing on limiting toxicities associated with current conditioning regimens.

Key Points

- DC is a disorder of telomere function characterized by the mucocutaneous triad of abnormal skin pigmentation, nail dystrophy, and leukoplakia, as well as BMF and predisposition to cancer.
- Patients with DC may present with BMF, in the absence of the mucocutaneous triad.
- A high index of suspicion and telomere length testing are essential for making the diagnosis of DC.
- HSCT and androgens are the therapeutic interventions available to treat BMF.

Clinical Case 4.1 (*continued*)

Telomere length testing strongly suggests a diagnosis of DC/other telomere biology disorder as the underlying cause of BMF. Genetic testing and immediate HLA typing are recommended for the patient and his family to rule out DC and find a transplant donor. While awaiting these, the patient receives supportive transfusion therapy and undergoes evaluation of pulmonary and liver function, among others.

SHWACHMAN–DIAMOND SYNDROME

Clinical Case 4.2

An 8-month-old male with neutropenia was referred for evaluation. His history was significant for hypospadias, for which urology was planning corrective surgery, a hospitalization at 4 months of age for failure to thrive, and eczema. He was in the fifth percentile for weight and length at birth, but on presentation, he was below the third percentile for both. The mother reported he had not gained weight, and his stools were frothy, light colored, and oily, despite a well-balanced diet of both table foods and pureed foods. On exam, he had a narrow chest, short neck, and short legs. CBC demonstrated mild normocytic anemia and ANC ranged from 800 to 1,500 cells/μL. Liver enzymes were two to three times the upper limit of normal.

Introduction

Shwachman–Diamond syndrome (SDS) is an autosomal recessive IBMFS characterized by the triad of pancreatic insufficiency, skeletal abnormalities, and neutropenia that may progress to BMF; however, this disorder is a multisystem disease with a wide scope of clinical abnormalities and malformations. Patients generally present in infancy due to problems with malabsorption from pancreatic insufficiency, but some cases have been identified later on. SDS is the third most common IBMFS after FA and Diamond–Blackfan anemia (DBA) and it is the second leading cause of pancreatic insufficiency after cystic fibrosis.

Diagnosis

The diagnosis of SDS has classically relied on evidence of the following (12,13):

- *Exocrine pancreatic dysfunction*, which may improve over time
  - Clinically manifests as failure to thrive or steatorrhea
  - Diagnosis can established by demonstrating the following:
    - Low levels of trypsinogen (in patients under 3 years of age)
    - Low levels of isoamylase (in patients over 3 years of age)
    - Reduced levels of fat-soluble vitamins (A, D, E, K)
    - Elevated fecal fat excretion
    - Imaging studies showing a small and/or fatty pancreas
- *BMF*, which ranges from single (neutropenia being the most common) to multilineage cytopenias, and may progress to MDS or AML
  - Clinically manifests as recurrent infections, pallor, and/or easy bruising or bleeding
  - Diagnosis is established by monitoring the CBC, and baseline bone marrow aspirate and biopsy, with cytogenetic and/or FISH analysis, is usually recommended

The phenotypic spectrum of SDS is broad and the classic combination of pancreatic insufficiency and BMF may be absent in some patients.

Other clinical features that should raise suspicion and support a diagnosis of SDS are listed in Table 4.7.

Table 4.7 Clinical Features That Can Be Seen In Shwachman–Diamond Syndrome Patients

Skeletal	Metaphyseal dysostosis, small thorax, narrow chest, dysplastic hips, bow legs, short limbs, Legg–Calve–Perthes, short neck
Developmental	Low birth weight, developmental delay, neurocognitive deficits
Gastrointestinal	Malabsorption, hepatomegaly
Ophthalmologic	Hypertelorism, retinitis pigmentosum, esotropia
Dental	Dental carries, oral ulcers
Cardiac	Congenital heart disease (PDA, right aortic arch, transposition of the great vessel), myocardial fibrosis
Endocrine	Insulin-dependent diabetes, growth hormone deficiency, hypogonadotropic hypogonadism, hypothyroidism
Gonadal	Atrophic testes, hypospadias
Neurologic	Microcephaly, macrocephaly, cleft lip/palate, Chiari malformation, cerebellar tonsillar ectopia
Immunologic	Low number of circulating NK cells, B and T cells, decreased immunoglobulins

NK, natural killer; PDA, patent ductus arteriosus.

In patients in whom SDS is suspected, genetic testing for the *SBDS* gene can be utilized as a confirmatory testing. Mutations in the *SBDS* gene can be found in 90% of patients; however, a negative test does not rule out SDS as 10% of patients with clinical features consistent with SDS will lack *SBDS* gene mutations (12).

Key Diagnostic Dilemma

While most patients with SDS are diagnosed early in childhood, some have subtle symptoms and remain undiagnosed. Other diagnoses that should be considered include FA, cystic fibrosis, and Pearson syndrome.

Prognosis

Due to the rarity of this syndrome, the natural history of SDS remains poorly understood.

Management

Table 4.8 summarizes the recommendations for managing this multisystemic disease (9,12,13).

Table 4.8 Management of Shwachman–Diamond Syndrome Manifestations

Exocrine pancreatic insufficiency	Supplementation with fat-soluble vitamins
Hematologic abnormalities	• *GCSF* can be administered to treat neutropenia and reduce the risk of infections in patients with ANC persistently at <500 cells/μL • *Transfusions* of red cells and/or platelets may be administered to patients with severe anemia or thrombocytopenia, respectively • *HSCT* can be considered in patients with severe pancytopenia, MDS, or AML
Skeletal abnormalities	Surgical management may be required
Growth/endocrine	Frequent assessments of growth and nutrition, with appropriate referral to the endocrinologist when necessary

AML, acute myeloid leukemia; ANC, absolute neutrophil count; GCSF, granulocyte colony-stimulating factor; HSCT, hematopoietic stem cell transplant; MDS, myelodysplastic syndrome; SDS, Shwachman–Diamond syndrome.

Future Directions

Studies are needed to further characterize the subset of patients with SDS who remain genetically undefined. In addition, information obtained from studies that examine the development of MDS/AML in patients with SDS may guide future screening strategies for early detection of MDS/AML as well as to inform therapy choices. Trials regarding the use of HSCT in patients with SDS focus on strategies to improve outcomes and reduce toxicities.

Key Points

- SDS is an autosomal recessive disorder characterized by exocrine pancreatic dysfunction and BMF.
- Most SDS patients present early in life with growth failure, skeletal abnormalities, and recurrent infections; however, adult diagnoses are reported.
- Neutropenia is the most common hematologic abnormality, but patients may develop BMF, MDS, and AML.
- Treatment for the hematologic manifestations of SDS is limited to granulocyte colony-stimulating factor (GCSF) for patients with neutropenia and HSCT for those with progressive BMF, MDS, or AML.

DIAMOND–BLACKFAN ANEMIA

Clinical Case 4.3

A 5-month-old Caucasian male presented to his pediatrician with rhinorrhea and cough. A CBC revealed Hgb of 6.9 g/dL with an MCV of 107 fL. His platelet count was 258,000 cells/μL with a WBC count of 7.4 × 10³ cells/μL and an ANC of 2,100 cells/μL. Physical exam revealed hypertelorism and low-set ears without other evident abnormalities; his neurocognitive development was appropriate for age. Further laboratory evaluation revealed a decreased reticulocyte count, increased fetal Hgb level, and normal telomere lengths and chromosome fragility testing. Erythrocyte adenoside deaminase activity was increased, bone marrow biopsy revealed 90% cellularity with a paucity of erythroid cells, and no abnormalities were noted in other cell lines.

Introduction

DBA, otherwise known as congenital erythroid hypoplastic anemia, is an inherited red cell aplasia associated with congenital anomalies and a predisposition to malignancies. Patients usually present early in infancy (diagnosis by 3, 6, and 12 months of age is estimated to be 50%, 75%, and 92%, respectively), with a *macrocytic anemia and reticulocytopenia.* WBC and platelet counts are typically normal, though platelet counts may be increased. The incidence of DBA is estimated to be between two and seven per million live births, and there is no gender or ethnic association with the disease.

Diagnosis

A diagnosis of "classical" DBA is made if all of the diagnostic criteria are present (Box 4.1) (14). "Non-classical" DBA is considered in clinical cases consistent with DBA with family members who have DBA-associated genetic mutations.

Congenital anomalies are commonly seen in patients with DBA (Table 4.9), as 50% of patients have associated anomalies and 21% of patients have more than one anomaly (14). While short stature is common in DBA, the cause is likely multifactorial as chronic glucocorticoid treatment, iron overload, and chronic anemia also likely contribute to the reduction in height.

Laboratory Workup

When DBA is suspected, it is important to consider other causes of macrocytic anemia or pure red cell aplasia, such as transient erythroblastopenia of childhood (TEC), infection (particularly parvovirus), and erythroblastopenic crisis in a patient with

Box 4.1 Diamond–Blackfan Anemia Diagnostic Criteria

Diagnostic criteria

Age <1 year

Macrocytic anemia with no other significant cytopenias

Reticulocytopenia

Normal marrow cellularity with a paucity of bone marrow erythroid precursors

Major supporting criteria

"Classical" ***DBA*** gene mutation*

Positive family history

Minor supporting criteria

Elevated red cell erythrocyte adenosine deaminase activity

Congenital anomalies consistent with "classical" DBA

Elevated fetal hemoglobin

No evidence for another inherited bone marrow failure disorder

* *"Classical" DBA genetic mutations:* Fifty percent of patients have identifiable mutations in a ribosomal protein gene, often having a haploinsufficiency in one of the following genes: *RPS17, RPS19* (most commonly mutated gene, found in 25% of cases), *RPS24, RPL5, RPL11,* or *RPL35A.* Inheritance is autosomal dominant in 40% to 45% of cases with variable penetrance and expressivity. Mutations may be sporadic as well. There are no associations between the affected gene and outcome, congenital anomalies, or expected response to treatment.

DBA, Diamond–Blackfan anemia.

underlying chronic hemolytic anemia. Chromosome fragility and telomere length testing may be considered in some cases. Checking a CBC and bone marrow exam, fetal Hgb level, and erythrocyte adenosine deaminase activity (eADA) are important in approaching a patient with suspected DBA, and the characteristic findings are summarized in Table 4.10. In addition to the typical bone marrow findings listed in Table 4.10, patients who have been transfused may have increased iron deposition in the bone marrow. Renal imaging and echocardiogram are necessary to evaluate for congenital anomalies with subspecialty consultation as necessary.

Key Diagnostic Dilemma

TEC is a pure red cell aplasia that presents similarly to DBA. While DBA is diagnosed in 90% of cases by 1 year of age, TEC presents in older children (between 6 months of age and 4 years). TEC presents

Table 4.9 Congenital Anomalies Associated With Diamond–Blackfan Anemia

Craniofacial	Hypertelorism, cleft or high-arched palate, microcephaly, micrognathia, microtia, low-set ears, low hairline, ptosis, flat nasal bridge
Neck	Short or webbed neck, Sprengel deformity, Klippel–Feil deformity
Ophthalmologic	Congenital glaucoma, strabismus, congenital cataract
Urogenital	Absent kidney, horseshoe kidney, hypospadias, duplicated collecting systems
Cardiac	Ventricular septal defect, atrial septal defect, coarctation of aorta, tetralogy of Fallot, complex cardiac anomalies
Musculoskeletal	Triphalangial, bifid, or hypoplastic thumb, syndactyly, absent radial artery
Neuromotor	Learning difficulties
Short stature	

with a normocytic, normochromic anemia, normal fetal Hgb and eADA, and without associated congenital anomalies. TEC typically spontaneously resolves in 1 to 2 months.

Prognosis

Survival to age 40 in DBA patients is estimated at 86% for steroid-responsive patients and 57% for transfusion-dependent patients. Deaths are frequently treatment related, due to infections (including *Pneumocystis jiroveci*), complications from iron overload, and complications of HSCT.

Table 4.10 Laboratory Findings in Diamond–Blackfan Anemia

Complete blood count	Macrocytic anemia Normal platelets (may be increased) Normal white blood cells (though neutropenia is associated in some cases)
Fetal hemoglobin	Increased
Erythrocyte adenosine deaminase activity	Increased (may be falsely normal with RBC transfusions in the past 8 to 12 weeks, but may still remain elevated)
Bone marrow findings	Normal cellularity Paucity of erythroid progenitor cells

RBC, red blood cell.

Spontaneous hematologic remission occurs in 20% to 30% of cases (defined as a stable Hgb level, not requiring transfusions, without steroid treatment). Remission often occurs in the first or second decade of life in steroid-responsive patients, although it may occur in steroid-resistant patients as well. There are no phenotypic or genotypic predictors for those who will go into spontaneous remission.

Predisposition to malignancy: Up to 4% of DBA patients go on to develop a malignancy. AML with or without preceding MDS is most frequently seen, followed by osteosarcoma and Hodgkin lymphoma. The median age of cancer development is 15, and there is no genotype–phenotype correlation with an increased risk of malignancy in DBA. While growth hormone may be used to address the short stature associated with DBA and its associated treatments, the decision to use growth hormone should be carefully made due to the potential increased risk of osteosarcoma development. Bone marrow examinations to monitor for evolution to MDS or AML should be performed annually and upon development of new cytopenias.

Management

Therapeutic interventions include red blood cell transfusions, oral steroids, and HSCT (15).

Corticosteroids: Initial therapy is often prednisone, at a dose of 2 mg/kg/d. At this dose, the Hgb level is expected to increase within 2 to 4 weeks of treatment initiation. Response is defined as an elevation in Hgb to a stable level (8–9 g/dL) at which transfusions are not required. About 70 to 80% of patients respond to steroids initially. If transfusion independence is not achieved in 4 weeks, steroids should be discontinued. In cases of steroid failure, steroids may be reintroduced in 12 to 18 months as some children may later become responders. After a response is seen, a slow taper is recommended until the minimum dose required for transfusion independence is found, referred to as the maintenance dose (failure to taper from the initial dose is also considered a treatment failure). Target maintenance dose should not exceed 0.5 mg/kg/d or 1 mg/kg every other day. Frequently, patients require a small dose of corticosteroids every other day or two to three times a week to maintain a stable Hgb level. Initiating corticosteroid therapy is usually delayed in early infancy (first 6 months of life) due to adverse growth and neurocognitive effects. As chronic steroid therapy is associated with a number of adverse effects, *Pneumocystis jirovecii* prophylaxis, periodic bone density measurements, gastric protection, and periodic ophthalmologic exams are important for steroid-responsive individuals.

Transfusion therapy is used for steroid-resistant disease and in early infancy. Leukocyte-depleted red blood cells are transfused every 3 to 6 weeks to keep the Hgb level above 8 g/dL (transfusion volume: 10–15 mL/kg). During transfusion therapy, it is important to monitor for signs of iron overload, as patients may require iron chelation to prevent end-organ damage.

HSCT is the only curative option for DBA. HSCT is used in transfusion-dependent patients, those who progress to BMF, patients who have HLA-matched siblings, or in cases when AML or MDS develops. Matched related donor HSCT should be considered before 10 years, preferably between ages 2 and 5.

Future Directions

Genetic therapy is being evaluated in DBA, including with *RPS19* deficiency. The branched-chain amino acid leucine regulates protein metabolism through activation of mammalian target of rapamycin (mTOR). Animal models have demonstrated improvement of anemia with leucine treatment. Modulation of the p53 pathway is also being evaluated as a potential therapy for DBA.

Key Points

- DBA is an inherited red cell aplasia disorder, which typically develops in the first year of life, characterized by congenital anomalies (short stature, thumb anomalies, and congenital heart disease) and a predisposition to develop malignancy.
- Laboratory findings include macrocytic anemia with reticulocytopenia, increased fetal Hgb, and increased erythrocyte deaminase activity level.
- Bone marrow studies reveal normal cellularity with a paucity of erythrocyte precursors.
- Treatment includes steroids as the first-line treatment and chronic transfusion for steroid-resistant patients. HSCT is the only curative management for selected patients.

GATA2 DEFICIENCY SYNDROME

Clinical Case 4.4

A 23 year old male is referred to a hematologist for thrombocytopenia following a second hospitalization within the past 2 months for pneumonia. Bronchoalveolar lavage cultures obtained during bronchoscopy grew Mycobacterium avium complex. His current medications include azithromycin, ethambutol, and rifampin. Six months prior to this encounter, he was diagnosed with CMV esophagitis. He denies further medical history. He does not have siblings and both parents are alive and healthy. On physical exam, patient is noted to have warts on bilateral hands and forearms. Upon questioning, patient states that he has seen various dermatologists over the past 3 years for the warts but has not received successful treatment. The remaining physical exam is unremarkable. Leukocyte count is 3,500 cells/μL. The differential consistently shows a decreased absolute monocyte count. Hemoglobin is 10.5 g/dL and platelet count is 78,000 cells/μL. Bone marrow biopsy and next generation sequencing are obtained.

Introduction

Germline mutations in *GATA2*, a transcription factor required for the genesis and function of hematopoietic stem and progenitor cells, have been reported in patients with various phenotypes ranging from mild cytopenias to severe immunodeficiency. Clinical entities known to be caused by *GATA2* mutations include monocytopenia and *Mycobacterium avium* complex (MonoMac)/dendritic cell, monocyte, B, and natural killer (NK) cell deficiency (DCML), Emberger syndrome (immunodeficiency, congenital deafness, and lymphedema), and familial MDS/AML predisposition syndrome. A common feature of these clinical entities is the propensity for myeloid dysplasia (MDS, myeloproliferative neoplasms, chronic myelomonocytic leukemia, AML), with an overall prevalence of approximately 75% and a median age of 20 at onset. These entities are now recognized as a single disorder (*GATA2* deficiency syndrome) with variable clinical phenotype and high risk for myeloid neoplasia (16). Inheritance is often autosomal dominant, though cases may be sporadic as well.

Laboratory Workup and Diagnosis

Patients with *GATA2* deficiency often present with characteristic and recurrent infections, which are a result of the underlying immunodeficiency. Peripheral blood after the clinical disease onset reveals monocytopenia, as well as B, NK, and dendritic cell hypoplasia. Up to 10% of patients with congenital neutropenia and/or AA have been found to have a *GATA2* mutation after investigation. Bone marrow is often hypocellular with varying degrees of multilineage dysplasia. The most commonly seen cytogenetic abnormalities are monosomy 7 and trisomy 8. Atypical megakaryocytes are often seen in the marrow of patients with *GATA2* deficiency. Flow cytometry analysis may demonstrate inverted CD4:CD8 ratios as well. Interval bone marrow monitoring is important, and diagnosis is made by detecting a mutation in the *GATA2* gene.

Infections are common, with 82% of patients presenting with major infections. Common viral infections include human papilloma virus (HPV), affecting 63% of patients, often with recalcitrant warts, condylomata, or dysplasia. Severe herpes infections occur in

35% of patients (recurrent stomatitis, esophagitis, or genital infections). Other common viral infections include varicella, persistent Epstein–Barr viral infections, and CMV infections. Disseminated nontuberculous mycobacterial infections occur in 53% of patients. Invasive bacterial (including severe cases *Clostridium difficile* colitis) and fungal infections (aspergillosis and histoplasmosis) are also associated with *GATA2* deficiency.

Pulmonary characteristics include the development of pulmonary alveolar proteinosis (PAP), a condition resulting from abnormalities in pulmonary alveolar macrophage metabolism of granulocyte–macrophage colony-stimulating factor (GM-CSF), which may progress to alveolar hemorrhage.

Other clinical characteristics of *GATA2* deficiency include chronic lymphedema, sensorineural hearing loss, and hypothyroidism.

Prognosis

There is phenotypic heterogeneity among patients with *GATA2* deficiency, as the onset of disease varies from early childhood to late adulthood. Presentation ranges from clinically unaffected individuals to those affected by life-threatening infections, leukemia, and complications of respiratory disease (16,17). Half of the patients develop symptoms by the age of 20, with 84% developing symptoms by age 40. Survival declines after development of symptoms, with 84% survival reported 10 years after development of symptoms and 67% survival reported 20 years after the symptoms develop. Survival to 40 years of age is estimated to be 50% without receiving a bone marrow transplant.

Management

Initial treatment of *GATA2* deficiency focuses on control and treatment of infections as well as management of pulmonary or other system-based diseases as they develop (17). HSCT is curative of many of the clinical manifestations of *GATA2* deficiency, though optimal transplant timing has not been established.

Future Directions

GATA2 deficiency is a relatively newly discovered disease, with many aspects of the disease process unknown. Evaluations are ongoing to characterize the related myeloid neoplasms and clinical characteristics of the resultant immunodeficiency.

Key Points

- *GATA2* deficiency syndrome is a heterogeneous IBMFS characterized by susceptibility to infection and predisposition to myeloid neoplasia.

- Hematologic findings can range from single cytopenias to monocytopenia, decreased B and NK lymphocytes, dendritic cells, and regulatory T cells.
- HSCT cures many clinical characteristics including the hematologic and resultant immunodeficiency.

REFERENCES

1. Young NS, Calado RT, Schneiberg P. Current concepts in the pathophysiology and treatment of aplastic anemia. *Blood.* 2006;108(8):2509–2519. doi:10.1182/blood-2006-03-010777

2. West AH, Churpek JE. Old and new tools in the clinical diagnosis of inherited bone marrow failure syndromes. *Hematology Am Soc Hematol Educ Program.* 2017;2017(1):79–87. doi:10.1182/asheducation-2017.1.79

3. Höchsmann B, Moicean A, Risitano A, et al. Supportive care in severe and very severe aplastic anemia. *Bone Marrow Transplant.* 2013;48(2):168–173. doi:10.1038/bmt.2012.220

4. Bacigalupo A. How I treat acquired aplastic anemia. *Blood.* 2017;129(11):1428–1436. doi:10.1182/blood-2016-08-693481

5. Scheinberg P, Young NS. How I treat acquired aplastic anemia. *Blood.* 2012;120(6):1185–1196. doi:10.1182/blood-2011-12-274019

6. Townsley DM, Scheinberg P, Winkler T, et al. Eltrombopag added to standard immunosuppression for aplastic anemia. *NEJM.* 2017;376:1540–1550. doi:10.1056/NEJMoa1613878

7. Fanconi Anemia Research Fund. Fanconi anemia: Guidelines for diagnosis and management. 2014. http://fanconi.org/images/uploads/other/Guidelines_4th_Edition.pdf

8. Smith AR, Wagner JE. Current clinical management of Fanconi anemia. *Expert Rev Hematol.* 2012;5(5):513–522. doi:10.1586/ehm.12.48

9. Calado RT, Cle DV. Treatment of inherited bone marrow failure syndromes beyond transplantation. *Hematology Am Soc Hematol Educ Program.* 2017;2017(1):96–101. doi:10.1182/asheducation-2017.1.96

10. Savage SA, Cook EF. Dyskeratosis Congenita and Telomere Biology Disorders: Diagnosis and Management Guidelines. 2015. https://www.dcoutreach.org/sites/default/files/DC%20%26%20TBD%20Diagnosis%20And%20Management%20Guidelines.pdf

11. Dokal I. Dyskeratosis congenita. *Hematology Am Soc Hematol Educ Program.* 2011;2001:480–486. doi:10.1182/asheducation-2011.1.480

12. Huang JN, Shimamura A. Clinical spectrum and molecular pathophysiology of Shwachman-Diamond syndrome. *Curr Opin Hematol.* 2011;18:30–35. doi:10.1097/MOH.0b013e32834114a5

13. Dror Y, Donadieu J, Koglmeier, et al. Draft consensus guidelines for the diagnosis and treatment of Shwachman-Diamond syndrome. *Ann N Y Acad Sci.* 2011;1242:40–55. doi:10.1111/j.1749-6632.2011.06349.x

14. Vlachos A, Ball S, Dahl N, et al. Diagnosing and treating Diamond Blackfan anaemia: results of an international clinical consensus conference. *Br J Haematol.* 2008;142:859–876. doi:10.1111/j.1365-2141.2008.07269.x

15. Vlachos A, Muir E. How I treat Diamond-Blackfan anemia. *Blood.* 2010;116:3715–3723. doi:10.1182/blood-2010-02-251090

16. Spinner MA, Sanchez LA, Hsu AP, et al. GATA2 deficiency: a protean disorder of hematopoiesis, lymphatics, and immunity. *Blood.* 2014;123(6):809–821. doi:10.1182/blood-2013-07-515528

17. Hsu AP, McReynolds LJ, Holland SM. GATA2 deficiency. *Curr Opin Allergy Clin Immunol.* 2015;15(1):104–109. doi:10.1097/ACI.0000000000000126

5 Myeloproliferative Neoplasms

Hussein Hamad and Gustavo Rivero

MYELOPROLIFERATIVE DISORDERS

Introduction

William Dameshek first used the term "myeloproliferative disorders" in 1951 to describe a group of clonal stem cell disorders characterized by uncontrolled expansion of one or more of the myeloid cell line components. The year 1960 marked the discovery of Philadelphia (Ph) chromosome and subsequent studies in the 1960s and 1970s by Fialkow and colleagues, using X chromosome inactivation methodology, helped to establish the clonal nature of these disorders. Discovery of the Janus Kinase 2 (*JAK2*) mutation in 2005 represented an important step in our understanding of the origin of these diseases. The most recent World Health Organization (WHO) 2016 revision of myeloid neoplasm classification includes eight types of myeloproliferative neoplasms (MPNs) (Table 5.1). In this chapter, we discuss the classical Ph chromosome-negative MPNs, polycythemia vera (PV), essential thrombocytosis (ET), and primary myelofibrosis (PMF), reviewing the pathophysiology, diagnostic criteria and dilemmas, and common complications and providing an update on their current management.

Pathophysiology

The hallmark pathologic marker of MPNs is the constitutive activation of the JAK-Signal Transducers and Activators of Transcription (JAK-STAT) signaling pathway. The *JAK2* gene is located on chromosome 9p24; a point mutation resulting in a valine to phenylalanine substitution at codon 617 (*JAK2*V617F) is found in more than 95% of patients with PV and in 50% to 60% of patients with ET and PMF. The V617F mutation results in loss of inhibitory function of the pseudokinase domain (JH2) on the kinase domain (JH-1), resulting in constitutive activation of the JAK-STAT pathway. *JAK2* associates with the cytoplasmic portion of different growth factor and cytokine receptors, including the erythropoietin receptor (EPOR), the

Table 5.1 2016 World Health Organization Classification of Myeloproliferative Neoplasms

CML, BCR-ABL1+

CNL

PV

PMF
PMF, prefibrotic / early stage
PMF, overt fibrotic stage

ET

Chronic eosinophilic leukemia, not otherwise specified

MPN, unclassifiable

CML, chronic myeloid leukemia; CNL, chronic neutrophilic leukemia; ET, essential thrombocythemia; MPN, myeloproliferative neoplasm; PMF, primary myelofibrosis; PV, polycythemia vera.

thrombopoietin (TPO) receptor (c-MPL), and the granulocyte-macrophage colony stimulating factor receptor (G-CSFR), leading to downstream signaling. When mutated, *JAK2* activation results in ligand-independent proliferation and a pleiotropic phenotype with varying degrees of erythrocytosis, thrombocytosis, and, to a lesser extent, leukocytosis. Less common driver mutations in PV cases are mutations in *JAK2* exon 12, such as the K391I mutation, which leads to *JAK2* binding of EPOR (1).

The second major mutations leading to JAK-STAT pathway activation are those affecting the TPO receptor c-MPL, most commonly leading to amino acid changes at W515L and less frequently at S505N, which are observed in 5% to 10% of patients with ET and PMF.

In 2013, calreticulin gene (*CALR*) mutations were identified as the second type of recurrent non-*JAK2* mutations in MPNs. *CALR* mutations are encountered in 25% to 30% of ET and PMF and are mutually exclusive from *JAK2* and *MPL* mutations. Insertion or deletion mutations are most common, with the most frequent being a 52-base frameshift deletion affecting the C-terminus of the *CALR* gene. It is not completely understood how *CALR* mutations lead to ET and/or PMF, but *CALR* mutants are thought to directly and specifically activate thrombopoietin receptor (TPOR) via interaction between the novel C-terminal tail of mutant *CALR* and the N-glycosylated extracellular domain of TPOR (2).

Approximately one third of patients with MPNs carry a somatic mutation in other genes. Common mutated genes include those involved in epigenetic regulation such as DNA methylation (*DNMT3a*, *TET2*, *IDH1/2*) and histone modification (*ASXL1*, *EZH2*), spliceosome mutations (*SF3B1*, *SRSF2*, *U2AF1*, *ZRSR2*), and tumor suppressor genes (*TP53*). The presence of these mutations helps to establish the clonality in triple-negative cases, but more importantly carries a prognostic significance, especially in PMF cases, and aids in decision management.

POLYCYTHEMIA VERA

Clinical Case 5.1

A 26-year-old female was admitted with abdominal pain. Her physical exam demonstrated tenderness in her right upper quadrant. An abdominal CT demonstrated suprahepatic vein thrombosis, and her portal vein was dilated without intraluminal thrombi (Figures 5.1A and B). Complete blood count (CBC) showed the hemoglobin (Hgb) level as 16.9 g/dL, hematocrit (Hct) of 52%, white blood count 16,000 μ/L, and platelets 425,000 μ/L. Her ferritin level was 2 ng/mL and erythropoietin (EPO) was 1.9 mU/mL.

Introduction

PV is the most common MPN in the United States, with an annual incidence rate of 1.1 cases per 100,000 persons per year (3). The prevalence is around 44 to 57 per 100,000 persons (4). The median age of diagnosis is 60 to 65 years with a slight male predominance.

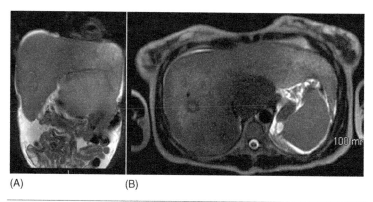

(A)   (B)

Figure 5.1 26-year-old female diagnosed with *JAK2* 617F-positive PV presenting with Budd–Chiari syndrome. (A) Abdominal CT demonstrates hepatomegaly and distended intrahepatic vessels. (B) Significant hepatomegaly and distended intrahepatic vessels associated with Budd–Chiari syndrome.

Patients may be asymptomatic and diagnosed by detection of abnormal blood tests or they may present with nonspecific symptoms. Fatigue is reported in a majority of patients with PV, ET, or PMF. Additional symptoms include pruritus (52%), bone pain (44%), and other constitutional symptoms (fever, night sweats, and weight loss), the latter being more common in myelofibrosis (5). Erythromelalgia (sensation of intense burning pain in extremities accompanied by erythema and warmth), ocular migraine, and vasomotor symptoms such as headaches, visual disturbances, dizziness, and lightheadedness are frequently present in PV. Physical examination shows variably elevated blood pressure and mild splenomegaly (<5 cm increase above normal) in 70% of patients with PV. Ruddy cyanosis (mucosal congestion along with cyanosis) and conjunctival plethora are manifestations of elevated red blood cell (RBC) mass observed in PV.

In addition to the these symptoms, thrombosis and bleeding are the major causes of morbidity and mortality in MPN. The incidence of thrombosis in different PV studies varied from 14% to 36%. In the large European Collaboration on Low-Dose Aspirin in Polycythemia Vera (ECLAP) study (6), major thrombosis was present in 36% of patients at diagnosis and an additional 10% developed thrombosis on follow-up. Approximately 70% to 75% of events were arterial. Twenty-five percent of deaths were attributed to thrombosis, with older age and a previous history of thrombosis being the major risk factors. Thrombosis in an unusual site should always prompt suspicion of an underlying MPN, particularly PV. Fifty percent of Budd–Chiari syndrome is due to PV, and hepatic vein thrombosis can be the presenting manifestation as illustrated in the case discussed here.

Diagnosis
Clinical Case 5.1 (*continued*)
Given the patient's high Hgb and low ferritin and EPO levels, a bone marrow (BM) was obtained, which showed panmyelosis with erythroid progenitor hyperplasia. JAK2 V617F mutation was positive with an allele frequency (relative frequency of the mutant gene) of 68%.

Laboratory Findings and Differential Diagnosis
PV is defined by the presence of elevated Hgb, Hct, and red cell mass (RCM). Hgb level required for diagnosis was lowered in the 2016 WHO diagnostic criteria (7) for MPN to >16.5 g/dL (or Hct >49%) in men and >16 g/dL (or Hct >48%) in women. PV cases usually have variable degrees of thrombocytosis and leukocytosis. Serum vitamin B12 and leukocyte alkaline phosphatase score (a test rarely used in the modern era) are usually elevated. Determination of

RCM and demonstration of endogenous colony-forming unit-erythroid (CFU-E) growth are no longer required for diagnosis. Mean corpuscular volume (MCV) and ferritin levels are low, and peripheral blood smear may also show microcytosis. Since Hgb, Hct, and RCM are dependent on plasma volume, the first clinical question when faced with an elevated Hgb/Hct is to ensure if absolute erythrocytosis is present. Relative erythrocytosis occurs in conditions of intravascular volume depletion, such as severe diarrhea, diuretic use, or third spacing. When true absolute polycythemia is present, serum EPO levels and testing for *JAK2* mutation in the peripheral blood help narrow the differential diagnosis. Secondary cases of polycythemia should be considered when the EPO level is normal or high in the absence of *JAK2* mutations (Table 5.2). Additional testing for secondary causes may include oxygen saturation, polysomnography, methemoglobin and carboxyhemogobin levels, and CT scans of the chest, abdomen, and pelvis.

Bone Marrow Biopsy (BMB) Findings

BMB is now included in the 2016 WHO diagnostic criteria of PV (Table 5.3). Typical BMB in PV shows panmyelosis with trilineage hyperplasia including granulocytic, erythroid, and megakaryocytic

Table 5.2 Secondary and Other Causes of Polycythemia

Appropriate EPO Production Secondary to Hypoxia	Inappropriate (Ectopic) EPO Production	Germline and Somatic Mutational Causes of Polycythemia	Other Causes
Chronic lung disease	Renal cell carcinoma	*EPOR* gene mutation	Use of anabolic steroids
Smoking (carboxy-hemoglobinemia)	Hepatocellular carcinoma	Chuvash polycythemia (*VHL* gene mutation)	Autologous blood transfusion (blood doping)
Right to left cardiac shunts	Cerebellar hemangio-blastoma	High oxygen affinity hemoglobins	POEMS syndrome
High altitude	Uterine fibroids		
Methemo-globinemia			

EPO, erythropoietin; POEMS, polyneuropathy, organomegaly, endocrinopathy, myeloma protein, and skin changes.

Table 5.3 2016 World Health Organization Diagnostic Criteria for Essential Thrombocytosis, Polycythemia Vera, and Pre-Primary Myelofibrosis

2016 WHO Criteria	PV	ET	Early/pre-PMF
Major criteria	1. Hgb >16.5 g/dL in men and >16 g/dL in women or Hct >49% in men and >48% in women or increased RCM (>25% mean normal predicted value) 2. BM biopsy showing hypercellularity for age with trilineage growth (panmyelosis) including prominent erythroid, granulocytic, and megakaryocytic proliferation with pleomorphic, mature megakaryocytes (differences in size) 3. Presence of JAK2V617F or JAK2 exon 12 mutation	1. Platelet count >450 × 10⁹/L 2. BM biopsy showing proliferation mainly of the megakaryocyte lineage with increased numbers of enlarged, mature megakaryocytes with hyperlobulated nuclei. No significant increase or left shift in neutrophil granulopoiesis or erythropoiesis and very rarely minor (grade 1) increase in reticulin fibers 3. Not meeting WHO criteria for BCR ABL CML, PV, PMF, MDSs, or other myeloid neoplasms 4. Presence of JAK2, CALR, or MPL mutation	1. Megakaryocytic proliferation and atypia, without reticulin fibrosis grade 1, accompanied by increased age-adjusted BM cellularity, granulocytic proliferation, and often decreased erythropoiesis 2. Not meeting WHO criteria for BCR-ABL 1 CML, PV, ET, MDS, or other myeloid neoplasms 3. Presence of JAK2, CALR, or MPL mutation or, in the absence of these mutations, presence of another clonal marker or absence of minor reactive BM reticulin fibrosis
Minor critera	1. Subnormal serum EPO level	1. Presence of a clonal marker or absence of evidence for reactive thrombocytosis	1. Anemia not attributed to a comorbid condition 2. Leukocytosis >11 × 10⁹/L 3. Palpable splenomegaly 4. LDH increase to above upper normal range
Criteria required for diagnosis	All three major or the first two major and the minor criteria	All four major or the first three major and the minor criteria	All three major and at least one minor criteria

BM, bone marrow; CML, chronic myeloid leukemia; EPO, erythropoietin; ET, essential thrombocytosis; Hct, hematocrit; Hgb, hemoglobin; LDH, lactate dehydrogenase; MDS, myelodysplastic syndrome; PMF, primary myelofibrosis; PV, polycythemia vera; RCM, red cell mass.

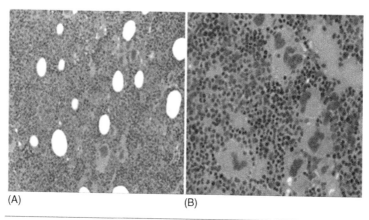

Figure 5.2 26-year-old female diagnosed with *JAK2* 617F-positive polycythemia vera presenting with Budd–Chiari syndrome. (A) Hematoxylin and eosin staining 10X microscopic BM examination demonstrating hypercellular marrow with significant erythroid hyperplasia. (B) Significant erythroid hyperplasia and small megakaryocyte clustering.

proliferation with pleomorphic, mature megakaryocytes (Figures 5.2A and B).

Diagnostic Criteria

The 2016 WHO criteria for diagnosis of MPN are summarized in Tables 5.3 and 5.4. Significant changes in PV diagnostic criteria as compared to the 2008 criteria include lowering of the Hgb threshold to 16.5 g/dL for men and 16 g/dL for women to help identify cases of masked PV in which iron deficiency or blood loss might disguise the expanded RCM. Additionally, BMB was included as a major criterion and the EPO-independent erythroid colony test was dropped. The International Working Group for Myeloproliferative Neoplasms Research and Treatment (IWG-MRT) developed its criteria to define progression from PV and ET to myelofibrosis (MF) (post-PV MF and post-ET MF), which are summarized in Table 5.5 (8).

Diagnostic Dilemmas

Despite the inclusion of BMB as a diagnostic criterion in the 2016 WHO guidelines, there is considerable variability in clinical practice. The WHO criteria allow omission of bone marrow (BM) examination in cases of sustained absolute erythrocytosis defined by Hgb >18.5 g/dL (Hct >55.5%) in men and >16.5 g/dL (Hct >49.5%) in women in the presence of *JAK2* mutation and a subnormal EPO level. In

Table 5.4 2016 World Health Organization Criteria for Overt Primary MF Diagnosis and MF Grading

WHO Criteria	Grading of Myelofibrosis
Major criteria 1. Presence of megakaryocytic proliferation and atypia, accompanied by either reticulin and/or collagen fibrosis grade 2 or 3 2. Not meeting the WHO criteria for ET, PV, BCR-ABL1[+] CML, myelodysplastic syndromes, or other myeloid neoplasms 3. Presence of JAK2, CALR, or MPL mutation or, in the absence of these mutations, presence of another clonal marker or absence of reactive myelofibrosis **Minor criteria** 1. Anemia not attributed to a comorbid condition 2. Leukocytosis >11 × 10^9/L 3. Palpable splenomegaly 4. LDH increased to above upper normal range 5. Leukoerythroblastosis Diagnosis of PMF requires all three major and at least one minor criteria	**MF-0:** Scattered linear reticulin with no intersections (crossovers) corresponding to normal BM **MF-1:** Loose network of reticulin with many intersections, especially in perivascular areas **MF-2:** Diffuse and dense increase in reticulin with extensive intersections, occasionally with focal bundles of thick fibers mostly consistent with collagen, and/or focal osteosclerosis **MF-3:** Diffuse and dense increase in reticulin with extensive intersections and coarse bundles of thick fibers consistent with collagen, usually associated with osteosclerosis

BM, bone marrow; CML, chronic myeloid leukemia; ET, essential thrombocytosis; LDH, lactate dehydrogenase; MF, myelofibrosis; PMF, primary myelofibrosis; PV, polycythemia vera; WHO, World Health Organization.

these situations, BM examination would be of prognostic significance as the presence of initial myelofibrosis (present in up to 20% of patients) predicts a more rapid progression to post-PV MF.

Prognosis and Risk Stratification

PV is a chronic disease and achieving cure is not realistic. However, more recent studies indicate median survival reaching near normal for patients diagnosed at age 60 to 65 years. The same does not hold true for patients diagnosed before the age of 40 years. One study involving 1,545 patients with WHO-defined PV identified three prognostic groups based on age, white blood cell (WBC) count, and history of prior thrombosis (Table 5.6) (9).

Table 5.5 International Working Group for Myeloproliferative Neoplasms Research and Treatment Criteria for Diagnosis of Post-Polycythemia Vera and Post-Essential Thrombocytosis Myelofibrosis

IWG-MRT Criteria	Post-PV MF	Post-ET MF
Required	1. Documentation of a previous diagnosis of PV as defined by the WHO criteria	1. Documentation of previous diagnosis of ET as defined by the WHO criteria
	2. BM fibrosis grade 2–3 (on 0–3 scale) or 3–4 (on 0–4 scale)	2. BM fibrosis grade 2–3 (on 0–3 scale) or 3–4 (on 0–4 scale)
Additional	1. Anemia or sustained loss of either phlebotomy or need for cytoreductive therapy for erythrocytosis	1. Anemia and >2 mg/mL decrease from baseline Hgb
	2. Leukoerythroblastic peripheral blood picture	2. Leukoerythroblastic peripheral blood picture
	3. Increasing splenomegaly defined as palpable spleen >5 cm from the left costal margin or newly palpable splenomegaly	3. Increasing splenomegaly defined as palpable spleen >5 cm from the left costal margin or newly palpable splenomegaly
	4. Development of one or more of three constitutional symptoms: >10% weight loss in 6 months, night sweats, unexplained fever (>37.5°C)	4. Increased LDH above the reference level
		5. Development of one or more of three constitutional symptoms: >10% weight loss in 6 months, night sweats, unexplained fever (>37.5°C)
Criteria required for diagnosis	All two required criteria and at least two additional criteria	All two required criteria and at least two additional criteria

BM, bone marrow; ET, essential thrombocytosis; Hgb, hemoglobin; IWG-MRT, International Working Group for Myeloproliferative Neoplasms Research and Treatment; LDH, lactate dehydrogenase; MF, myelofibrosis; PV, polycythemia vera; WHO, World Health Organization.

Table 5.6 Polycythemia Vera Prognostication

Age (years)	WBC (×10⁹/L)	Prior Thrombosis	Risk Group (sum)
<57: 0 point 57 to 66: 2 points >67: 5 points	<15: 0 point >15: 1 point	No: 0 point Yes: 1 point	**Low risk:** 0 point (median overall survival 27.8 years)
			Intermediate risk: 1 to 2 points (median overall survival 18.9 years)
			High risk: ≥3 points (median overall survival 10.9 years)

WBC, white blood cell.

Risk of Thrombosis

Arterial and venous thrombosis events remain the most common cause of morbidity and mortality in PV and ET. Prevention of thrombosis is, therefore, a major goal of therapy in MPN. The Italian group for PV investigation (10) reported that the risk of thrombosis increases with age from 1.8% per year for patients with PV diagnosed at <40 years of age to 5.1% per year for patients >60 years old. A prior history of arterial or venous thrombosis is the second major risk for recurrence of an arterial or a venous event, respectively (11). Age and prior thrombosis form the most common clinically used risk stratification (Table 5.7). Leukocytosis (>15 × 10⁹) has been variably reported to correlate with increased thrombosis, leukemic transformation, and post-PV thrombosis.

Risk of Acute Myeloid Leukemia (AML) Transformation

Transformation of PV or ET into AML or MF is the most common late complication of PV and ET. Direct transformation to AML without an intervening MF phase is uncommon. Table 5.8 summarizes the IWG-MRT criteria for progression to MPN-blast phase (MPN-BP). The rate of progression from PV is around 1% to 3% for patients

Table 5.7 Risk Stratification of Polycythemia Vera and Essential Thrombocytosis

Risk category	
Low	≤60 years and no history of thrombosis
High	>60 years and/or history of thrombosis

Table 5.8 International Working Group for Myeloproliferative Neoplasms Research and Treatment Criteria for Progression to Acute Myeloid Leukemia

Criteria	
Bone marrow	>20% blasts
Peripheral blood	>20% blasts with absolute blast count >1 × 10⁹/L sustained for >2 weeks

treated only with phlebotomy. This risk increases up to 15-fold for patients treated with phosphorus-32 (^{32}P), busulfan, and alkylating agent combinations previously used to treat PV (12). In the ECLAP study, the rate of AML development was 1.3% after 8.4 years of follow-up (6). Risk of leukemic transformation was not increased with hydroxyurea (HU) despite concern from earlier observational studies.

Risk of Fibrotic Transformation

Post-PV MF typically develops in late stages of disease. Disease duration >10 years is associated with 15-fold higher risk of transformation to MF compared to a shorter disease duration (0–2 years). The rate of transformation is approximately 2% to 10% in different studies. Around 25% to 30% will go on to progress to AML after transformation, and the median survival after transformation to MF is around 5 years (13). Markers of transformation include development of anemia or decreased need for phlebotomy in the absence of iron deficiency, decreasing platelet count, increasing WBC count, worsening of splenomegaly, and constitutional symptoms. Diagnostic criteria of IWG-MRT are summarized in Table 5.7.

Management
Clinical Case 5.1 (*continued*)

A diagnosis of Budd–Chiari syndrome associated with JAK2 617F mutation was considered for this patient. Transjugular intrahepatic portosystemic shunt resulted in improvement of abdominal pain and distention. Enoxaparin at 1 mg/kg was administered subcutaneously every 12 hours. After 10 days of enoxaparin, rivaroxaban was initiated at 20 mg orally daily.

Establishing the goals of treatment is important for patients and physicians who may have discrepant views. While cure might not be reasonable with current therapies, the European Leukemia Network (ELN) identified prevention of thrombosis and bleeding complications, minimizing the risk of progression to MF and AML, and symptom management as goals of treatment for PV and ET.

Lowering the Hct has long been shown to reduce thrombosis risk. Early PV trials showed mixed results with regard to targeting an Hct goal until the cytoreductive therapy in PV (CYTO-PV) trial demonstrated that Hct <45% conferred a fourfold lower risk of major thrombotic events as compared to a target of 45% to 50% (14). In CYTO-PV, achieving Hct <45% resulted in 1.1 major cardiovascular (CV) or thrombotic events per 100 patient-years compared with 4.4 events per 100 patient-years with higher targets. Therefore, Hct should be maintained at <45% in men and 42% in women.

Low-dose aspirin (81–100 mg) is the other evidence-based intervention to lower thrombotic risk. The 2004 ECLAP trial (6) demonstrated a 60% reduction in nonfatal major CV events (composite endpoint of myocardial infarction, stroke, pulmonary embolism, and major venous thrombosis) when low-dose aspirin was compared to placebo. There was no significant reduction in CV mortality or overall mortality and no significant increase in major bleeding episodes. Higher doses of aspirin or a combination of aspirin and dipyridamole increased the risk of gastrointestinal bleeding.

The role of anticoagulation is not well studied following thrombosis events in PV. It is unclear whether anticoagulation guidelines for the general population can be applied to patients with PV. Oral anticoagulants including vitamin K antagonists (VKA) are generally indicated for prevention of recurrence of venous thrombosis events. In the absence of controlled prospective trials, a retrospective analysis (15) of 206 patients with MPN-associated venous thromboembolic events (deep venous thrombosis of the legs and/or pulmonary embolism) assessed the optimal duration and efficacy of oral VKA. The study found a double risk of recurrence among patients who stopped VKA compared to those on long-term treatment, with incidence rate of 5.3 per 100 patient-years compared to 12.8 per 100 patient-years, respectively. In addition, the incidence, risk factors, and effects of various interventions on recurrence of thrombosis were retrospectively analyzed by the Italian GIMEMA group (16). Age >60 years was an independent risk factor for recurrence on multivariate analysis (5.9% vs. 8.9%). Cytoreductive therapy (majority receiving HU) nearly halved the risk of recurrence, but the effect was most pronounced for patients who had acute coronary syndrome as their index thrombotic event with 70% reduction. The effect was modest when the cerebrovascular event was the initial thrombosis site, with only 30% reduction of risk with cytoreductive therapy alone. Conversely, in this setting, antiplatelet (aspirin) treatment showed high efficacy with 67% risk reduction. In the setting of venous thromboembolism as a first event, long-term treatments with both antiplatelet and oral VKA were independently effective in preventing re-thrombosis, thus demonstrating that oral VKA are highly effective for prevention of re-thrombosis following a first MPN-related venous thromboembolism (VTE). Interestingly, aspirin was effective in prevention of venous VTE recurrences, hence warranting prospective trials to define the optimal prevention strategy. Of note, preliminary data from limited number of patients with PV and ET suggest that direct oral anticoagulants (DOACs) are safe and effective in these patients (17).

High-risk patients as defined by age >60 years and prior episodes of thrombosis should receive cytoreductive therapy in addition to phlebotomy to achieve count control. HU and interferon (IFN) are the two most frequently used agents and the choice of initial cytoreductive agent between the two depends on the patient's individual characteristics such as age or pregnancy. Chemotherapy, alkylating agents, ^{32}P, and pipobroman should generally be avoided due to their leukemogenic effect. Data for HU are derived from retrospective and single-arm studies. An uncontrolled PVSG study (18) demonstrated lower incidence of thrombosis with HU compared to historical controls treated with phlebotomy alone (6.6% vs. 14% at 2 years) and lower rates of leukemic transformation when compared to historical patients treated with chlorambucil and ^{32}P (5.9% vs. 10.6% and 8.3%, respectively). Whether HU is leukemogenic or not has long been debated, but most data do not implicate HU in increasing leukemia (1%–17% in different studies with different follow-up periods). However, many experts recommend IFN treatment as the initial therapy instead of HU, an off-label use, for younger patients (<40 years) who are expected to survive for longer periods. The recommended starting dose of HU is 500 mg BID (around 15 mg/kg/d). Dosage adjustments are not recommended more frequently than once weekly and should be done for renal but not for hepatic impairment. Adverse effects with HU include cytopenias, mucosal and cutaneous toxicities including ulcers, gastrointestinal toxicity, non-melanoma skin cancers, fever, interstitial pneumonitis, and teratogenic potential.

IFN is a biologic modifier that retains antiangiogenic, antiproliferative, proapoptotic, and immunomodulatory properties. Pegylated IFN alfa-2 (peg-IFN) has a more favorable toxicity profile than the shorter acting formula and is administered once weekly. Peg-IFN achieves blood count control and reduction in spleen size and pruritus. Peg-IFN has the potential to induce molecular remissions, an advantage over HU; however, the influence on thrombotic outcomes and survival is unclear. A phase 2 trial of peg-IFN (19) in patients with PV or ET showed sustained hematologic and molecular responses in 79% and 63% of patients, respectively. Rates of thrombotic events (10%), MF (7%), and AML (1.2%) were similar to historical matched cohorts. HU remains the preferred agent by

Table 5.9 European Leukemia Network Criteria for Hydroxyurea Resistance/Intolerance

ELN Consensus Criteria for Resistance and Intolerance to HU

1. Need for phlebotomy to keep Hct <45% after 3 months of at least 2 g/d of HU *OR*

2. Uncontrolled myeloproliferation, i.e., platelets >400 × 10^9/L and WBC >10 × 10^9/L after 3 months of at least 2 g/d of HU *OR*

3. Failure to reduce massive splenomegaly (i.e., extending .10 cm from the left costal margin) by 50% as measured by palpation *OR* failure to completely relieve symptoms related to splenomegaly, after 3 months of at least 2 g/d of HU *OR*

4. Absolute neutrophil count <1.0 × 10^9/L or platelets <100 × 100^9/L or hemoglobin <10 g/dL at the lowest dose of HU required to achieve a complete or partial clinicohematologic response *OR*

5. Presence of leg ulcers or other unacceptable HU-related nonhematologic toxicities such as mucocutaneous manifestations, gastrointestinal symptoms, pneumonitis, or fever at any dose of HU

ELN, European Leukemia Network; Hct, hematocrit; HU, hydroxyurea.

most U.S. physicians for first-line cytoreduction, with peg-IFN being reserved for young and pregnant patients. Final analysis of phase 3 trials comparing the two medications may warrant a change in practice. Peg-IFN alfa-2a is given at 45 mcg/wk subcutaneously as the starting dose and is increased to maximum of 180 mcg/wk as tolerated. Common side effects that may lead to treatment discontinuation include flu-like symptoms, fever, mood changes, nausea, vomiting, and malaise.

Approximately 10% of patients develop HU intolerance and/or resistance (Table 5.9). ELN has developed criteria to define these circumstances, which require shifting to second-line therapies. However, it is to be noted that occasional phlebotomies while on optimal HU doses are not associated with adverse outcomes and do not necessarily require change of therapy.

Second-line options include HU or IFN if the other agent was used as the first-line option. Busulfan is an alkylating agent acceptable as a second-line agent for patients not responding to or tolerating HU or IFN; however, it should be reserved for older individuals (>60 years) since its long-term use has been linked to leukemia transformation and long-term cytopenias, especially when used in combination with other agents.

The *JAK1/2* inhibitor ruxolitinib is frequently used in the setting of refractoriness or intolerance to HU. The RESPONSE and RESPONSE-2 trials compared ruxolitinib to best available therapy

(BAT). Ruxolitinib was superior in terms of Hct control after 32 weeks (21% vs. 1%) (20). Ruxolitinib also induced complete hematologic responses (control of Hct, platelets, and WBC) in 24% of patients versus 9% with BAT, induced at least a 35% spleen reduction in 38% versus 0.9% with BAT, and caused significant reduction in symptom burden in 49% versus 5% with BAT. Grade 3 and 4 anemia and thrombocytopenia were uncommon with ruxolitinib, occurring in 2% and 5%, respectively. However, ruxolitinib treatment was associated with 6% herpes zoster infection and an increased incidence of non-melanoma skin cancers. Notably, ruxolitinib did not modify the natural course of the disease in regard to reducing the risk for fibrotic or leukemia transformation nor did it induce molecular remissions.

Key Points

- MPNs are clonal BM stem cell disorders characterized by abnormal proliferation of platelets, RBCs, WBCs, and/or marrow fibrosis.
- Constitutional JAK-STAT pathway activation is the hallmark feature of these disorders, and their diagnosis is guided by the 2016 WHO criteria.
- Thrombosis and bleeding are the major complications of PV; progression to MF and leukemia are less common late complications.
- Hct should be maintained below 45% in PV with phlebotomy ± cytoreductive therapy.
- High-risk features include age >60 years and history of thrombosis.
- Generally, low-dose aspirin is the mainstay treatment for thrombosis prevention in low-risk patients, while high-risk patients require additional cytoreductive therapy with HU or IFN.

ESSENTIAL THROMBOCYTOSIS

Clinical Case 5.2

A 40-year-old female was seen in clinic with headaches and platelet count of 1,300,000/µL. She had a 10-year history of uncontrolled hypertension. Her Hgb was 13 g/dL and WBC count was 7,600/µL. Her BCR-ABL RT PCR and JAK 617F mutation were negative. BM showed megakaryocytic hyperplasia. Her CALR and MPL mutations were negative. Her brain MRI showed chronic white matter changes.

Introduction

ET has a prevalence similar to PV (38–57 per 100,000) with only a slightly lower incidence (incidence rate of 9.6 per million/year). However, it has a female to male predominance of 1.5- to 2-fold.

ET is most frequently diagnosed when elevated platelets are found on routine blood count check. Fatigue is the most common symptom (72%) (5). The high platelet count leads to vasomotor symptoms such as dizziness, headaches, erythromelalgia, and acral paresthesia. Physical examination shows variably elevated blood pressure and mild splenomegaly (<5 cm increase above normal) in 40% of patients.

The prevalence of thrombosis at the time of diagnosis of ET is 10% to 29%. Bleeding in ET especially occurs in cases of extreme thrombocytosis at a platelet count of $>1.5 \times 10^6/\mu L$ and is associated with acquired von Willebrand factor (VWF) deficiency.

Diagnosis

Laboratory Findings and Differential Diagnosis

CBC in ET shows thrombocytosis (platelets $>450,000/\mu L$) typically in the absence of polycythemia. Moderate leukocytosis may be seen in 50% of cases. Peripheral blood smear shows large or giant platelets and occasional circulating megakaryocyte fragments. Howell–Jolly bodies on peripheral smear indicate post-splenectomy state, a common cause of secondary thrombocytosis. Other causes of secondary thrombocytosis are summarized in Table 5.10.

BM Examination

BMB evaluation in ET typically shows only megakaryocytic proliferation with an increased number of mature megakaryocytes with hyperlobated nuclei (Figure 5.3), absence of trilineage hyperplasia or dysplasia, and minor (grade 1) increase in reticulin fibrosis.

Table 5.10 Secondary Causes of Thrombocytosis

Nonmalignant Hematologic Conditions	Malignant Conditions	Acute and Chronic Inflammatory Diseases	Infections	Tissue Damage	Other Causes
Iron deficiency anemia	Lymphoma	Rheumatologic diseases	Tuberculosis	Trauma	Asplenia
Acute hemorrhage	Metastatic carcinoma	Celiac disease	Chronic infections	Burns	Rebound thrombocytopenia
		Inflammatory bowel disease	Acute bacterial and viral infections	Acute pancreatitis	Reaction to medications
			Post-surgical period		

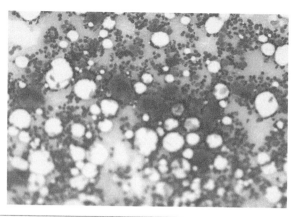

Figure 5.3 Hematoxylin and eosin stain from bone marrow biopsy from a patient with ET showing mature megakaryocytic hyperplasia.

ET, essential thrombocytosis.

Differentiating ET from early or prefibrotic myelofibrosis may be difficult. BMB in MF shows megakaryocytic proliferation and atypia, accompanied by increased age-adjusted BM cellularity, granulocytic proliferation, and often decreased erythropoiesis, in the absence of reticulin fibrosis above grade 1 (Table 5.3).

Diagnostic Criteria

The 2016 WHO criteria are used for ET diagnosis. Some significant updates in these criteria are the inclusion of *CALR* mutation as part of the major criteria for diagnosis and the distinction of pre-PMF as a separate entity from ET and overt PMF. ET and pre-PMF are distinguished by morphologic assessment of BM megakaryocytes and the overall morphology, which displays abnormal maturation in cases of pre-PMF, accompanied by increased cellularity and leukocytes and often decreased erythrocytosis, as opposed to large mature megakaryocytes in ET accompanied by normal age-adjusted cellularity. This distinction is of prognostic significance, as demonstrated in a series of 278 patients (21) showing a hazard ratio for death of 2.7 for pre-PMF as compared to ET.

Diagnostic Dilemmas

The distinction between ET and prefibrotic stage of PMF represents a major challenge for pathologists and requires careful examination of BM biopsy. As stated earlier, BMB in ET should only show increased numbers of mature megakaryocytes with no or minor grade (grade 1) fibrosis.

Another dilemma that clinicians encounter is the distinction between *JAK2*-positive cases of ET and "masked PV." The latter is characterized by lower Hgb levels and higher platelet count. In addition, ferritin levels are significantly lower in masked PV than ET. The lowered Hgb threshold in the 2016 WHO criteria combined with thorough BM examination should help address this distinction.

Prognosis and Risk Stratification
The International Prognostic Score of Thrombosis for Essential Thrombocythemia (IPSET) includes three risk factors: age, WBC count, and history of prior thrombosis (Table 5.11).

Risk of Thrombosis
The traditional two-tiered risk stratification for thrombosis classifies patients as high risk based on the presence of either age >60 years or prior history of thrombosis. *CALR* mutation was found to be associated with fewer thrombotic events as compared with *JAK2* mutation. The IPSET score was revised to include the presence of *JAK2* mutation as a variable, thus forming a four-category risk score (Table 5.12) (22). CV risk factors (diabetes, hypertension, and smoking) are also the risk factors of thrombosis, and some experts consider ET patients having one or more of these risk factors to be at intermediate risk of thrombosis even if younger than 60 years with no prior history of thrombosis.

Risk of AML Transformation
The cumulative incidence of AML transformation is 2.1% to 3.8% in different studies and increases with age. Table 5.13 summarizes the IWG-MRT criteria for progression to MPN-BP.

Table 5.11 International Prognostic Score of Thrombosis for Essential Thrombocythemia Prognosis Model

Age (years)	WBC (×10⁹/L)	Prior Thrombosis	Risk Group (sum)
<60: 1 point >60: 2 points	<11: 0 point >11: 1 point	No: 0 point Yes: 1 point	**Low risk**: 0 point (median overall survival not reached)
			Intermediate risk: 1–2 points (median overall survival 24.5 years)
			High risk: 3–4 points (median overall survival 13.8 years)

Table 5.12 Revised International Prognostic Score of Thrombosis for Essential Thrombocythemia Risk Stratification of Essential Thrombocythemia

Risk Category	
Very low	No thrombosis, age <60 years, and *JAK2* unmutated
Low	No thrombosis, age <60 years, and *JAK2* mutated
Intermediate	No thrombosis, age >60 years, and *JAK2* unmutated
High	Thrombosis history or age >60 years, and *JAK2* mutated

Risk of Fibrotic Transformation

Features of transformation into PMF in ET are similar to those in PV, including development of anemia, decreasing platelet count, increasing WBC count, worsening of splenomegaly, and constitutional symptoms. The probability for MF increases with time and is 8% to 9% at 15 years. Caution must be exercised with careful examination of marrow at diagnosis for proper identification of early/prefibrotic PMF cases that have higher risk to progress to PMF and a shorter overall survival (21).

Management

Very Low-Risk Patients

Contrary to PV in which ECLAP established the benefit of low-dose daily aspirin, no prospective randomized trial of aspirin in ET has been conducted, and its use is extrapolated from the ECLAP trial and expert recommendations. The use of aspirin should not be automatic for the very low-risk population in the absence of

Table 5.13 Secondary Causes of Myelofibrosis

Myeloid Disorders	Malignant Disorders	Infections	Autoimmune Disorders
Acute megakaryoblastic leukemia	Hodgkin and non-Hodgkin lymphoma	Tuberculosis	Systemic lupus erythematosis
Myelodysplasia with fibrosis	Hairy cell leukemia	Fungal infections	Sjogren's syndrome
Chronic myelomonocytic leukemia	Metastatic carcinoma		Primary autoimmune myelofibrosis
Systemic mastocytosis	Plasma cell dyscrasias		

CV risk factors (young patients with no history of thrombosis and without *JAK2/MPL* mutations). This population may display extreme thrombocytosis and aspirin may increase the risk of bleeding.

Very low-risk patients should be observed without treatment or offered a daily low-dose aspirin in the presence of CV risk factors and absence of extreme thrombocytosis or contraindications to antiplatelet therapy.

Low-Risk Patients

Patients with *JAK2* mutations and CV risk factors seem to derive benefit from low-dose aspirin. Hence, for other risk groups, a daily low-dose aspirin is generally prescribed.

Intermediate Risk Patients

Intermediate risk is defined by age >60 years, but no *JAK2/MPL* mutations and no history of thrombosis. Age alone would have merited a classification as high risk; however, in the revised IPSET, the annual risk of thrombosis in these patients was 1.44% compared to 4.17% in the presence of *JAK2* mutation or CV risk factor, and this seems to be similar to that in low-risk patients. Management in these cases does not necessarily include cytoreductive therapy, but it should be considered in the presence of CV risk factors.

High-Risk Patients

High-risk ET patients, as in PV, require cytoreductive treatment. The evidence dates back to the Bergamo trial (23) in which 114 high-risk ET patients were randomized to receive HU to maintain platelets at <600 × 10^9/L versus no cytoreductive therapy. HU resulted in an absolute 20.4% reduction in thrombotic events.

Second-line agents include peg-IFN alfa-2a, anagrelide, and less commonly busulfan. Peg-IFN is effective in inducing clinical responses as detailed earlier; in addition, it can induce molecular responses in around 10% to 20% in a subset of patients, particularly with *CALR* mutations.

Anagrelide was compared to HU in the ANAHYDRET trial. This trial of high-risk ET patients showed that anagrelide was non-inferior to HU in reducing major arterial and venous thrombosis and had similar severe bleeding events (24). However, patients taking anagrelide had higher number of cardiac events (hypertension, tachycardia) and no data were provided on the rates of progression to myelofibrosis or leukemia. The initial dose of anagrelide is 0.5 mg administered two to four times daily, titrated to optimize platelet count to a maximum of 1 to 4 mg/d. The most common side effects are headaches, tachycardia, and fluid retention.

Ruxolitinib was evaluated in a phase 2 trial of 110 patients resistant and/or intolerant to HU versus BAT (HU continuation, anagrelide, or IFN) (25). There was no difference in thrombohemorrhagic events or transformation at 1 year. Ruxolitinib was associated with more grade 3 and 4 anemia and thrombocytopenia and grade 3 infections. Ruxolitinib was superior in some aspects of symptom control, including pruritus.

The considerations for anticoagulation treatment in patients with history of thrombosis are similar to those in patients with PV.

Special Situations

Extreme Thrombocytosis

Extreme thrombocytosis, defined by platelet count >1,000 × 10^9/L, is not necessarily an indication for cytoreductive therapy in otherwise asymptomatic patients. However, extreme thrombocytosis is associated with acquired VWF deficiency and an increased risk of bleeding, especially when aspirin is given. Although different opinions exist, a general consensus is to screen for VWF deficiency and avoid aspirin, especially if the ristocetin cofactor level is <30%. Cytoreductive therapy is also suggested in this setting and warranted if a rapid decline in platelet count is needed, such as in situations like ongoing bleeding, recent thrombosis, or severe neurologic symptoms due to microvascular disturbances.

Lifestyle and CV Risk Factors

Generic CV risk factors (hypertension, smoking, obesity, diabetes) should be aggressively managed. Of special note, smoking and obesity in ET were shown to be thrombogenic and smoking is stated to antagonize aspirin activity; therefore, smoking cessation should be emphasized.

Role of Plateletpheresis

In selected cases, plateletpheresis can be used for rapid reduction of platelet counts in conjunction with cytoreductive therapy. These cases include severe or life-threatening organ dysfunction, such as digital limb ischemia, severe stroke, massive pulmonary embolus, or ongoing bleeding due to acquired VWF deficiency.

Pregnant Patients

Very low- or low-risk young pregnant patients can be given low-dose aspirin once daily. High-risk patients with history of thrombosis should receive both aspirin and cytoreductive therapy with IFN-alpha, which has been shown to be safe during pregnancy and may lower the rates of miscarriages in ET. The role of heparin products is not established.

Key Points

- ET has slightly lower incidence than PV and can present with incidental findings of high platelets, vasomotor symptoms, or a thrombotic event.
- Extreme thrombocytosis (platelets >1,000 × 10^9/L) increases the risk of bleeding and predisposes to acquired VWF deficiency.
- Cytoreductive therapy is generally required for high-risk patients.

PRIMARY MYELOFIBROSIS

Clinical Case 5.3

A 46-year-old man presented to emergency room with fatigue, decreased appetite, and weight loss of a few months duration. His physical exam showed splenomegaly 7 cm below the costal margin, and his CBC showed pancytopenia with WBC 2,900/μL, Hgb 6.6 g/dL, and platelet count 99,000/μL. BMB showed a cellular marrow with trilineage hematopoiesis, mild megakaryocytic dyspoeisis, and increased reticulin fibrosis (grade 2 or 3). JAK2 mutation was negative. He received multiple supportive transfusions and developed secondary iron overload. He was not interested in pursuing allogeneic hematopoietic stem cell transplantation (HSCT). Ruxolitinib was initiated with Hgb improvement; he became transfusion independent and continues to receive iron chelation therapy.

Introduction

PMF is less common than ET and PV with an annual incidence of 0.2 to 0.5 cases per 100,000 persons per year and prevalence of 4 to 6 per 100,000 persons. Median age is 65 years, and 70% of patients are diagnosed after the age of 60 years.

Constitutional symptoms (fever, weight loss, night sweats) are more common in PMF than PV and ET, and physical exam may reveal hepatosplenomegaly or signs of extramedullary hematopoiesis.

Diagnosis

Laboratory Findings and Differential Diagnosis

The major hematologic finding in myelofibrosis is anemia. Progression from polycythemia to anemia in PV marks fibrotic progression. Approximately 50% to 70% of MF patients have anemia at presentation and a quarter have Hgb <8 g/dL. Anemia is caused by hematologic failure, ineffective erythropoiesis, portal hypertension with bleeding, and hypersplenism. Thrombocytopenia develops in around 40% of PMF cases; however, leukocytosis is more common than leukopenia and is seen in half of the cases. Serum lactate dehydrogenase (LDH) and uric acid are commonly elevated.

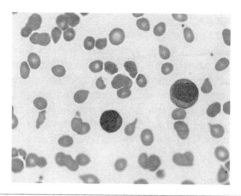

Figure 5.4 Primary myelofibrosis smear showing teardrops and immature myeloid cells.

Peripheral blood smear may show a leukoerythroblastic picture of immature myeloid precursors, teardrops, nucleated RBCs, and large platelets (Figure 5.4). Diagnosis of PMF can be challenging, and it is important to consider secondary causes of bone marrow fibrosis when dealing with ambiguous cases. Table 5.13 summarizes the secondary causes of myelofibrosis.

BMB Findings

BM aspiration in PMF may be hindered by advanced fibrosis resulting in a "dry tap." The biopsy will show megakaryocytic proliferation and atypia with reticulin and collagen fibrosis grade 2 or 3 (Figure 5.5). Osteosclerosis may develop in some cases.

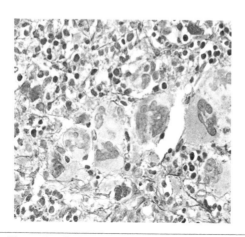

Figure 5.5 Reticulin stain demonstrating fibrosis.

Diagnostic Criteria

The 2016 WHO criteria for PMF diagnosis requires the presence of high-grade (grades 2 and 3) fibrosis on BMB and the presence of one of three MPN common mutations (*JAK2, CALR, MPL*) or other clonal mutations, as well as the absence of causes of reactive myelofibrosis. In addition, patients should have at least one of the following minor criteria: anemia, leukocytosis, palpable splenomegaly, elevated LDH, or leukoerythroblastosis (Table 5.4). The IWG-MRT criteria for post-PV and post-ET MF are summarized in Table 5.5.

Diagnostic Dilemmas

Distinguishing prefibrotic PMF from ET is sometimes difficult. In addition, it is important to keep PMF in the differential diagnosis of patients with pancytopenia or in patients with PV who develop anemia. Establishing clonality through next-generation sequencing to detect myeloid mutations can help support the diagnosis in triple-negative cases when PMF is suspected.

Prognosis and Risk Stratification

The three common risk prognostication models used for PMF are the International Prognostic Scoring System (IPSS), Dynamic International Prognostic Scoring System (DIPSS), and DIPSS-plus (Table 5.14). IPSS was designed to be used at diagnosis, while DIPSS and DIPSS-plus (if the karyotype is available) can be used at any point during the disease course. Studies on the prognostic relevance of specific mutations in PMF showed the *CALR* mutation was associated with the longest survival (median overall survival 17.7 years) as compared to *JAK2* mutation, *MPL* mutations, and "triple-negative" cases that were associated with the shortest survival (median overall survival 2.3 years) (26). *ASXL1*, *TET2*, *EZH2*, *SRSF2*, *IDH1/2*, and *TP53* mutations are termed high molecular risk mutations and predict a worse overall survival and higher risk of leukemic transformation. This molecular risk stratification, in addition to DIPSS, helps in decision-making and selection of patients for stem cell transplantation as discussed in the "Management" section. More sophisticated risk assessment tools that take into consideration the mutation profile include the MIPSS70 (Mutation-Enhanced IPSS for patients with PMF ≤70 years old) and MIPSS70-plus which adds unfavorable karyotype into risk stratification.

Risk of AML Transformation

PMF is characterized by higher propensity for leukemic transformation. Although most patients with PMF die while they are in MF

Table 5.14 Primary Myelofibrosis Prognostication

IPSS Risk Factor	DIPSS Risk Factor	DIPSS-Plus Risk Factor
Age >65 years: 1 point	Age >65 years: 1 point	DIPSS low: 0 point
Constitutional symptoms: 1 point	Constitutional symptoms: 1 point	DIPSS int-1: 1 point
Hgb <10 g/dL: 1 point	Hgb <10 g/dL: 2 points	DIPSS int-2: 2 points
WBC >25 × 10^9/L: 1 point	WBC >25 × 10^9/L: 1 point	DIPSS high: 3 points
Blood blasts >1%: 1 point	Blood blasts >1%: 1 point	RBC transfusion dependence: 1 point
		Thrombocytopenia (<100 × 10^9/L): 1 point
		Unfavorable karyotype: 1 point
Risk group	**Risk group**	**Risk group**
Low: 0 point (MOS 11.3 years)	**Low**: 0 point (MOS not reached)	**Low**: 0 point (MOS 15.4 years)
Intermediate-1: 1 point (OS 7.9 years)	**Intermediate-1**: 1 to 2 points (OS 14.4 years)	**Intermediate-1**: 1 point (OS 6.5 years)
Intermediate-2: 2 points (MOS 4.4 years)	**Intermediate-2**: 3 to 4 points (MOS 4 years)	**Intermediate-2**: 2 to 3 points (MOS 2.9 years)
High: >=3 points (MOS 2.3 years)	**High**: 5 to 6 points (MOS 1.5 years)	**High**: 4 to 6 points (MOS 1.3 years)

DIPSS, Dynamic International Prognostic Scoring System; IPSS, International Prognostic Scoring System; MOS, median overall survival; OS, overall survival.

phase, AML is the cause of death in 5% to 30% of patients. Anemia, RBC transfusion dependency, WBC >30 × 10^9/L, blast count >10%, platelet count <50 × 10^9/L, select "high-risk" cytogenetic abnormalities, and low *JAK2* allele burden are all the reported risk factors for shorter blast phase (BP)-free survival. Although DIPSS was designed to predict survival at any point of time in PMF patients, a study performed on behalf of the IWG-MRT (27) demonstrated that DIPSS could also predict BP transformation. In fact, patients with intermediate-2 DIPSS had 2.6 per 100 patient-years risk of transformation and patients with high-risk DIPSS had 8.6 per 100 patient-years risk. These numbers represented 7.8- and 24.9-fold higher risk, respectively, when compared with low-risk patients.

Management

Allogeneic HSCT is currently the only curative option for PMF. However, it comes at the cost of high transplant-related mortality (TRM) and morbidity. Selection for transplant should, therefore, be selective and justified. DIPSS score (and DIPSS-plus when the karyotype is available) and molecular stratification help to make these decisions.

Low- and Intermediate-1–Risk Patients

In the absence of high-risk molecular mutations, asymptomatic patients do not require any treatment. Surveillance is appropriate for these patients with history and physical examinations, symptom assessment, and laboratory monitoring. The goal of therapy in the presence of symptoms is symptom control and improved quality of life. Potential indications for therapy include symptomatic anemia, splenomegaly, severe constitutional symptoms, and extramedullary hematopoiesis. Treatment for MF-related anemia includes erythropoietin stimulating agents (ESA), androgens (e.g., danazol), steroids (e.g., prednisone), and immunomodulatory agents (IMiDS; lenalidomide ± prednisone or thalidomide ± prednisone), which induce various response rates, but generally 20% to 30% of patients would have response. IMiDS can also produce response in platelet counts in the setting of thrombocytopenia in approximately 30% of patients. Treatment for MF-induced splenomegaly includes HU as the preferred agent which can induce spleen size reduction by half in approximately 40% of patients, but its use requires careful monitoring for development of cytopenias. Splenectomy may be considered in select patients with mechanical discomfort along with recurrent infarcts, refractory, transfusion-dependent anemia, refractory thrombocytopenia, or portal hypertension. Splenic irradiation could also be considered in poor surgical candidates, but it comes at the risk of severe pancytopenia, and the responses are usually transient. Radiation therapy is successful in controlling symptoms related to extramedullary hematopoiesis, including severe extremity bone pain, paraspinal sites, MF-related pulmonary hypertension and ascites, and symptomatic hepatomegaly.

The presence of high-risk mutations in low- and intermediate-1–risk group presents a challenging management decision. They confer a worse prognosis independent of DIPSS with a shortened expected survival (e.g., 2.3 years in *ASXL-1* mutated/*CALR* wild type); thus, early search for a suitable donor for HSCT is appropriate.

Intermediate-2– and High-Risk Patients

Allogeneic HSCT is indicated for suitable patients, as it is the only curative treatment. Intermediate-2– and high-risk patients derive

Table 5.15 Investigational Therapy for Primary Myelofibrosis

JAK2 inhibitors	Memolitinib, pacritinib
Telomerase inhibitor	Imetelstat
HDAC inhibitor	Panobinostat
PI3K/mTOR inhibitor	BEZ235
TGF-beta monoclonal antibody	Fresolimumab
Activin receptor antagonist	Luspatercept
Antifibrosis agent	PRM-151
Hypomethylating agents	Azacitidine, decitabine

HDAC, Histone deacetylase; mTOR, Mammalian Target of Rapamycin; TGF, Tumor growth factor beta.

survival benefit when compared to low- and intermediate-1–risk groups and the recommendation for HSCT is supported by the ELN.

The use of reduced intensity conditioning (RIC) has allowed a wider application of HSCT to older age groups. In one large analysis by the Center for International Bone Marrow Transplant Research (CIBMTR) involving 289 patients, long-term relapse-free survival was achieved in about one third of patients with a 100-day TRM of 18% in HLA-matched siblings and 35% in transplants from unrelated donors (28).

For patients who are not candidates for HSCT, ruxolitinib is indicated for relief of symptoms and reduction of spleen size and associated symptoms as established by COMFORT-1 and COMFORT-2 trials (29,30). The two trials demonstrated that ruxolitinib is superior to placebo or BAT, inducing >35% spleen size reduction and improvement in control of symptoms. Common side effects include anemia and thrombocytopenia in a third of patients and increased risk of opportunistic infections. Ruxolitinib should not be stopped abruptly as this can cause a "withdrawal syndrome" characterized by rapid relapse of symptoms, worsening of splenomegaly, and cytopenias. Ruxolitinib does not seem to modify the natural course of PMF, and although some studies showed survival benefit, the crossover nature of the COMFORT trials and use of historical controls for comparison may have confounded these results.

Investigational therapies for PMF are presented in Table 5.15.

Key Points

• PMF risk stratification is guided by DIPSS and DIPSS-plus scores, as well as by the presence of high molecular risk mutations.

- Low- and intermediate-1–risk patients are usually managed with surveillance and symptomatic treatment for anemia, splenomegaly, and constitutional symptoms.
- Allogenic HSCT is the only curative treatment for eligible high- and intermediate-2–risk patients.
- *JAK1/2* inhibitor ruxolitinib is beneficial for non–transplant-eligible patients.

REFERENCES

1. Scott LM, Tong W, Levine RL, et al. JAK2 exon 12 mutations in polycythemia vera and idiopathic erythrocytosis. *N Engl J Med.* 2007;356(5):459–468. doi:10.1056/NEJMoa065202

2. Chachoua I, Pecquet C, El-Khoury M, et al. Thrombopoietin receptor activation by myeloproliferative neoplasm associated calreticulin mutants. *Blood.* 2016;127(10):1325–1335. doi:10.1182/blood-2015-11-681932

3. Srour SA, Devesa SS, Morton LM, et al. Incidence and patient survival of myeloproliferative neoplasms and myelodysplastic/myeloproliferative neoplasms in the United States, 2001-12. *Br J Haematol.* 2016;174(3):382–396. doi:10.1111/bjh.14061

4. Mehta J, Wang H, Iqbal SU, Mesa R. Epidemiology of myeloproliferative neoplasms in the United States. *Leuk Lymphoma.* 2014;55:595–600. doi:10.3109/10428194.2013.813500

5. Mesa RA, Niblack J, Wadleigh M, et al. The burden of fatigue and quality of life in myeloproliferative disorders (MPDs): an international Internet-based survey of 1179 MPD patients. *Cancer.* 2007;109:68–76. doi:10.1002/cncr.22365

6. Landolfi R, Marchioli R, Kutti J, et al. Efficacy and safety of low-dose aspirin in polycythemia vera. *N Engl J Med.* 2004;350(2):114–124. doi:10.1056/NEJMoa035572

7. Arber DA, Orazi A, Hasserjian R, et al. The 2016 revision to the World Health Organization classification of myeloid neoplasms and acute leukemia. *Blood.* 2016;127(20):2391–2405. doi:10.1182/blood-2016-03-643544

8. Barosi G, Mesa RA, Thiele J, et al. Proposed criteria for the diagnosis of post-polycythemia vera and post-essential thrombocythemia myelofibrosis: a consensus statement from the International Working Group for Myelofibrosis Research and Treatment. *Leukemia.* 2008;22(2):437–438. doi:10.1038/sj.leu.2404914

9. Tefferi A, Rumi E, Finazzi G, et al. Survival and prognosis among 1545 patients with contemporary polycythemia vera: an international study. *Leukemia.* 2013;27(9):1874–1881. doi:10.1038/leu.2013.163

10. Gruppo Italiano Studio Policitemia. Polycythemia vera: The natural history of 1213 patients followed for 20 years. *Ann Intern Med.* 1995;123:656–664. doi:10.7326/0003-4819-123-9-199511010-00003

11. Barbui T, Carobbio A, Rumi E, et al. In contemporary patients with polycythemia vera, rates of thrombosis and risk factors delineate a new clinical epidemiology. *Blood.* 2014;124:3021–3023. doi:10.1182/blood-2014-07-591610

12. Kiladjian JJ, Gardin C, Renoux M, et al. Long-term outcomes of polycythemia vera patients treated with pipobroman as initial therapy. *Hematol J.* 2003;4(3):198–207. doi:10.1182/blood-2014-07-591610

13. Cerquozzi S, Tefferi A. Blast transformation and fibrotic progression in polycythemia vera and essential thrombocythemia: a literature review of incidence and risk factors. *Blood Cancer J.* 2015;5(11):e366. doi:10.1038/bcj.2015.95

14. Marchioli R, Vannucchi AM, Barbui T. Treatment target in polycythemia vera. *N Engl J Med.* 2013;368(16):1556. doi:10.1056/NEJMc1301262

15. De Stefano V, Ruggeri M, Cervantes F, et al. High rate of recurrent venous thromboembolism in patients with myeloproliferative neoplasms and effect of prophylaxis with vitamin K antagonists. *Leukemia.* 2016;30:2032–2038. doi:10.1038/leu.2016.85

16. De Stefano V, Za T, Rossi E, et al. GIMEMA CMD-Working Party. Recurrent thrombosis in patients with polycythemia vera and essential thrombocythemia: incidence, risk factors, and effect of treatments. *Haematologica.* 2008;93:372–380. doi:10.3324/haematol.12053

17. Ianotto JC, Couturier MA, Galinat H, et al. Administration of direct oral anticoagulants in patients with myeloproliferative neoplasms. *Int J Hematol.* 2017;106:517–521. doi:10.1007/s12185-017-2282-5

18. Fruchtman SM, Mack K, Kaplan ME, et al. From efficacy to safety: a Polycythemia Vera Study group report on hydroxyurea in patients with polycythemia vera. *Semin Hematol.* 1997;34(1):17–23.

19. Masarova L, Patel KP, Newberry KJ, et al. Pegylated interferon alfa-2a in patients with essential thrombocythaemia or polycythaemia vera: a post-hoc, median 83 month follow-up of an open-label, phase 2 trial. *Lancet Haematol.* 2017;4(4):e165–e175. doi:10.1016/S2352-3026(17)30030-3

20. Vannucchi AM, Kiladjian JJ, Griesshammer M, et al. Ruxolitinib versus standard therapy for the treatment of polycythemia vera. *N Engl J Med*. 2015;372(5):426–435. doi:10.1056/NEJMoa1409002

21. Guglielmelli P, Pacilli A, Rotunno G, et al. Presentation and outcome of patients with 2016 WHO diagnosis of prefibrotic and overt primary myelofibrosis. *Blood*. 2017;129(24):3227–3236. doi:10.1182/blood-2017-01-761999

22. Barbui T, Vannucchi AM, Buxhofer-Ausch V, et al. Practice-relevant revision of IPSET-thrombosis based on 1019 patients with WHO-defined essential thrombocythemia. *Blood Cancer J*. 2015;5:e369. doi:10.1038/bcj.2015.94

23. Cortelazzo S, Finazzi G, Ruggeri M, et al. Hydroxyurea for patients with essential thrombocytosis and a high risk of thrombosis. *N Engl J Med*. 1995;322(17):1132–1136. doi:10.1056/NEJM199504273321704

24. Gisslinger H, Gotic M, Holowiecki J, et al. Anagrelide compared with hydroxyurea in WHO-classified essential thrombocythemia: the ANAHYDRET Study, a randomized controlled trial. *Blood*. 2013;121(10):1720–1728. doi:10.1182/blood-2012-07-443770

25. Harrison CN, Mead AJ, Panchal A, et al. Ruxolitinib vs best available therapy for ET intolerant or resistant to hydroxycarbamide. *Blood*. 2017;130(17):1889–1897. doi:10.1182/blood-2017-05-785790

26. Rumi E, Pietra D, Ferretti V, et al. JAK2 or CALR mutation status defines subtypes of essential thrombocythemia with substantially different clinical course and outcomes. *Blood*. 2014;123(10):1544–1551. doi:10.1182/blood-2013-11-539098

27. Passamonti F, Cervantes F, Vannucchi AM, et al. Dynamic International Prognostic Scoring System (DIPSS) predicts progression to acute myeloid leukemia in primary myelofibrosis. *Blood*. 2010;116(15):2857–2858. doi:10.1182/blood-2010-06-293415

28. Ballen KK, Shrestha S, Sobocinski KA, et al. Outcome of transplantation for myelofibrosis. *Biol Blood Marrow Transplant*. 2010;16(3):358–367. doi:10.1016/j.bbmt.2009.10.025

29. Verstovsek S, Mesa RA, Gotlib J, et al. A double-blind, placebo-controlled trial of ruxolitinib for myelofibrosis. *N Engl J Med*. 2012;366(9):799–807. doi:10.1056/NEJMoa1110557

30. Harrison C, Kiladjian JJ, Al-Ali HK, et al. JAK inhibition with ruxolitinib versus best available therapy for myelofibrosis. *N Engl J Med*. 2012;366(9):787–798. doi:10.1056/NEJMoa1110556

6 Hypoproliferative Anemia

Patrick E. Prath and Courtney Miller-Chism

INTRODUCTION

Bone marrow stem cells proliferate and differentiate along a committed erythroid cell lineage that ends with expulsion of the nucleus to create mature erythrocytes. Mature red blood cells (RBCs) survive for up to 120 days in circulation prior to removal by the splenic macrophages and other cells in the system. At steady state, the rates of production and destruction are equivalent. This process is tightly controlled by erythropoietin (EPO), a hormone produced primarily in the periglomerular cells of the kidneys in a tightly regulated fashion and, to a lesser extent, in the liver cells in a constitutive fashion. Tight regulation in the kidneys is mediated by oxygen-sensing cells. RBC mass changes during an individual's life span. Females reach their adult level of hemoglobin (Hgb) around puberty, compared to age 18 in males. Higher Hgb in males is a result of androgens and a difference of 1 to 2 g/dL persists until late adult life. After the age of 70, Hgb values decline by about 1g/dL in males and 0.2 g/dL in females (1).

Anemia is defined by low red cell mass by laboratory evaluation. Iron deficiency anemia (IDA) accounts for over half of all the cases with predominance in the very young and menstruating females.

The most common way to describe anemia is by etiology and red cell size. The primary etiologies are acute blood loss, decreased production, and increased destruction. Red cell sizes can be small (microcytic), normal (normocytic), or large (macrocytic). This chapter focuses on hypoproliferative anemia.

Hypoproliferative anemia is defined by the production of an inadequate number of erythrocytes to maintain homeostasis. The hallmark is low reticulocyte count, which may be due to bone marrow failure, bone marrow replacement, inflammation, or nutritional deficiencies. Iron deficiency is the most common hypoproliferative anemia, followed by anemia of chronic inflammation and renal disease.

A careful history, including diet, and a thorough physical examination often provide clues to the cause of anemia. Typical examination findings in anemia include pallor, scleral icterus, and tachycardia with systolic murmurs. The presence of Janeway lesions and subtle murmurs may reveal underlying infective endocarditis. Angular cheilitis and koilonychia may be observed in iron-deficient patients. Splenomegaly may be observed in patients with diseases with increased RBC turnover, liver disease, or splenic infiltration. Neurologic findings may be seen in patients with vitamin B12, copper, and zinc deficiencies.

Reticulocyte count is an important laboratory test to evaluate for anemia and is usually reported as reticulocyte percent. A reticulocyte production index (RPI) corrects for the patient's hematocrit, accounting for the increased life span of the reticulocyte, which develops into a mature erythrocyte within 24 hours of entrance into peripheral circulation when the hematocrit is normal. The formula is RPI = (%retic × [patient's hematocrit/normal hematocrit])/ maturation correction. The maturation correction estimates the life span in days of a reticulocyte in the bloodstream based on the degree of anemia.

Normal range is 0.5% to 2.5%. RPI <2% in the context of anemia usually indicates an inadequate bone marrow response. RPI >3% in the context of anemia excludes hypoproliferative anemia.

No correction is needed if absolute counts are reported. Normal absolute count in nonanemic patients is 25,000 to 75,000 cells/μL. An absolute reticulocyte count of <75,000 cells/μL in anemic patients suggests a component of hypoproliferation, while a count of >100,000 cells/μL excludes the diagnosis.

In addition to reticulocyte count, mean corpuscular volume (MCV) and red cell distribution width (RDW), which assess the average size of the erythrocyte and heterogeneity of the red cell volume, respectively, should be analyzed. MCV is measured in femtoliters. Though RDW may be reported in femtoliters, it is more commonly expressed as % (standard deviation of MCV/MCV × 100). Low reticulocyte count with MCV <70 fL usually signifies iron deficiency, while MCV >120 fL is observed in vitamin B12 and folate deficiency. Anemia of chronic inflammation may also be associated with microcytosis. Though hemoglobinopathies may cause microcytosis, reticulocytosis is often present unless there is a concurrent marrow-suppressing process. In nutritional deficiencies, the RDW is often elevated due to variable red cell sizes that result from inefficient erythropoiesis.

A peripheral blood smear should be reviewed as there are classic findings associated with the various etiologies of hypoproliferative anemias. Bone marrow examination should be considered when the diagnosis is inconclusive following analysis of peripheral blood and laboratory indices and/or if bone marrow pathology is suspected. Observation may be a reasonable alternative to a bone marrow biopsy for asymptomatic mild anemia.

IRON DEFICIENCY ANEMIA

Clinical Case 6.1

A 55-year-old nulliparous female presents to her primary care physician with progressive fatigue over the past 3 months. Her past medical history is significant for gastroesophageal reflux disease (GERD) and she takes omeprazole daily. Her surgical, family, and social histories are unremarkable. She is postmenopausal and denies a history of heavy menstrual bleeding. Her review of systems is negative for pica, change in weight, abdominal pain, bowel changes, or dark or bloody stools. Her reflux symptoms have resolved with daily omeprazole use. She eats a well-balanced diet, which includes iron-rich foods. Her laboratory profile shows Hgb 10.3 g/dL, MCV 75fL, platelet count 400,000, ferritin 10, total iron-binding capacity (TIBC) 435, and iron saturation 8%.

Introduction

IDA is the most common cause of anemia worldwide with a prevalence of at least 50% in developing countries, largely due to endemic gastrointestinal (GI) parasitic infections and vegetarian diet (1). The most common etiologies for IDA in developed countries include restrictive diets that exclude iron-rich foods, chronic blood loss, and decreased absorption. Normal daily iron loss is about 1.0 mg/d in men and 1.5 mg/d in premenopausal women. Shedding of enterocytes in the GI tract accounts for most of the iron loss and is typically balanced with iron absorption from the gut. Any pathology that impairs iron homeostasis will result in iron deficiency. Menorrhagia and pregnancy are the most likely causes of iron deficiency in premenopausal women. Women lose approximately 1 g of iron with each pregnancy. Men and postmenopausal women should undergo a thorough GI evaluation to identify a potential source for bleeding (i.e., occult malignancy, angiodysplasia). Dietary iron is absorbed mostly in the duodenum and proximal jejunum with the aid of gastric acid which reduces ferric to ferrous iron. Therefore, stomach or bowel resections, as well as GI bypass surgeries often result in IDA. Moreover, *Helicobacter pylori* infection and proton pump inhibitors may also impair iron absorption.

IDA may rarely be explained by a condition known as iron-refractory iron deficiency anemia (IRIDA). This autosomal recessive disorder is caused by a mutation in *TMPRSS6* gene, which results in increased hepcidin production and subsequently, decreased gut absorption of iron (2).

IDA occurs in a stepwise fashion following depletion of total body iron storage. Iron-deficient erythropoiesis occurs once the iron stores are fully depleted, and leads to microcytosis and hypochromia.

Absolute IDA should be distinguished from functional IDA. The former refers to diminished iron storage, while the latter condition refers to adequate iron storage, but insufficient circulating iron to maintain effective erythropoiesis. The most common causes of functional IDA are inflammation and chronic renal disease, discussed in greater detail in this chapter.

Diagnosis

A diagnosis of anemia typically triggers a diagnostic evaluation that should include serum ferritin and iron profile, which includes serum iron, serum transferrin (or TIBC), and transferrin saturation. Though microcytosis is usually present, a normal or elevated MCV should not discourage testing for iron deficiency.

In the absence of inflammation, serum ferritin reflects body iron stores. The optimal "cutoff" for iron deficiency is unclear, but clearly a ferritin level <15 ng/mL is diagnostic. A ferritin level <30 ng/mL has 92% sensitivity and 98% specificity in correlation with absent bone marrow stores. In the absence of inflammation, a ferritin level >100 ng/mL generally excludes the diagnosis of IDA. Serum transferrin level (or TIBC) is typically elevated and transferrin saturation is typically <20%, though the cutoff may be slightly higher in functional iron deficiency (2).

Low MCV and mean corpuscular Hgb concentration (MCHC) are typical, given the restrictive erythropoiesis that occurs with limited iron stores. The RDW is typically elevated, especially at the onset of IDA, due to coexistence of newly formed smaller erythrocytes with older normal erythrocytes. These lab abnormalities affecting the erythrocytes are not routinely seen in anemia of chronic inflammation.

Thrombocytosis is present in up to 50% of patients with IDA. The mechanism is not completely elucidated, but a recent abstract demonstrated increased EPO and thrombopoietin levels in patients with IDA compared to normal subjects (3).

Peripheral smear findings in IDA include microcytosis (erythrocyte is smaller than the nucleus of a lymphocyte) and hypochromia (central pallor >1/3 the diameter of the erythrocyte) (Figure 6.1). Anisocytosis may be present, with pencil-shaped erythrocytes, teardrop cells, and target cells.

Historically, the gold standard for evaluation of IDA was a Prussian blue stain of the bone marrow aspirate. However, this

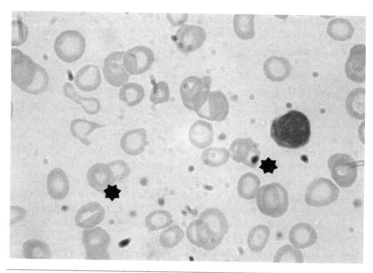

Figure 6.1 Peripheral smear of a patient with iron deficiency anemia. The erythrocytes surrounding the right asterisk demonstrate hypochromia, along with anisocytosis and poikilocytosis with variable sizes and shapes. The left asterisk highlights microcytosis, in which the erythrocyte is smaller than the nucleus of the neighboring lymphocyte.

invasive procedure is typically unnecessary with the use of the previously referenced laboratory tests and perhaps a trial of oral iron in the event that laboratory studies are non-confirmatory.

Key Diagnostic Dilemmas

Serum iron and transferrin saturation may be low in both IDA and anemia of chronic inflammation. Therefore, these lab indices should not be used in isolation for evaluation of anemia.

Serum ferritin is an acute phase reactant, thus interpretation in the context of acute inflammation may be challenging. Patients with inflammatory conditions, such as cancer infection, rheumatologic diseases, and inflammatory bowel disease, follow different diagnostic criteria for IDA. Ferritin <100 ng/mL or transferrin saturation <20% supports a diagnosis of IDA in the setting of inflammation. If ferritin level is between 100 and 300 ng/mL, a transferrin saturation <20% may still diagnose IDA (4).

Use caution with interpretation of iron studies in the setting of a recent packed RBC transfusion or recent iron intake (i.e., IV iron), as these may cause spurious elevations in serum iron, transferrin saturation, and ferritin levels. Following iron infusion, ferritin levels peak within a week and then gradually decline over several months. Therefore, it is recommended to re-evaluate the iron status approximately a month after completion of IV iron therapy to obtain a true reflection of iron stores.

Management

The goal of treatment is twofold: repletion of iron storage and identification and management of the underlying etiology. Though oral iron is generally well tolerated, GI toxicity, including nausea, vomiting, changes in bowel habit, and epigastric discomfort, may limit use in some patients. As a result, titration of oral iron to maximal dose should be considered to assess tolerance. Oral iron also causes black, sometimes tarry stools which may mimic melena.

Historically, the recommended dose of oral iron is 150 to 200 mg of elemental iron daily, often administered in two to three doses per day. However, recent data have challenged this practice. A Swiss group demonstrated decreased iron absorption amid increased serum hepcidin levels in young, healthy, normal-weight females with low iron stores and mild to no anemia who received more frequent dosing of oral iron, suggesting that less-frequent dosing (i.e., alternate daily dosing or at the most single daily dosing) may be more effective than twice or thrice daily dosing (5). The small study population and minimal to no anemia in healthy female patients in these studies do not yet support a definitive change in the standard approach to iron-deficient patients, yet invite more robust studies with patients with moderate-to-severe IDA to determine if these more scientific outcomes translate clinically to a more diverse patient population.

Parenteral iron supplementation can be considered in cases where rapid improvement is required, malabsorption exists, or if patients are unable to tolerate oral iron. Though parenteral iron overcomes impaired GI absorption and decreased tolerance, it may be costly of both time and money. These factors should be considered when IV iron is prescribed, and are reviewed in Table 6.1. Infusion reactions, including anaphylaxis, are potential adverse effects, but are now quite rare with newer formulations. Low-molecular-weight (LMW) iron dextran is safe and effective and has the convenience of delivering a single 1-g dose (6). A test dose is required for LMW iron dextran; other IVformulations do not require a test dose. Premedication (i.e., diphenhydramine, corticosteroids, or acetaminophen) is not routinely recommended, unless there is a history of infusion reactions with iron formulations or a history of inflammatory arthritis. In fact, premedication with diphenhydramine likely accounts for some of the adverse effects attributed to parenteral iron.

In addition to replacement of iron losses, the source of iron deficiency should be addressed. Gynecology referral for menorrhagia

Table 6.1 Oral and IIV Iron Formulations

Formulation	Brand Name	Dose	Recommended Frequency	Cost	Special Considerations
Oral					
Ferrous sulfate		• 325 mg tablet (65 mg Fe) • 220 mg/5 mL (44 mg Fe) • 75 mg/mL (15 mg Fe)	Two to three times daily (alternate day dosing is now being considered)	• $.01 to $.11 per tablet • $.01/5 mL • $.21/mL	
Ferrous gluconate		• 240 mg (27 mg Fe) • 324 mg (38 mg Fe)	Two to three times daily (alternate day dosing is now being considered)	• $.02 per tablet • $.06 to $.11 per tablet	
Ferrous fumarate		• 325 mg (106 mg Fe)	Two to three times daily (alternate dosing is now being considered)	• $0.35 per tablet	
IV					
LMW iron dextran	Infed	• 50 mg/mL (off-label dosing up to 1,000 mg dose over 1 hour)	One to three single doses, depending on the infusion dose and iron deficit	• $16.69 per 50 mg/mL ($333.80 per 1 g)	• 25 mg test dose required 1 hour prior to therapeutic dose • Larger doses associated with delayed (24–48 hours) infusion reactions

(continued)

Table 6.1 Oral and IV Iron Formulations (continued)

	Brand name	Dose	Recommended frequency	Cost	Special considerations
Ferric gluconate	Ferrlicit	• 12.5 mg/mL (125 mg dose over 1 hour)	• Requires numerous infusion appointments, at least eight to replace a 1-g deficit	• $7.63/mL ($76.30 per 125 mg)	• Does not require test dose • Serial infusions account for additional costs with each infusion visit
Iron sucrose	Venofer	• 20 mg/mL (100 mg dose over 15 minutes)	• Requires numerous infusion appointments, at least 10 to replace a 1-g deficit	• $8.64/mL ($43.20 per 100 mg)	• *Similar profile to ferric gluconate • *Both may be more appropriate in patients who already require frequent infusion appointments (i.e., dialysis, chemotherapy)
Ferric carboxymaltose	Injectafer	• 750 mg/15 mL (750 mg dose over 15 minutes)	• Two doses, 1 week apart • Can repeat another dose if needed	• $86.91/mL ($1,303.65 per dose)	• May be associated with hypophosphatemia
Ferumoxytol	Feraheme	• 510 mg/17 mL (510 mg dose over 15 minutes)	• Two doses, 3–8 days apart • Can repeat another dose 30 days after the second dose if needed	• $68.55/mL ($1,165.35 per dose)	

LMW, low molecular weight.

Source: From Camaschella C. Iron-Deficiency Anemia. *N Engl J Med.* 2015;372(19):1832–1843. doi:10.1056/NEJMra1401038; Auerbach M, Macdougall I. The available intravenous iron formulations: history, efficacy, and toxicology. *Hemodial Int.* 2017;21:S83–S92. doi:10.1111/hdi.12560; Lexicomp Online. *Lexi-Drugs Online.* Hudson, OH: Wolters Kluwer Clinical Drug Information, Inc.; 2019.

or gastroenterology referral for GI bleeding or unexplained iron deficiency to exclude an occult malignancy is warranted in an attempt to completely resolve the iron deficiency. Patients with menorrhagia or dysmenorrhea with no clear gynecologic etiology for abnormal bleeding should be considered for underlying von Willebrand's disease. Similarly, patients without apparent GI pathology should be considered for absorptive disorders such as celiac disease or tropical sprue.

Prognosis

Restoration of normal erythropoiesis occurs within 5 days with adequate iron replacement. Hematocrit rises approximately 1 g/dL after 7 days and peaks around 40 days. MCV gradually normalizes over 3 to 4 months. Ferritin is the last to rise as replenishment of total body iron storage occurs last in the sequence of events. Medication compliance should be assessed in cases of treatment failure.

Future Directions

As explained earlier, the less-frequent dosing of oral iron may more effectively increase the iron stores and Hgb, with potentially fewer side effects. Larger randomized studies will help determine if the standard twice to three times daily dosing of oral iron will become obsolete.

Key Points

- IDA in developed countries includes restrictive diets that exclude iron-rich foods, chronic blood loss, and decreased absorption (i.e., bariatric surgeries, bowel resection, *H. pylori* infection, antacid use).
- Serum iron level alone is not adequate for assessing IDA and should only be used in conjunction with ferritin and other iron parameters.
- The optimal cutoff for the diagnosis of IDA remains unclear. Though ferritin levels <15 ng/mL definitively diagnose iron deficiency, levels as high as 50 ng/mL are often diagnostic. In the setting of inflammation, ferritin levels may also be higher and should be analyzed in conjunction with serum transferrin and transferrin saturation levels.
- A trial of oral iron is recommended in the initial treatment of IDA. Less-frequent dosing may be more efficient and less toxic, but further studies are needed to confirm.
- IV iron is an alternative to oral iron if there is an inadequate response or intolerance to oral iron.

ANEMIA OF CHRONIC DISEASE

Clinical Case 6.2

A 32-year-old female is referred for evaluation of anemia. Her past medical history is significant for recently diagnosed rheumatoid arthritis. Her menstruation is light on a progesterone-based contraceptive. Her laboratory evaluation is significant for Hgb of 9.8 g/L, MCV 77 fL, RDW 18%, platelet count 250/mL, erythrocyte sedimentation rate (ESR) >120 mm/hr, C-reactive protein (CRP) >20 mg/L, ferritin 2,100 ng/mL, TIBC 150 mcg/dL, and transferrin saturation of 6%.

Introduction

Anemia of chronic disease (ACD), also referred to as anemia of chronic inflammation, is the second most common form of anemia after IDA. It can be seen in up to 40% of cancer patients and 60% of rheumatoid arthritis patients (7). ACD is caused by functional iron deficiency (failure to absorb or traffic iron), resulting in inhibition of RBC production and mildly decreased RBC life span.

Macrophages supply >95% of the daily iron requirements through recycling of iron from senescent erythrocytes. Increased inflammation causes disruption of iron homeostasis via increased production of hepcidin by the liver. Hepcidin binds to ferroportin, an iron export protein, and sets off a sequence of events resulting in internalization and degradation of the protein. This leads to decreased macrophage iron export and intestinal absorption, resulting in functional iron deficiency, despite adequate iron stores.

Erythropoiesis inhibition and relative EPO deficiency have been attributed to inflammatory cytokines. In rheumatoid arthritis, for example, there is an inverse relationship between serum tumor necrosis factor (TNF) level and burst forming unit-erythroid (BFU-Es). EPO expression is generally decreased or inappropriately normal. The degree of anemia is directly proportional to the degree of elevation of inflammatory markers such as ESR, CRP, or interleukin (IL)-6 (8).

Diagnostic Criteria

As described, the reticulocyte count, iron studies, ferritin, complete blood count (CBC), and peripheral smear are typically adequate for diagnosis of ACD. The anemia is generally normocytic and normochromic, with the Hgb between 8 and 9.5 g/L. Up to one third of patients can have a more severe form with hypochromia and microcytosis, mimicking IDA. In this functionally iron deficient state, iron stores are adequate, often resulting in **elevated ferritin**, which is also elevated as an acute phase reactant in the setting of inflammation. Reduced iron transport and reduced erythropoiesis result in **low transferrin levels with low to low-normal transferrin saturation** and **low reticulocyte count**, respectively.

Key Diagnostic Dilemma

ACD remains largely a clinical diagnosis. An unequivocal ACD diagnosis can be challenging as anemia in these patients may have other coexisting etiologies. For example, up to 70% of anemia in patients with rheumatoid arthritis has multifactorial etiologies. A combination of true and functional iron-deficient states may coexist and should be suspected in patients with inflammation and low-normal serum ferritin level. Meta-analyses showed iron deficiency in 6.7% of 1,842 patients with ferritin above 45 ng/mL and 3.5% of 1,368 patients with ferritin above 100 ng/mL. Conversely, an absence of bone marrow iron storage has been observed in patients with serum ferritin above 3,500 ng/mL during an acute inflammation. Moreover, a ferritin level above 8,000 ng/mL has also been observed in a patient with an acute liver failure with the bone marrow showing absent iron stores (8). Serum soluble transferrin receptors and hepcidin may be helpful in detecting absolute iron deficiency in the setting of inflammation, but are costly and not readily available in clinical practice. Therefore, if serum transferrin saturation is low (<16%–20%), it may be reasonable to undertake a trial of oral iron in the setting of ACD, bearing in mind that intestinal absorption may be thwarted by increased hepcidin. Bone marrow aspirate in patients with pure anemia usually adds little to the diagnosis, except in cases where bone marrow pathology is suspected.

Prognosis

The prognosis of ACD depends on the underlying disease. Hgb of <9 g/dL has been found to independently predict prolonged hospital stay and mortality (9).

Treatment

Treatment of ACD should be directed toward the underlying disease. Treatment of anemia itself is not recommended in asymptomatic patients. Moreover, there is not a standard Hgb target that indicates when ACD should be treated. In asymptomatic hospitalized patients, the general approach is to transfuse packed RBCs when the Hgb drops below 7 to 8 g/dL. This restrictive strategy is also applied to critically ill patients and is supported by clinical evidence. The transfusion threshold is generally higher in cardiac patients with acute ischemia (10).

In the setting of chronic inflammatory conditions, effective treatment of the underlying disease should improve the Hgb. However, anemia may persist after initiation of treatment, perhaps due to inadequate control of the primary disease and/or myelosuppression from the treatment. If transfusion support is needed, then EPO replacement may be considered to avoid complications related to serial transfusions. However, EPO replacement has its own toxicity profile, and thus, caution must be exercised, particularly in the setting of malignancy and renal disease. Routine EPO replacement in these scenarios is discussed later in the chapter.

Future Directions

Novel therapies targeting hepcidin and ferroportin pathways are under investigation. NOX-H94 binds to and inactivates hepcidin. Its safety, tolerability, and efficacy were evaluated in a study of cancer patients with ACD, supporting hepcidin blockade as a treatment target in ACD (8).

Key Points

- ACD is caused by a functionally iron-depleted state.
- Treatment of ACD should be directed to underlying inflammatory causes.
- Blood transfusions are not recommended in asymptomatic patients.

MEGALOBLASTIC ANEMIA

Clinical Case 6.3

A 72-year-old female is referred for evaluation of her anemia. Her past medical history is significant for well-controlled hypothyroidism and diabetes mellitus (DM) type 2. Her medications include levothyroxine and metformin. Pertinent laboratory evaluation shows Hgb of 8.5 g/dL, MCV 107 fL, RDW 17%, platelet count 160/mL, WBC 4.0 × 10⁹ cells/L, ferritin 150 ng/mL, TIBC 150 mcg/dL, transferrin saturation 26%, folate >20 ng/mL, and B12 level 245 pg/mL.

Introduction

Megaloblastosis is the result of defective DNA synthesis, which leads to impaired cell division from S phase arrest. These cells tend to have two to four times the amount of DNA with the resultant enlarged nuclei. The transcription and translation processes, on the other hand, remain relatively functional. Anemia is a common finding in megaloblastosis, which affects all proliferating cells. The most common causes are nutritional deficiencies such as vitamin B12 and folate. Megaloblastosis starts to develop after the body has depleted the stored nutrients.

In the United States, it is estimated that up to 20% of elderly patients have vitamin B12 deficiency. In India, a developing country with prevalent vegetarian diet, the prevalence is estimated to be up to 75% of the population (11).

Diagnostic Criteria

Serum cobalamin, folate, and reticulocyte count are now standard studies in the routine evaluation of anemia. These tests should be especially considered in patients with macrocytic anemia (MCV >100), normocytic anemia with elevated RDW, or anemic patients at risk for nutritional deficiencies.

Peripheral blood smear analysis often shows abnormal morphology of erythrocytes and granulocytes. The earliest manifestation is increase in MCV, coinciding with macroovalocytes on the peripheral smear. Dyssynchrony between the maturation of cytoplasm and that of nuclei leads to macrocytosis, immature nuclei, and hypersegmentation (greater than five or six lobes) in granulocytes in the peripheral blood (Figure 6.2). Poikilocytosis and

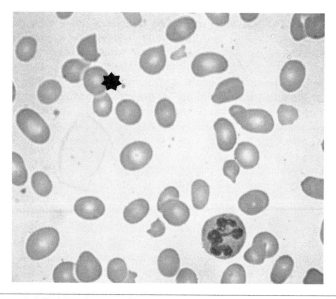

Figure 6.2 Peripheral smear of a patient with cobalamin deficiency. Macroovalocytes are present, along with RBC fragments (upper asterisk) that are a result of ineffective erythropoiesis and marrow hemolysis and a hypersegmented neutrophil (lower right field). Peripheral smear findings in vitamin B12 deficiency can sometimes mimic microangiopathic hemolytic anemia.

RBC, red blood cell.

anisocytosis may be present as a result of ineffective erythropoiesis and resultant intramedullary hemolysis in the bone marrow, resulting in increased hemolytic parameters in the serum (i.e., lactate dehydrogenase [LDH], total and indirect bilirubin).

Sensitivity of cobalamin level below 200 is 95%. In the case of cobalamin deficiency, patients should be tested for pernicious anemia. Elevated serum anti-intrinsic factor antibody has a 50% sensitivity and 100% specificity for pernicious anemia. Serum antiparietal cell antibodies historically had lower specificity until the advent of newer-generation enzyme-linked immunosorbent assay (ELISA) targeting gastric H+/K+ ATPase. Combination of the two tests results in sensitivity of 73% and specificity of 100%. Other coexisting autoimmune diseases should also be evaluated. Referral for endoscopy is recommended in patients diagnosed with pernicious anemia, given the increased risk of gastric malignancies (12).

In equivocal cases where cobalamin levels are between 200 and 400 pg/dL, serum homocysteine and methylmalonic levels should be obtained. Normal values of both completely exclude cobalamin deficiency. Increase in serum homocysteine alone is seen in folate deficiency. Patients with combined deficiency have elevation in both methylmalonic acid (MMA) and homocysteine levels. In clinical practice, patients are frequently empirically treated with vitamin B12 replacement without obtaining a definitive diagnosis. Though vitamin B12 replacement in this situation likely carries little to no risk, this could be an additional unnecessary medication that will contribute to polypharmacy which is increasingly a concern in the elderly population. Empiric treatment is strongly recommended when neurologic symptoms are present while waiting for the MMA levels to return.

Serum folate testing in the Western world is done by indirect immunoassays, which have a high specificity with low sensitivity. A serum folate level >4 ng/mL is considered normal and does not require further evaluation. A serum folate level <2 ng/mL supports a diagnosis of folate deficiency and warrants folate replacement. A serum folate level of 2 to 4 ng/mL is borderline and may benefit from RBC folate testing versus empiric folate supplementation. An RBC folate level is useful in this scenario (12).

History and physical examination are important in assessing the presence of clinical symptoms in the setting of cobalamin and/or folate deficiency. The severity of symptoms may impact management, especially in cobalamin deficiency, in the decision to treat with oral versus parenteral vitamin B12 replacement. Patients may have low-grade fever. Dermatologic examination may show diffuse brown hyperpigmentation or blotchy tanned spots. Premature graying of hair is reversible within 6 months of supplementation. Patients with pernicious anemia may also present with typical physical examination of autoimmune thyroid disorders, mimicking hyperthyroidism and hypothyroidism. Glossitis, thyromegaly, jugulovenous distention, cardiac summation gallop, pericardial or pleural effusions, hepatosplenomegaly, or myxedema may be observed. In prolonged cobalamin deficiency, careful neurologic examination may reveal evidence of loss of position and vibratory senses in early cases. Upper motor neuron signs may include progressive spasticity, increased muscle tone, hyperreflexia, extensor plantar response, and spastic paraplegia. Lower motor neuron signs, such as flaccidity and hyporeflexia, may also be observed. Reduced cerebral functions, delirium, and catatonia can also be observed in more severe cases (12).

Key Diagnostic Dilemma

As described, patients with low-normal vitamin B12 and/or folate levels are frequently started on empiric vitamin replacement. Because MMA and homocysteine levels normalize within 1 week of supplementation, an opportunity to definitively diagnose vitamin B12 and/or folate deficiency may be lost once empiric supplementation is started.

Several conditions, including liver disease, autoimmune disease, and hematologic malignancies, can surreptitiously elevate cobalamin levels in patients with actual cobalamin deficiency. High titers of serum anti-intrinsic factor (anti-IF) antibody may have cross-reactivity with older assays used to measure vitamin B12 levels, causing spuriously high levels in patients with cobalamin deficiency. However, evaluation of newer assays shows that this pitfall has been overcome (12).

Cobalamin deficiency may falsely raise serum folate level by up to 30%, while hypovolemia and renal failure can cause elevated homocysteine and MMA levels.

Prognosis

Upon initiation of vitamin replacement, normal hematopoiesis is re-established within 2 days. Physical complaints of fatigue and pain also tend to improve within the first couple of days of supplementation. Serum MMA and homocysteine can normalize within 1 week. Reticulocytosis can be seen within 2 days and peaks at about a week. Cytopenias typically normalize within 2 months. Further neurologic damage is usually halted, with the resolution of symptoms seen in over weeks to months. Extent of recovery depends on the extent and duration of neurologic symptoms. Further recovery after 12 months is unlikely (12).

Management

Cyanocobalamin may be replaced via oral or parenteral adminis-tration. Recommended oral dose is 1,000 to 2,000 mcg daily and has been shown to be effective even in patients with pernicious anemia, as even a small degree of absorption in these patients is adequate to satisfy the recommended daily requirement from this high dose. This may apply to patients with gastritis and bowel sur-gery as well. However, it is important to monitor the serum levels and clinical symptoms closely to ensure that oral replacement is sufficient. Parenteral administration (intramuscular or subcuta-neous) is typically started with daily injection of 1,000 mcg for approximately 1 week, followed by weekly dosing for 1 month, and then indefinite monthly injections. In patients with neurologic symptoms, parenteral administration is most appropriate at the onset of treatment.

Oral folic acid replacement is effectively achieved with 1 mg daily. Once vitamin B12 or folate deficiency is diagnosed, it is imperative to educate patients that this is lifelong treatment. Noncompliance with vitamin replacement may result in return of hematologic and neuropsychiatric symptoms, often with the onset of neurologic deficits at 6 months following discontinuation of cyanocobalamin replacement (see Table 6.2) (2,11–13).

Key Points

- Pernicious anemia should be investigated in every patient with vitamin B12 deficiency.
- Serum methylmalonic acid and homocysteine should be obtained in cases where the vitamin B12 level is unequivocal (200–400 pg/dL).
- Daily folate supplementation of 1 mg is more than adequate.
- There is no single correct way to replete vitamin B12. Consider parenteral supplementation in symptomatic or critically ill patients.

ANEMIA IN PREGNANCY

Clinical Case 6.4

A 19-year-old female is referred for evaluation of her anemia. She is currently 22 weeks pregnant. Her past medical, surgical, and family histories are unre-markable. Her laboratory evaluation is significant for Hgb of 10.4 g/L, MCV 85 fL, RDW 13%, platelet count 300/mL, ferritin 250 ng/mL, TIBC 200 mcg/dL, and transferrin saturation of 30%.

Table 6.2 Nutritional Deficiencies

Vitamin/Mineral	Dietary Source	Recommended Daily Intake	Site of Gut Absorption	Critical Requirements for Gut Absorption	Etiologies for Vitamin Deficiency	Clinical Manifestations Associated With Deficiency

Iron	• Breakfast cereals (fortified)
	• Oysters
	• Beans
	• Dark chocolate
	• Beef liver
	• Lentils
	• Spinach, cooked
		Newborn (0–6 months)
		• 0.27 mg 7 months to 13 years
		• 8 to 11 mg
		14 to 18 years
		• Male: 11 mg
		• Female: 15 mg
		19 to 50 years
		• Male: 8 mg
		• Female: 18 mg
		51+ years
		• Male: 8 mg
		• Female: 8 mg
		Pregnant female
		• 27 mg
		Lactating female
		• 20 mg
			Duodenum	• **Acidic environment to reduce ferric iron to ferrous iron**	• **Blood loss**
					  Heavy menses
					  GI bleeding
					  GU bleeding
					  Frequent blood donations
					  Inadequate diet
					• **Bariatric surgery**
					• **Pregnancy/lactation**
					• **Gut malabsorption**
					  Inflammatory bowel disease
					  Celiac disease
					  Helicobacter pylori
					  Antacids/proton pump inhibitors
					• **IRIDA**
						• Most commonly asymptomatic
						• Pagophagia (craving for ice)
						• Koilonychia (spoon-shaped nails)
						• Restless legs syndrome
						• Fatigue
						• Shortness of breath/exertional dyspnea (severe)
						• Chest pain (severe)

(continued)

Table 6.2 Nutritional Deficiencies (*continued*)

Vitamin/ Mineral	Dietary Source	Recommended Daily Intake	Site of Gut Absorption	Critical Requirements for Gut Absorption	Etiologies for Vitamin Deficiency	Clinical Manifestations Associated With Deficiency
Copper	• Liver • Seafood • Beans • Nuts • Whole grains	Newborn/children (0–10 years) • 0.4 to 2 mg Adolescents/ adults • 1.5 to 3 mg	Unknown in humans, though animal studies suggest mainly duodenum, as well as stomach/ileum	• Gastric acidity (to release copper from food)	• Gastric surgery • Zinc overload (large quantities interfere with copper absorption) • Copper-chelating agents • Long-term parenteral nutrition	• Sideroblastic anemia • Neutropenia • Demyelinating disease (paresthesias, weakness, ataxia)

(*continued*)

Table 6.2 Nutritional Deficiencies (*continued*)

Vitamin/ Mineral	Dietary Source	Recommended Daily Intake	Site of Gut Absorption	Critical Requirements for Gut Absorption	Etiologies for Vitamin Deficiency	Clinical Manifestations Associated With Deficiency
Cobalamin (vitamin B12, Cbl)	Animal products • Meat (**clams, liver**) • Fish • Dairy products • Eggs	Newborn/children (0–13 years) • 0.4 to 1.8 mcg Adolescents/adults (14+ years) • 2.4 mcg Pregnant female • 2.6 mcg Lactating female • 2.8 mcg *May take several **years** for deficiency to develop upon withdrawal of vit B12 from diet	Ileum	• **Gastric acidity** (to release vitamin B12 from food) • **Intrinsic factor** (secreted by gastric parietal cells to bind vitamin B12, so that vitamin B12–IF complex is later absorbed in the ileum) • **Pancreatic proteases** to cleave binding proteins from vitamin B12 prior to binding IF	• **Pernicious anemia** (autoantibodies to parietal cells or IF) • Inadequate diet • Bariatric surgery (total gastrectomy > subtotal gastrectomy, gastric bypass) • *H. pylori* infection • Medications • PPI/H2 blockers • **Metformin** (reduces calcium which is required for vitamin B12–IF absorption) • Pancreatic insufficiency • Small bowel disease	Neuropsychiatric • SCD of dorsal/lateral columns of spinal cord (classic, but may not be present early) – demyelination • **Symmetric paresthesia, ataxia** → impaired vibration/proprioception in lower extremities → autonomic dysfunction (orthostasis, impaired gut motility) • Depression, mood changes, cognitive dysfunction, dementia, psychosis

(*continued*)

Table 6.2 Nutritional Deficiencies (continued)

Vitamin/ Mineral	Dietary Source	Recommended Daily Intake	Site of Gut Absorption	Critical Requirements for Gut Absorption	Etiologies for Vitamin Deficiency	Clinical Manifestations Associated With Deficiency
Folate (vitamin B9)	Animal products • Meat (clams, **liver**) • Dairy products • Eggs • Seafood • Plants • Green leafy vegetables (**spinach**) • **Asparagus** • **Brussel sprouts** • Fruits/fruit juices • Nuts • Beans Cereal/grain products (fortification program required by FDA)	Newborn/children (0–15 years) • 65 to 300 mcg Adolescents/adults (14+ years) • 400 mcg Pregnant female • 600 mcg Lactating female • 500 mcg *May take **weeks to months** for deficiency to develop upon withdrawal of folate from diet	Jejunum	Intact carrier system – PCFT transports dietary folate into enterocytes **Acidic** environment Normal reduction/ methylation to form 5-methyl-tetrahydrofolate	• Inadequate diet • Increased requirement for rapid cell proliferation (chronic hemolysis, exfoliative skin conditions, hemodialysis) • Small bowel disease/surgery • Medications that interfere with acidity of folate metabolism (methotrexate, trimethoprim, pyrimethamine, antiepileptics)	• Historically not associated with neurologic deficits, but recent data suggest otherwise, particularly with cognitive impairment, depression, and dementia • Less commonly associated with SCD of the spinal cord • Neural tube defects during embryogenesis

Note: Bold text represents high yields.

FDA, U.S. Food and Drug Administration; GI, gastrointestinal; IF, intrinsic factor; IRIDA, iron-refractory iron-deficiency anemia; PCFT, proton coupled folate transporter; SCD, subacute combined degeneration.

Source: From Camaschella C. Iron-deficiency Anemia. *N Engl J Med.* 2015;372(19):1832–1843. doi:10.1056/NEJMra1401038; Hannibal L, Lysne V, Bjørke-Monsen A, et al. Biomarkers and algorithms for the diagnosis of vitamin B12 deficiency. *Front Mol Biosci.* 2016;3:27. doi:10.3389/fmolb.2016.00027; Antony AC. Chapter 39 – Megaloblastic anemias. In: Hoffman R, Benz EJ, Silberstein LE, et al., eds. *Hematology.* 7th ed. New York, NY: Elsevier; 2018:514–545.e7; Fuller SJ, Wiley JS. Chapter 38 – Heme biosynthesis and its disorders: Porphyrias and sideroblastic anemias. In: Hoffman R, Benz EJ, Silberstein LE, et al., eds. *Hematology.* 7th ed. New York, NY: Elsevier; 2018: 497–513.e6.

Introduction

Anemia is observed in half of all pregnancies, with higher incidence and prevalence in developing countries at approximately 35% to 60%, compared to <20% in developed countries (14). Physiologic (dilutional) anemia occurs due to disproportionate increase in plasma volume as compared to RBC mass. Plasma volume increases by >50% during pregnancy with a 25% increase in RBC mass, resulting in dilutional anemia. Iron deficiency accounts for 75% of all pathologic anemias in pregnancy. Folate deficiency has historically been the second leading cause of anemia in pregnancy, with vitamin B12 deficiency far less common due to large stores which typically take years to deplete. However, the nationwide folate fortification programs have resulted in a decline in folate deficiency in the United States, and an increase in bariatric surgeries has increased the prevalence of cobalamin deficiency in pregnant women (15). Hemoglobinopathies also contribute to anemia in pregnancy and may require a different management approach in the peripartum setting.

Diagnostic Criteria

The Centers for Disease Control and Prevention (CDC) and the American College of Obstetricians and Gynecologists (ACOG) define anemia in pregnancy as Hgb <11 g/dL in the first and third trimesters and <10.5 g/dL in the second trimester (15). This definition accounts for the physiologic changes seen in pregnancy. If anemia is diagnosed, further evaluation for iron deficiency, vitamin B12, and folate, as described in iron deficiency anemia and megaloblastic anemia sections, is warranted.

Key Diagnostic Dilemma

Despite the definition for anemia provided by the CDC and the ACOG, dilutional anemia may be seen with lower Hgb values than the cutoffs established in the definition. This was demonstrated in a prospective study in Israel. Of 686 women diagnosed with anemia according to the current definition, 78% of women with singleton pregnancies and Hgb between 10 and 10.5 g/dL, as well as 73.8% of women with twin pregnancies and Hgb between 10 and 10.5 g/dL had a negative anemia workup (16).

Prognosis

Pathologic anemia poses risks upon the mother and developing fetus. Thus, correction of underlying causes for anemia is imperative. Iron, vitamin B12, and folate deficiencies are major risk factors for preterm and low-birth-weight babies. Iron and vitamin B12 deficiency have been implicated in neurocognitive deficits, including learning and memory impairments, in infants and children born to iron-deficient mothers. Folic acid deficiency is associated with neural tube defects. In addition to anemia-related symptoms, the anemic mother is at increased risk for preeclampsia, placental abruption, and cardiac failure (15).

Management

The CDC and the ACOG recommend oral iron supplementation of 15 to 30 mg/day of elemental iron, 400 mcg/day of folate, and 2.6 mcg/day of cobalamin from beginning of gestation to 3 months postpartum for all pregnant women (15). If iron deficiency is diagnosed, prompt iron supplementation is warranted, given the deleterious effects of low iron on the mother and the fetus. If iron deficiency is diagnosed in the first trimester, a trial of oral iron supplementation is reasonable. However, the adverse GI effects associated with oral iron formulations may be exacerbated by progesterone's effect on gut motility that results in indigestion, nausea, vomiting, and constipation. If oral iron is not tolerated or a more rapid correction of anemia is desired (i.e., inadequate response to oral iron, severe anemia, second or third trimesters), then IV iron is safe and should be administered.

Key Points

- Dilutional anemia is a physiologic response to pregnancy and should be considered prior to pathologic etiologies.
- Iron deficiency, followed by folate and cobalamin deficiencies account for the majority of pathologic anemias in pregnancy.
- All pregnant patients should receive iron, vitamin B12, and folic acid supplementation, and all nutritional deficiencies should be corrected rapidly to avoid developmental and neurocognitive risks to the fetus.
- IV iron should be considered in pregnant women who do not tolerate oral iron or require rapid correction of Hgb.

ANEMIA OF RENAL DISEASE

Clinical Case 6.5

A 72-year-old male is referred for evaluation of anemia. His past medical history is significant for uncontrolled DM type 2 with resulting neuropathy and nephropathy. His medications include venlafaxine and insulin neutral protamine hagedorn (NPH). Pertinent laboratory evaluation shows Hgb of 9.0 g/L, MCV 85 fL, RDW 13%, platelet count 120/mL, WBC 4.0 × 10⁹ cells/L, ferritin 150 ng/mL, TIBC 350 mcg/dL, transferrin saturation 8%, folate 15 ng/mL, B12 700 pg/mL, and creatinine 2.2 mg/dL.

Introduction

Anemia can be seen in up to 50% of patients with chronic kidney disease (CKD). Relative EPO deficiency largely accounts for anemia in these patients, as EPO is produced in the kidney and regulated by the hypoxia inducible factor (HIF) system which is stimulated by hypoxia. Hsu et al. showed that anemia as defined by an Hgb concentration of <12 g/dL in men and <11 g/dL in women was more common with creatinine clearance <70 and <50 mL/min in men and women, respectively. Over time, the degree of anemia parallels the decline in creatinine clearance. Another interesting finding is that patients with both DM and CKD are at higher risk for developing anemia than non-diabetic counterparts with CKD. Approximately one quarter of diabetics already have anemia with Stage III CKD, compared to 8% of non-diabetics with CKD (17).

Other contributors to anemia in CKD include absolute and functional iron deficiency, inflammation, hyperparathyroidism, hemolysis, nutritional deficiencies, and reduced erythrocyte survival. CKD patients have a high incidence of iron deficiency due to occult bleeding, blood loss during frequent phlebotomy and hemodialysis, inflammatory states from infections and surgery, and impaired gut absorption due to upregulation of hepcidin. Therefore, frequent assessment of iron stores is key in the initial evaluation and management of anemia in CKD patients.

Diagnostic Criteria

Anemia of CKD is multifactorial and essentially a diagnosis of exclusion. There are really no specific laboratory findings that support the diagnosis. Initial evaluation of anemia in CKD patients should include complete metabolic profile, CBC, serum reticulocyte count, peripheral blood smear, transferrin, transferrin saturation, ferritin, vitamin B12, and folate. If not already included in CKD evaluation, serum protein electrophoresis with immunofixation and serum light chains should be considered to exclude plasma cell dyscrasias. Optional studies include serum EPO and parathyroid levels. Given that there is a relative EPO deficiency, these levels rarely aid in diagnosis or alter management.

Diagnosis of iron deficiency in patients with CKD is important with slightly different criteria compared to non–CKD-related anemia. Prior to considering treatment with EPO-stimulating agents (ESAs), it is imperative to replenish the iron stores as ESAs are not effective without adequate iron stores. In fact, iron supplementation alone may improve the Hgb in anemia of CKD. According to the Kidney Disease Improving Global Outcome (KDIGO) Clinical Practice Guidelines, iron deficiency should be considered when transferrin saturation is ≤30% and ferritin is ≤500 ng/mL (18). This liberal threshold should be limited to patients who require treatment of the anemia.

Key Diagnostic Dilemma

Because anemia of CKD is a diagnosis of exclusion, the inability to corroborate the diagnosis with specific lab indices may be unsettling. Bone marrow biopsy is not frequently recommended and will not confirm this diagnosis. A small decline in creatinine clearance may result in mild anemia. Bear in mind that the degree of anemia often correlates with the degree of renal failure. Discordance between the degree of anemia and renal failure should prompt further investigation for an alternative diagnosis. Abnormalities in other cell lineages should also raise concern for an alternative diagnosis.

Plasma cell dyscrasias, most commonly monoclonal gammopathy of undetermined significance (MGUS), are often detected in the setting of CKD and anemia. Determining if the anemia is related to plasma cell dyscrasia versus anemia of CKD may be challenging, especially given the difficulty with interpretation of serum light chains in the setting of renal failure. If there is no identifiable etiology for CKD (i.e., poorly controlled DM or hypertension), bone marrow biopsy is warranted. The evaluation for MGUS does not routinely involve a bone marrow biopsy unless the M-protein is ≥1.5 g/dL, serum free light chain (FLC) ratio is abnormal, or there is evidence of end-organ damage. A patient with anemia of CKD and MGUS may often fulfill these criteria and would be subject to the invasiveness of a bone marrow biopsy. To account for the impaired renal clearance of serum light chains in CKD, which may result in higher kappa FLC levels, a revised reference serum light chain ratio of 0.37 to 3.1 (vs. 0.26–1.65) should be used for CKD patients (19). This may prevent unnecessary bone marrow biopsies for patients with anemia of CKD. However, once diagnosed with MGUS, these patients are at risk for progression to multiple myeloma and must be monitored carefully.

Management

The decision to treat anemia of CKD should consider the risks and benefits of iron and/or ESA therapy (i.e., symptoms, quality of life, transfusion requirement, and comorbidities that may be negatively affected by ESA therapy – active or history of malignancy, history of stroke, uncontrolled hypertension). Prior to initiation of ESA therapy, all correctable etiologies of anemia, including iron deficiency (transferrin saturation is ≤30% and ferritin is ≤500 ng/mL), should be addressed first. Because of impaired gut absorption of iron, mediated by increased hepcidin, IV iron is recommended in all dialysis patients. However, in non-dialysis patients, a trial of oral iron is reasonable. Iron status should be evaluated every 3 months with transferrin saturation and ferritin.

In non-dialysis patients, ESA therapy should not be considered unless the Hgb is <10 g/dL. In dialysis patients, it is recommended to start ESA therapy when the Hgb is between 9 and 10 g/dL. Suggested starting doses are as follows:

- Epoetin alfa: 50 to 100 U/kg three times weekly (dialysis) or every 1 to 2 weeks (non-dialysis)
- Darbopoetin alfa: 0.45 mcg/kg once weekly (dialysis) or every 2 to 4 weeks (non-dialysis) (12)

The target Hgb should not exceed 11.5 g/dL, as numerous studies have shown increased cardiovascular and thrombotic risks with higher Hgb targets. Moreover, caution is recommended in the use of ESAs in CKD in patients with a history of malignancy, given concerns for increased mortality in this subset of patients (17).

Initial and acquired ESA hyporesponsiveness is defined as no increase in Hgb from baseline after the first month of ESA therapy on appropriate weight-based dosing or following two increases in ESA dose beyond the previous dose which had initially stabilized the Hgb, respectively. Escalations beyond double the initial weight-based dose are not recommended in initial ESA hyporesponsiveness. Moreover, it is not advised to increase the dose beyond double the dose of the original stable dose if there was initially a response. Consider potential etiologies for ESA hyporesponsiveness, including treatment compliance, iron status, active bleeding, vitamin B12 and folate deficiencies, hyperparathyroidism, infection, inadequate dialysis, or angiotensin converting enzyme inhibitor/angiotensin receptor blocker (ACE/ARB) use (18).

Antibody-mediated pure red cell aplasia (PRCA) is a rare, but well-recognized complication of ESAs in which antibodies develop to both synthetic and endogenous EPO. The risk of this complication is rare and has decreased since removal of a prior epoetin-alfa formulation from the market. Antibody-mediated PRCA should be considered if there is a sudden decrease in Hgb at the rate of 0.5 to 1.0 g/dL per week, decreased reticulocyte count, and normal platelet and white blood cell count. ESA therapy should be stopped immediately if the patient develops antibody-mediated PRCA, and peginesatide, a synthetic, peptide-based EPO receptor agonist, should be administered (18).

Prognosis

Observational studies have shown that anemia may have a negative impact on quality of life, as well as mortality and left ventricular hypertrophy (LVH). In randomized clinical trials, however, ESA therapy has not been proven to reduce mortality or improve LVH (17). In fact, overcorrection of anemia to normal Hgb increased the cardiovascular and mortality risks. Nonetheless, improving the quality life (i.e., decreasing fatigue, reducing blood transfusions) with higher Hgb supports treatment of anemia in patients with CKD.

Future Directions
Numerous trials are ongoing to investigate alternatives to ESAs to improve erythropoiesis in patients with anemia of CKD. HIF stabilizers prevent HIF-alpha degradation, promoting endogenous EPO synthesis in the kidneys. The potential advantage of this medication class over ESAs is its oral administration. And also, physiologic EPO levels are less likely harmful than the surge in EPO received with ESA therapy. Roxadustat, an HIF stabilizer, has been approved in China to treat anemia of CKD in dialysis patients. In two phase 3 clinical trials, roxadustat met the primary efficacy endpoints in improving Hgb in both non-dialysis and dialysis patients (20).

Key Points
- Anemia can be observed in >50% of patients with CKDs.
- The decision to treat anemia of CKD should consider the risks and benefits of therapy, with the initiation of iron supplementation done when ferritin is <500 ng/mL and transferrin saturation is <30% and initiation of ESA therapy done once the Hgb levels become <9 to 10 g/dL in dialysis patients.
- Initiation of ESA therapy should not be considered in non-hemodialysis patients until the Hgb is <10 g/dL.
- Target Hgb during ESA therapy should not exceed 11.5 g/dL.

ANEMIA OF ENDOCRINE DISORDERS

Clinical Case 6.6
A 77-year-old male is referred for evaluation of anemia. His past medical history is significant for well-controlled hypertension. He is compliant with his medications, which include aspirin and carvedilol. He is up-to-date on all cancer screenings. He is not sexually active. His laboratory evaluation reveals Hgb 11 g/dL, MCV 83 fL, RDW 14%, ferritin 175 ng/mL, TIBC 200 mcg/dL, transferrin saturation 30%, B12 700 pg/mL, folate >20 ng/mL, and testosterone level of 184 ng/dL.

Introduction
Anemia is a common coexisting disease in patients with endocrine disorders; however, it is not well defined. Thyroid

hormones exert their effects on numerous targets, including the bone marrow, where there is direct stimulation of erythrocyte precursors, as well as effects on transcription of the *EPO* gene and EPO synthesis in the kidneys. The diminished metabolism in hypothyroidism reduces the body's oxygen requirement and likely resets the HIF system, resulting in a decline in EPO synthesis. The underlying mechanism for anemia in the thyrotoxic state, on the other hand, is more conspicuous. It is hypothesized that a combination of coexisting nutritional deficiencies, immune-mediated hemolysis, and increased susceptibility to oxidative stress may result in shortened erythrocyte survival. Another consideration is a dilutional state induced by increased plasma volume in the setting of hyperthyroidism. A cohort study identified anemia in 40.9% of patients with overt hyperthyroidism and 57.1% of patients with overt hypothyroidism. Data for subclinical hypothyroidism are conflicting. An interesting finding is the association of subclinical hypothyroidism and IDA. Numerous studies have shown that concomitant iron and thyroid supplementation produces the best results in treating iron deficiency, even in the setting of subclinical hypothyroidism. Iron plays an essential role in thyroid peroxidase activity, and thus thyroid production synthesis. Therefore, anemia refractory to adequate iron supplementation should elicit a further diagnostic evaluation that includes thyroid studies (21).

Testosterone stimulates burst forming unit (BFU) and colony forming unit (CFU) nuclear receptors and enhances their proliferation. It is also hypothesized that testosterone stimulates EPO production. There are consistent findings in the literature that androgens have a positive effect on erythropoietic activity, suggesting that low testosterone level is a risk factor for anemia (16).

Diagnostic Criteria

Thyroid function studies should be considered in the initial evaluation of hypoproliferative anemia. Though it is not clear if subclinical hypothyroidism alone accounts for anemia, thyroid replacement may be appropriate when iron deficiency exists. Thyroid-related anemia may be microcytic, normocytic, or macrocytic. RDW may also be increased in anemia associated with thyroid disease.

Anemia secondary to testosterone deficiency is typically normocytic. Free and total testosterone levels should be obtained in males with negative results in the initial anemia evaluation. A definite cutoff does not exist, though a recent trial used a testosterone level of 275 ng/dL as a threshold to initiate testosterone replacement in the management of anemia (16).

Key Diagnostic Dilemma

Normalization of thyroid and testosterone levels may not improve anemia. Nonetheless, if the evaluation for anemia is otherwise unrevealing, it is reasonable to treat the underlying endocrine disorder to determine if there is a therapeutic effect on anemia. There are no well-established thresholds for the Hgb to determine when to initiate treatment. Often, the anemia is mild and incidentally found on routine CBC. If there is no absolute indication to treat the endocrine disorder (i.e., subclinical hypothyroidism) and the anemia is mild and asymptomatic, an alternative approach could be observation.

Prognosis

In thyroid disorders–related anemia, restoration of euthyroid state may improve anemia. Successful treatment of Graves' disease improves anemia in nearly 90% of patients, with the anemia attributed to Graves' disease.

A recent small study has shown that over 50% of older men (age >65) with testosterone level below 275 ng/dL show improvement in Hgb of at least 1 g/dL when treated with testosterone gel compared to <20% of patients treated with placebo after 12 months. Testosterone supplementation is also associated with statistically significant improvement in general health and energy sections of the questionnaire in the study. There are reported improvements in walking ability, sexual desire, and memory, but they do not reach statistical significance (16).

Management

Patients with suspected thyroid-related anemia should be investigated for coexisting iron deficiency. Iron and thyroid replacement can be done concurrently. Of note, patients with anemia may have an increased risk for developing palpitations and anxiety with concurrent thyroid replacement; thus, treatment of iron deficiency should be considered prior to restoration of euthyroid state (21).

Future Directions

Large, prospective, randomized studies to evaluate the treatment effect of endocrine disorders on anemia may provide guidance to identify those patients who will benefit from treatment of underlying endocrine disorder.

Key Points

- Anemia secondary to endocrinologic disorders is often overlooked.
- Thyroid disorders and low testosterone levels in men should be considered and addressed if present in the setting of anemia.

- Patients with endocrine disorders often have coexisting iron deficiency.
- Therapeutic benefit has been demonstrated in restoration of euthyroid states and testosterone replacement. Further studies are needed to look at the side effects.

ANEMIA IN HIV/AIDS

Clinical Case 6.7

A 45-year-old male is referred for evaluation of anemia. His past medical history is significant for recently diagnosed HIV with CD4 count of 150. He was recently started on highly active antiretroviral therapy (HAART). Laboratory evaluation is significant for Hgb of 8.5 g/dL, MCV 82 fL, RDW 14%, platelet count 150/mL, WBC 4.0 × 10⁹ cells/L, ferritin 210 ng/mL, TIBC 150 mcg/dL, and transferrin saturation of 26%.

Introduction

Patients with HIV infection have an increased risk of acquiring opportunistic infections, autoimmune diseases, and malignancies. Hematologic abnormalities including cytopenias are common in untreated disease. Anemia is the second most common hematologic aberration in patients with HIV (after CD4 lymphopenia) with inflammation from HIV and/or associated infections and malignances as the most common etiologies. Direct HIV replication in the bone marrow environment likely accounts for suppressed hematopoiesis via the release of inflammatory cytokines, including transforming growth factor (TGF)-beta, TNF-alpha, and IL-1. Patients have blunted production of and response to EPO. In addition, direct marrow infiltration from malignancies (lymphoma or, less likely, Kaposi sarcoma) or infections (parvovirus, mycobacterial infections, histoplasma, and cytomegalovirus) and medications that may induce myelosuppression or hemolysis may also contribute to anemia in the HIV patient. Anemia is an independent negative predictive factor, regardless of the CD4 count (22).

Diagnostic Criteria

An evaluation for anemia in the HIV-infected patient should mimic the approach in patients without HIV infection, including CBC with differential, peripheral smear, and evaluation for nutritional deficiencies. Close inspection of blood counts in relation to the timing of initiation of myelosuppressive medications commonly used in HIV patients (i.e., HAART, trimethoprim–sulfamethoxazole, ganciclovir, amphotericin B) may identify the drug triggers. The anemia is generally normocytic and normochromic (22).

If severe reticulocytopenia is detected, parvovirus B-19–induced PRCA should be suspected and can be seen even with low levels of B19 antibodies, thus rendering parvovirus IgG and IgM levels unreliable and nondiagnostic. PCR for parvovirus DNA or hybridization is recommended. Pronormoblasts with the arrest of erythrocyte maturation in the bone marrow is the diagnostic hallmark of parvovirus B-19 infection.

Though a bone marrow examination is not indicated in anemia alone, it should be obtained in patients with unexplained fever, multiple cytopenias, suspected bone marrow infection, or malignancy. Leukoerythroblastosis on the peripheral blood smear suggests an infiltrative process in the bone marrow and should also prompt a bone marrow biopsy.

Key Diagnostic Dilemmas

Anemia of chronic inflammation will likely arise after analysis of iron indices. However, patients with HIV may have multiple inflammatory etiologies that warrant further investigation and treatment beyond HAART. Careful inspection for other inflammatory etiologies is warranted when the clinical presentation is not explained by HIV alone.

HIV-associated changes in the bone marrow may have features similar to myelodysplastic syndrome (MDS). Dysplastic changes and altered architecture with variable cellularity are often observed. The main differences between MDS and HIV-associated change, however, are the lack of collagen fibrosis (vs. reticulin fibrosis) and preserved myeloid-to-erythroid ratio in HIV-associated marrow. Eosinophilia and polyclonal plasmacytosis are more commonly seen in HIV-associated bone marrows (22).

A direct Coombs test is frequently included in the diagnostic evaluations for anemia, even when there is no clinical evidence of hemolysis. Though a positive test may occur, autoimmune hemolytic anemia in HIV patients is rare.

Prognosis

Anemia is an independent risk factor for clinical disease progression and mortality in patients with HIV, with Hgb <8 g/dL associated with a threefold increase in disease progression or death compared to less-severe anemia, and a fourfold increase in mortality found in patients with Hgb <6.5 g/dL (18). However, this finding likely reflects the severity of the HIV infection and associated comorbidities and is not solely due to anemia.

Management

The first priority in treatment of HIV-associated anemia is adequate control of HIV replication through HAART initiation and compliance.

Improvement in anemia can be seen as early as 2 to 3 months, with the maximal response seen after 12 months. Other inflammatory etiologies driving the anemia, as well as all nutritional deficiencies, should be addressed. Though EPO therapy can be considered in symptomatic patients with lower Hgb levels (<9–10 g/dL), this is often not necessary and does not improve survival or reduce transfusion requirement.

Treatment of parvovirus-induced PRCA should start with IV immunoglobulin (IVIG) 0.4 g/kg daily for 5 days. Relapses are common if the immunodeficiency is left untreated. Monthly maintenance IVIG may be needed in relapsed cases. Immune reconstitution after HAART is the ultimate treatment for this disease (22).

Key Points

- Anemia in HIV is multifactorial.
- Coexisting nutritional deficiencies should be treated.
- HAART is the ultimate treatment in the management of anemia associated with HIV.

ACQUIRED RED CELL APLASIA

Clinical Case 6.8

A 42-year -old male with HIV is referred for evaluation of anemia. His past medical history is significant for HIV, well controlled on HAART, with a CD4 count of 350. His laboratory evaluation is significant for Hgb of 5.5 g/dL, MCV 80 fL, RDW 13%, platelet count 180/mL, WBC 4.2 × 10⁹ cells/L, ferritin 210 ng/mL, TIBC 150 mcg/dL, transferrin saturation 26%, B12 600 pg/mL, folate >20 ng/mL, and undetectable reticulocyte count. Three weeks prior to presentation, his Hgb value was 11.2 g/dL.

Introduction

PRCA is characterized by a complete absence of erythropoiesis. Primary PRCA is mostly autoimmune in origin. Proposed immune-mediated mechanisms include antibody or direct cytotoxic T lymphocyte (CTL)-mediated destruction of erythrocyte precursors, as well as cytokine production from CTLs, which inhibit erythrocyte differentiation (23).

Secondary PRCA is associated with thymoma, hematologic malignancies (most notably, large granular lymphocyte [LGL] leukemia), solid tumors (i.e., renal cell carcinoma, thyroid cancer) infections, autoimmune diseases, drugs, and pregnancy. In parvovirus B19, the virus directly attacks the blood group P antigen, resulting in maturation arrest beyond proerythroblast stage. Infected individuals tend to have lifelong immunity to parvovirus after transient red cell reduction during an acute infection. Transient aplastic crisis can be seen in patients with other conditions which increase red cell turnover (e.g., sickle cell disease, hereditary spherocytosis). Chronic aplasia can be seen in immunocompromised patients, as described in HIV-infected patients. Several other viruses such as Epstein–Barr virus (EBV), cytomegalovirus (CMV), human T-cell leukemia virus type 1 (HTLV-1), and hepatitis viruses have also been associated with PRCA. Pregnancy-related PRCA is self-limiting and tends to resolve postpartum, with a high chance of relapse during subsequent pregnancies. PRCA may be observed post-allogeneic stem cell transplantation due to ABO incompatibility and inhibition of donor erythroid precursors by residual recipient T cells in non-myeloablative cases (23).

Diagnostic Criteria

Blood count and peripheral blood smear generally reveal normocytic and normochromic anemia with absence of reticulocytes and normal WBC and platelet count. Reticulocyte count must be <1%. A reticulocyte count >2% excludes the diagnosis (23).

Bone marrow examination generally reveals absent or greatly diminished numbers of erythroid cells (few proerythroblasts) with normal granulocytic, monocytic, and megakaryocytic cell lines. A clonal lymphoproliferative process, such as LGL leukemia, should be excluded.

Once a diagnosis of PRCA is established, attention should focus on the etiology. Patients should be screened for parvovirus, EBV, CMV, HTLV-1, and HIV infections. Parvovirus polymerase chain reaction (PCR) has a high negative predictive value, with negative values completely excluding parvovirus-mediated disease. Chest x-ray (CXR) and CT of the chest may reveal the presence of thymoma. Pregnancy test should be obtained in females of childbearing age. Anti-EPO antibodies, anti-nuclear antibodies, and complement levels should be considered to evaluate for coexisting autoimmune diseases in the appropriate clinical setting.

Key Diagnostic Dilemma

Though PRCA can typically be differentiated from most bone marrow failure syndromes, idiopathic PRCA and MDS with erythroid hypoplasia may be more difficult. Cytogenetics and fluorescence in situ hybridization (FISH) analysis may be helpful in such cases (23).

Prognosis

Prognosis of PRCA depends on the underlying disease. Overall, complete remission is observed in 70% of patients, with spontaneous remission in 5% to 10% of cases. Relapses are common and generally occur within the first year. Rechallenge with remitting regimen is recommended. Evolution to aplastic anemia or acute leukemia is very rare. Most patients in second remission will stay on low-dose immunosuppressive therapies (23).

Management

Immunosuppression is the cornerstone of treatment of most cases of PRCA. Prednisone at 1 mg/kg/d can induce remission in 40% of patients after 6 weeks of treatment. Slow steroid taper over 12 weeks is recommended to minimize the risk of relapse. Prednisone should be withdrawn if no response is observed within 8 weeks.

Treatment of relapsed or refractory PRCA or secondary PRCA include cyclosporine (especially in the setting of LGL leukemia), oral cyclophosphamide, azathioprine, antithymocyte globulin, rituximab (especially in B-cell malignancies, EBV infection, or post-allogeneic stem cell transplants), and alemtuzumab. Concurrent prednisone and cyclosporine may increase the response rates to 60% to 80%. Cyclosporine should be continued for 6 months with a slow taper in responsive cases. Cyclosporine should be discontinued if there is no response after 3 months (23).

In the setting of drug-induced PRCA, remission can be observed within 1 month after withdrawal of the offending drugs without initiation of immunosuppression. Thymectomy can induce remission in 30% to 40% of thymoma-associated PRCA cases (23).

Key Points

- PRCA should be suspected when anemia is associated with severe reticulocytopenia.
- Immunosuppression, often prednisone as the first-line therapy, is primarily used in the treatment of primary and most cases of secondary PRCA.
- Thymectomy may induce remission in 30% to 40% of all thymoma-associated PRCA cases.

ANEMIA OF LIVER DISEASE

Clinical Case 6.9

A 56-year-old male is referred for evaluation of anemia. His past medical history is significant for alcoholism and cirrhosis. His medications include furosemide and spironolactone. Spleen is palpable 3 cm below the left costal margin. Pertinent laboratory evaluation shows Hgb of 10.2 g/dL, MCV 105 fL, RDW 17%, platelet count of 100 K/µL, WBC 4.0 × 10⁹ cells/L, ferritin 150 ng/mL, TIBC 150 mcg/dL, transferrin saturation 26%, folate 15 ng/mL, and B12 445 pg/mL. Aspartate transaminase (AST) is 52 U/L and ALT is 20 U/L. Total bilirubin is 2.5 mg/dL with a direct bilirubin of 2.0 mg/dL. Serum albumin is 2.5 g/dL. Peripheral smear shows ovalocytes with occasional target cells and acanthocytes. Platelets are reduced with occasional large forms.

Introduction

Normal liver function is essential for hematopoiesis, as it harbors the site for the production of numerous hematopoietic growth factors. Seventy-five percent of patients with liver disease have cytopenias. Anemia in liver disease is multifactorial, often attributed to portal hypertension, which leads to acute and chronic GI blood loss and splenic sequestration, alcohol toxicity, which may cause direct marrow suppression, nutritional deficiencies, and spur cell anemia, which is a form of extravascular hemolysis in which abnormal lipid metabolism causes alteration in shape and size of the RBC membrane, resulting in damage and/or clearance by the spleen (24).

Diagnostic Criteria

Standard diagnostic evaluation for anemia, including reticulocyte count and assessment for vitamin deficiencies, and thyroid function tests are warranted. Peripheral blood smear evaluation to assess for target cells, macroovalocytes, and/or acanthocytes is the most sensitive diagnostic study to correlate the liver disease with anemia, as there is no specific laboratory abnormality to confirm the diagnosis (Figure 6.3). Social history is also very important, particularly to evaluate alcohol intake, as this will not be detected in laboratory workup. If GI blood loss is suspected, gastroenterology referral is warranted.

Key Diagnostic Dilemma

Macrocytic anemia due to liver failure is generally a diagnosis of exclusion following a thorough history and physical and anemia evaluation. Peripheral smear analysis is the key. A frequent concern in anemic patients with liver disease is hemolysis. As part of an anemia evaluation, low haptoglobin and increased LDH may be detected in patients with anemia and liver disease. This may prompt further evaluation with a direct antiglobulin test (DAT). A negative DAT essentially rules out immune-mediated hemolysis. However, weak or moderately positive DAT, which may be observed in normal subjects, may confuse the picture. Haptoglobin is produced in the liver and is often suppressed in patients with hepatic dysfunction. Furthermore, spur cell hemolysis may occur in advanced cirrhosis, and thus may cause a mild-to-moderate elevation of LDH. If there is a positive DAT, peripheral smear is crucial in differentiating immune-mediated hemolysis (presence of spherocytes on peripheral smear) from spur cell hemolysis. Autoimmune hemolytic anemia related to hepatitis B or C is rare. However, as with other autoimmune diseases, immune-mediated hemolysis should be considered in the setting of autoimmune hepatitis or primary biliary cirrhosis.

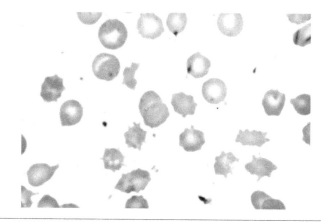

Figure 6.3 Peripheral smear of a patient with liver disease. Acanthocytes are noted throughout the smear.

Management

Treatment should be directed toward the underlying causes of liver disease, including cessation of hepatotoxic agents, vitamin supplementation for vitamin deficiencies, identification and management of GI bleeding, management of hepatitis B and C, and liver transplantation for spur cell anemia associated with severe liver disease. Iron deficiency should be corrected, and standard principles of transfusion should be applied.

Key Points

- Hematologic problems can be observed in up to 75% of patients with liver disease.
- Demonstration of acanthocytes, target cells, and/or macroovalocytes supports liver disease as the etiology for anemia.
- Spur cell anemia is a form of extravascular hemolysis anemia found in severe liver disease.
- Treatment should be directed toward the underlying causes of liver disease, along with any associated vitamin or mineral deficiencies.

ANEMIA OF MALIGNANCY

Clinical Case 6.10

A 37-year-old woman with newly diagnosed metastatic estrogen receptor (ER)-positive breast cancer and diffuse bone metastases is referred for anemia.

Medical history is significant for depression. Several family members have a BRCA2 mutation. She takes sertraline. Laboratory evaluation shows Hgb of 9.0 g/dL, MCV 85 fL, RDW 14%, platelet count of 180 K/μL, WBC 4.0 × 10^9 cells/L, ferritin 700 ng/mL, TIBC 100 mcg/dL, transferrin saturation 4%, folate 15 ng/mL, B12 700 pg/mL, and creatinine 1.2 mg/dL.

Introduction

Some studies suggest that anemia can be seen in up to 30% of patients with early-stage cancers. This number increases to 90% in patients with advanced-stage cancers. Pathogenesis is generally multifactorial and includes blood loss, inadequate erythrocyte production, and increased RBC destruction. Bone marrow invasion, nutritional deficiencies, inflammatory states, hormonal deficiencies, and iatrogenic blood loss can all contribute to hypoproliferative anemia in cancer patients.

Marrow fibrosis, chemotherapy, and tumor invasion can reduce the bone marrow's ability to produce erythrocytes. In terms of nutritional deficiencies, iron deficiency is the most common abnormality, which can be seen in up to 60% of all cancer patients. As in ACD, cancer patients have elevated serum cytokines and hepcidin due to ongoing systemic inflammation. Cytokines such as IL-6 and TNF-$\alpha\lambda\pi\eta\alpha$ inhibit erythropoiesis both directly and indirectly. Hepcidin also indirectly inhibits erythropoiesis by decreasing the level of physiologically available iron. Lastly, therapies for cancer have hematologic side effects. Most of the conventional chemotherapeutic agents suppress bone marrow production, often in a cumulative, dose-dependent fashion (25).

Diagnostic Criteria

A routine anemia evaluation to exclude coexisting nutritional deficiencies, renal or liver disease, and endocrine disorders is warranted. Special attention should be directed to treatment history and chronicity of anemia. Bleeding or RBC destruction should be considered in patients with either an abrupt or rapidly declining hematocrit. Peripheral smear evaluation is again important, particularly in cancer patients with skeletal metastases, as leukoerythroblastosis may be observed in the setting of bone marrow infiltration (Figure 6.4). Lung cancer, breast cancer, prostate cancer, and sarcoma are the most common solid tumors associated with myelophthisis (26). Microangiopathic hemolytic anemia (MAHA), due to direct endothelial damage or disseminated intravascular coagulation (DIC), should also be considered particularly in the setting of concomitant thrombocytopenia in patients with disseminated mucin-producing adenocarcinomas, such as pancreatic cancer and gastric cancer. Peripheral smear would show

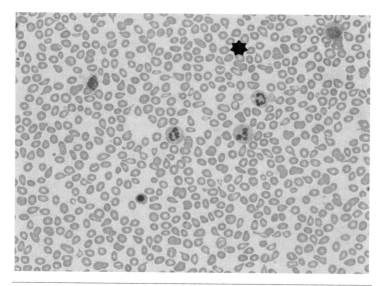

Figure 6.4 Peripheral smear of a patient with metastatic breast cancer and bone metastases with leukoerythroblastosis. The bottom blue cell highlights a nucleated red blood cell. The left upper asterisk is above a teardrop cell. The right upper asterisk highlights a myelocyte.

schistocytes. Hemolysis markers, along with evaluation for DIC (coagulation profile, fibrinogen, and fibrin split products [i.e., D-dimer]) should be ordered. DIC may also be accompanied by thrombosis and/or bleeding, though a subclinical case may only reveal lab derangements.

Key Diagnostic Dilemma

Identification of an etiology for anemia may be challenging, particularly after cancer treatment is initiated. An anemia evaluation at the time of diagnosis to document a cause for the anemia is recommended. Correctible causes of anemia may be addressed prior to or concurrently with cancer treatment. Though it may be tempting to blame underlying cancer inflammation or myelotoxic therapy for the anemia, the clinician should remain vigilant for less-common etiologies such as myelophthisis or MAHA, as these diagnoses carry prognostic implications that could alter treatment decisions.

Prognosis

Anemia is rarely directly prognostic in cancer patients. However, it may affect the quality of life, which is indeed prognostic and may impact the patient's tolerance of and eligibility for cancer treatment.

In addition, the anemia may reflect the severity of disease, such as in myelophthisis, which signifies advanced stages and correlates with a poorer prognosis.

Management

Treatment of malignancy-associated anemia depends on the underlying mechanisms. For symptomatic or actively bleeding patients, RBC transfusions remain the most effective treatment. In hemodynamically stable patients with vitamin deficiencies, such as iron deficiency, adequate nutritional supplementation (i.e., iron supplementation) is recommended.

The role of EPO-stimulating agents for cancer-associated anemia has been challenged by reports of increased rate of cardiac events, thromboembolic events, cancer progression, and lower overall survival, despite their efficacy in increasing Hgb level and decreasing transfusion requirements by 50%. The American Society of Clinical Oncology and the American Society of Hematology have recently updated clinical practice guidelines to resolve some of the concerns about the safety of ESAs in cancer-associated anemia and they are outlined as follows (27). Discussion with patients about the risks and benefits of ESA therapy remains paramount.

- ESAs may be offered to patients with **non-curative** cancers with chemotherapy-associated anemia and Hgb <10 g/dL. RBC transfusions are an acceptable alternative.
- ESAs are not appropriate in most cases of cancer-associated anemia not associated with myelosuppressive therapy, excluding low-risk MDS with serum EPO level <500 IU/L.
- In patients with hematologic malignancies (i.e., multiple myeloma, non-Hodgkin lymphoma, chronic lymphocytic leukemia), ESAs should not be considered until anemia has not appropriately responded to cancer-directed therapy first.
- Address all reversible causes of anemia prior to consideration of ESAs.
- All available formulations of ESAs, including biosimilars, are equally effective and safe.
- ESAs are associated with an increased risk of thromboembolism.
- ESA dosing should follow U.S. Food and Drug Administration (FDA) guidelines.
- ESAs should be discontinued if a hematologic response is not achieved within 6 to 8 weeks.
- Adequate iron supplementation complements the effect of ESAs in cancer-associated anemia, warranting baseline and periodic iron studies.

Key Points

- The mechanisms underlying malignancy-associated anemia are multifactorial and include bone marrow pathology from the cancer itself and/or treatment, nutritional deficiencies, inflammatory states, and hormonal deficiencies.
- Identification of reversible causes of anemia at diagnosis is recommended.
- ESAs may be offered in cancer-associated anemia in non-curative cancers and in the setting of myelosuppressive therapy; however, the risks should be considered and discussed with each patient.

REFERENCES

1. Lin JC. Chapter 34 - Approach to anemia in the adult and child. In: Hoffman R, Benz EJ, Silberstein LE, et al., eds. *Hematology*. 7th ed. Elsevier; 2018:458–467.
2. Camaschella C. Iron-deficiency anemia. *N Engl J Med*. 2015;372(19):1832–1843. doi:10.1056/NEJMra1401038
3. Kawasugi K, Yamamoto T, Shirafuji N, Oka Y. Increased levels of thrombopoietin and IPF in patients with iron deficiency anemia [abstract]. *Blood*. 2014;124:5018.
4. Dignass A, Farrag K, Stein J. Limitations of serum ferritin in diagnosing iron deficiency in inflammatory conditions. *Int J Chronic Dis*. 2018;2018:1–11. doi:10.1155/2018/9394060
5. Stoffel NU, Cercamondi CI, Brittenham G, et al. Iron absorption from oral iron supplements given on consecutive versus alternate days and as single morning doses versus twice-daily split dosing in iron-depleted women: two open-label, randomised controlled trials. *Lancet Haematol*. 2017;4(11):e524. doi:10.1016/S2352-3026(17)30182-5
6. Auerbach M, Macdougall I. The available intravenous iron formulations: history, efficacy, and toxicology. *Hemodial Int*. 2017;21:S83–S92. doi:10.1111/hdi.12560
7. Lexicomp Online. *Lexi-Drugs Online*. Hudson, OH: Wolters Kluwer Clinical Drug Information, Inc.; 2019.
8. Nayak L, Gardner LB, Little JA. Chapter 37 - Anemia of chronic diseases. In: Hoffman R, Benz EJ, Silberstein LE, et al., eds. *Hematology*. 7th ed. New York, NY: Elsevier; 2018:491–496.
9. Fraenkel PG. Understanding anemia of chronic disease. *Hematology*. 2015;2015(1):14–18. doi:10.1182/asheducation-2015.1.14

10. Hébert PC, Wells G, Blajchman MA, et al. A multicenter, randomized, controlled clinical trial of transfusion requirements in critical care. *N Engl J Med.* 1999;340(6):409–417. doi:10.1056/NEJM199902113400601

11. Hannibal L, Lysne V, Bjørke-Monsen A, et al. Biomarkers and algorithms for the diagnosis of Vitamin B12 deficiency. *Front Mol Biosci.* 2016;3:27. doi:10.3389/fmolb.2016.00027

12. Antony AC. Chapter 39 - Megaloblastic anemias. In: Hoffman R, Benz EJ, Silberstein LE, et al., eds. *Hematology.* 7th ed. New York, NY: Elsevier; 2018:514–545.e7.

13. Fuller SJ, Wiley JS. Chapter 38 - Heme biosynthesis and its disorders: Porphyrias and sideroblastic anemias. In: Hoffman R, Benz EJ, Silberstein LE, et al., eds. *Hematology.* 7th ed. New York, NY: Elsevier; 2018:497–513.e6.

14. Di Renzo GC, Spano F, Giardina I, et al. Iron deficiency anemia in pregnancy. *Womens Health.* 2015;11(6):891–900. doi:10.2217/whe.15.35

15. Achebe MM, Gafter-Gvili A. How I treat anemia in pregnancy: iron, cobalamin, and folate. *Blood.* 2017;129(8):940. doi:10.1182/blood-2016-08-672246

16. Roy CN, Snyder PJ, Stephens-Shields A, et al. Association of testosterone levels with anemia in older men: a controlled clinical trial. *JAMA Intern Med.* 2017;177(4):480–490. doi:10.1001/jamainternmed.2016.9540

17. Fishbane S, Spinowitz B. Update on anemia in ESRD and earlier stages of CKD: core curriculum 2018. *Am J Kidney Dis.* 2018;71(3):423–435. doi:10.1053/j.ajkd.2017.09.026

18. Kidney Disease: Improving Global Outcomes (KDIGO) Anemia Work Group. KDIGO clinical practice guideline for anemia in chronic kidney disease. *Kidney Int Suppl.* 2012;2(4):279–335.

19. Hutchison CA, Harding S, Hewins P, et al. Quantitative assessment of serum and urinary polyclonal free light chains in patients with chronic kidney disease. *Clin J Am Soc Nephrol.* 2008;3(6):1684–1690. doi:10.2215/CJN.02290508

20. Coyne DW, Goldsmith D, Macdougall IC. New options for the anemia of chronic kidney disease. *Kidney Int Suppl.* 2017;7(3):157–163. doi:10.1016/j.kisu.2017.09.002

21. Szczepanek-Parulska E, Hernik A, Ruchała M. Anemia in thyroid diseases. *Pol Arch Intern Med.* 2017;127(5):352–360. doi:10.20452/pamw.3985

22. Liebman HA, Tulpule A. Chapter 157 - Hematologic manifestations of HIV/AIDS. In: Hoffman R, Benz EJ, Silberstein LE, et al., eds. *Hematology.* 7th ed. NewYork, NY: Elsevier; 2018:2262–2277.

23. Maciejewski JP, Thota S. Chapter 32 - Acquired disorders of red cell, white cell, and platelet production. In: Hoffman R, Benz EJ, Silberstein LE, et al., eds. *Hematology*. 7th ed. New York, NY: Elsevier; 2018:425–444.e5.

24. Hillis C, Lim W. Chapter 153 - Hematologic manifestations of liver disease. In: Hoffman R, Benz EJ, Silberstein LE, et al., eds. *Hematology*. 7th ed. New York, NY: Elsevier; 2018:2238–2243.

25. Widick P, Brunner AM, Schiffman F. Chapter 155 - Hematologic manifestations of malignancy. In: Hoffman R, Benz EJ, Silberstein LE, et al., eds. *Hematology*. 7th ed. New York, NY: Elsevier; 2018:2247–2252.

26. Makoni SN, Laber DA. Clinical spectrum of myelophthisis in cancer patients. *Am J Hematol*. 2004;76(1):92–93. doi:10.1002/ajh.20046

27. Bohlius J, Bohlke K, Castelli R, et al. Management of cancer-associated anemia with erythropoiesis-stimulating agents: ASCO/ASH clinical practice guideline update. *Blood Adv*. 2019;3(8):1197. doi:10.1182/bloodadvances.2018030387

Approach to Hemolytic Anemias

Iberia Romina Sosa, Harish Madala, and Mark Udden

HEMOLYTIC ANEMIA

Introduction

Hemolytic anemias are proliferative anemias, characterized by a shortened red blood cell (RBC) life span and normal bone marrow function. The bone marrow can increase red cell production substantially in some circumstances, such as hereditary elliptocytosis (HE), where there is hemolysis with a normal hemoglobin (Hgb) and hematocrit (HCT)—a compensated hemolytic anemia. The human RBC is remarkably durable and enjoys a life span of 120 days. A shortened RBC life span may be caused by intrinsic defects, which include disorders of the RBC membrane, mutations affecting enzymatic function, or abnormalities of Hgb. Extrinsic causes of premature RBC destruction include immunologic conditions such as autoimmune hemolytic anemia (AIHA); disorders which cause fragmentation hemolysis such as microangiopathic hemolytic anemia (MAHA), and a wide variety of exposures to physical agents such as heat, toxins, and microbial infection. Intrinsic defects are generally hereditary and extrinsic defects are often acquired, with exceptions. For example, thrombotic thrombocytopenic purpura (TTP), a MAHA caused by deficiency of the metalloproteinase ADAMST13, is most often due to an acquired antibody inhibitor of this enzyme, but can be due to a germline mutation affecting the function or production of the metalloproteinase. Response to transfusion therapy differs among the hemolytic anemias. Transfused RBCs have a longer effect in intrinsic disorders, whereas transfused red cells fall prey to environmental factors in extrinsic hemolytic disorders. Only about 30% of anemia is attributable to hemolysis—iron deficiency, thalassemia, and anemia of chronic inflammation are much more common.

Diagnosis

The presence of young RBCs or reticulocytosis is the primary laboratory abnormality in hemolytic anemias. Reticulocytes are increased when RBC production in the marrow is increased. On Wright Giemsa stain, reticulocytes have bluish cytoplasm, or polychromasia, and are often larger than mature RBCs and persist approximately 1 day in the circulation. Given the 120-day life span of the mature RBC, approximately 1% of cells need to be replaced each day, accounting for the normal range for reticulocytes of 1% to 2%. Knowing the RBC count and the percent of reticulocytes, one can calculate the absolute reticulocyte count, which is typically 40 to 70,000/μL. The reticulocyte production index (RPI) is a handy assessment of the reticulocyte response in hemolytic disorders. This index takes into account two reasons for the reticulocytes to increase: A normal number of reticulocytes released each day will result in a higher percent when there is a decreased RBC count, and reticulocytes emerge up to 3 days earlier when there is a very high erythropoietin level. The calculation is:

$$RPI = \% \text{ reticulocytes} \times \frac{(HCT)}{45} \times \frac{1}{MF}$$

where the maturation factor (MF) is 1.0 for an HCT of 45 and increases by 0.5 for each drop in the HCT by 10% (i.e., 1.5 for an HCT of 35, 2.0 for an HCT of 25, and 2.5 for an HCT of 15). The MF adds half a day to the reticulocyte life span for every drop in the HCT by 10%. If the HCT is 15% and the reticulocyte count is 15%, the RPI will be 2. An RPI of 2 or greater is consistent with an adequate bone marrow response in proliferative anemias. The reticulocyte count should be high in hemolytic anemia, except in situations where hemolysis coexists with problems that blunt the erythropoietic response. These may include renal failure, iron or folate deficiency, or anemia of inflammation.

Hemolysis can be categorized as being extravascular (macrophages in spleen, liver, or bone marrow) and/or intravascular (within blood vessels). In extravascular hemolysis, the reticulocyte count is elevated and indirect bilirubin may be increased. The increase in bilirubin reflects the increased turnover of RBC, manifested by cleavage of the heme ring by heme oxygenase (HO), resulting in release of iron (Fe^{2+}), water, and carbon monoxide (CO), along with biliverdin. Biliverdin is converted to bilirubin by biliverdin reductase, which is conjugated in the liver to monoglucuronide and diglucuronide forms, which are then excreted in the bile. In a healthy liver, hemolysis increases the total bilirubin up to 5.0 mg/dL and usually 80% to 90% of this is indirect and not water soluble. Hemolysis may result in jaundice without changes in the urine color—so-called acholuric jaundice. In intravascular hemolysis, the RBC perishes in the bloodstream, Hb disperses into dimers, and the dimers are bound by haptoglobin and cleared. The heme ring is also released and bound by hemopexin. Red cells contain lactate dehydrogenase (LDH), which is released in intravascular hemolysis. The hallmark of intravascular hemolysis is an increase in serum LDH and low haptoglobin, in addition to increased indirect bilirubin and elevated reticulocyte count.

Examination of the peripheral blood smear is key in the evaluation of hemolytic anemias—most often, there is a clue to the disorder in the RBC morphology. The presence of polychromatophilic RBCs is an indication that RBC production is increased. Specific abnormalities are covered in this chapter. Normal RBC morphology and a high reticulocyte count should prompt a search for bleeding.

Personal and family histories are essential to diagnosing hemolytic anemias. The patient may give a history of intermittent jaundice, suggesting prior hemolysis and a congenital reason for hemolytic anemia. A history of gallstones in a younger patient or a family history of gallstones or splenectomy may also be clues. Mild icterus and splenomegaly are clinical clues during physical exam. A rule of thumb is that a drop in the Hgb of more than one gram per week suggests the presence of hemolysis. Increased indirect bilirubin often occurs and when there is intravascular hemolysis, there will also be elevation of LDH and a low haptoglobin. Low haptoglobins may also be seen in patients with liver disease and in those with ineffective erythropoiesis.

Key Diagnostic Dilemma

Hemolysis is associated with a constellation of labs that may be seen in other conditions. A high reticulocyte count is characteristic of hemolysis, but may also be seen in response to blood loss; nutritional replacement with B12, folate, or iron in the deficient individual with anemia also causes a high reticulocyte count. A high reticulocyte count can be seen when the marrow sinusoidal barrier is disordered by fibrosis (myelofibrosis) or other myelophthisic process. Indirect hyperbilirubinemia may be seen in Gilbert's syndrome, a benign disorder associated with a mutation in *UGT1A1*. Ineffective erythropoiesis in pernicious anemia and other disorders also results in lab values suggestive of hemolysis: elevated indirect bilirubin, LDH (can be in the thousands), and a low haptoglobin.

Management

Treatment of hemolytic anemias can range from supportive care to immunosuppression and depends on the underlying mechanism for hemolysis.

Key Points

1. Examination of the peripheral smear is essential in the workup of hemolysis. The finding of spherocytes, elliptocytes, stomatocytes, blister cells, and fragmented RBCs or sickle forms can focus the workup.
2. An elevated reticulocyte count and indirect bilirubin are the main findings supporting hemolysis, both extravascular and intravascular. Extravascular hemolysis is associated with the additional findings of increased LDH and low haptoglobin.

RBC MEMBRANE DISORDERS

Clinical Case 7.1

A 27-year-old woman presents with mild fatigue for a few weeks. She reports intermittent jaundice and a cholecystectomy for gallstones. Laboratory shows an Hgb of 9 g/dL, with a mean corpuscular volume (MCV) of 84 fL and mean cell Hgb concentration (MCHC) of 37 g/dL. On physical exam, she has mild pallor and mild splenomegaly. Her father and paternal cousin also had anemia. Peripheral blood smear is shown in Figure 7.1.

Diagnosis: hereditary spherocytosis

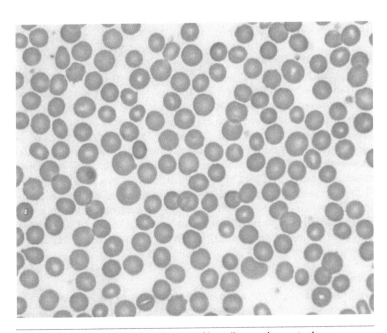

Figure 7.1 Peripheral smear of hereditary spherocytosis.

Overview

The normal RBC is very deformable and can navigate small blood vessels and pores in the splenic pulp. The cell is strong enough to withstand shearing forces in the arterioles. These properties are possible due to the lipid bilayer and the RBC cytoskeleton as depicted in Figure 7.2. The structural integrity of the RBC membrane is provided by the cytoskeletal proteins, band 3, glycophorin C, and RhAG, that link the bilayer to the spectrin-based membrane cytoskeleton. Vertical interactions are perpendicular to the plane of the membrane and involve a spectrin–ankyrin–band 3 association facilitated by protein 4.2 and attachment of spectrin–actin–protein 4.1 junctional complexes to glycophorin C (Figure 7.2) (1). Horizontal interactions, which are parallel to and underlying the plane of the membrane, involve the assembly of alpha- and beta-spectrin chains into heterodimers, which self-associate to form tetramers (Figure 7.2). Distal ends of spectrin bind to actin, with the aid of protein 4.1 and other minor proteins.

Hemolytic anemias due to abnormalities of the erythrocyte membrane comprise an important group of inherited disorders. These include hereditary spherocytosis (HS), HE, hereditary pyropoikilocytosis (HPP), and hereditary stomatocytosis (HSt) syndromes. The involved membrane and skeleton proteins are described in Table 7.1. Mutations in the vertical associations typically result in loss of the lipid bilayer and spherocytosis, while mutations in the horizontal interaction typically result in loss of membrane plasticity and elliptocytosis.

HEREDITARY SPHEROCYTOSIS

Introduction

The HS syndromes are a group of autosomal dominant inherited disorders characterized by the presence of spherical erythrocytes

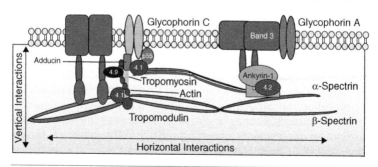

Figure 7.2 RBC membrane cytoskeleton.

RBC, red blood cell.

Table 7.1 Mutations in Inherited Human Red Cell Membrane Disorders

Spherocytosis	
Ankyrin	50% to 60%
Spectrin	20%
Band 3	15% to 20%
Protein 4.2	5%
Elliptocytosis	
Alpha-spectrin	65%
Beta-spectrin	30%
Protein 4.1	5%
Ovalocytosis	
Band 3	100%

on blood smear. In HS, there is loss of membrane surface compared to volume, which is the result of defective anchoring of the lipid bilayer to the cytoskeleton due to mutations in proteins responsible for the vertical interactions depicted in Figure 7.2 (1). A common cause is a defect in production of the protein, ankyrin. The lipid bilayer is untethered to the cytoskeleton and is unstable, leading to small losses of membrane surface. This loss of lipid membrane is accentuated by unfavorable conditions in the spleen ("splenic conditioning"), where with each passage, cells become more spherical until they are finally retained there by macrophages. HS is an extravascular hemolytic disorder. The spleen is a key player in RBC destruction, thus splenectomy may normalize the Hgb, although the RBC morphology remains spherocytic.

Diagnosis

HS is characterized by anemia, splenomegaly, jaundice, and gallstones. A family history of anemia, gallstones, and splenectomy may be present. About 10% of newly diagnosed patients represent new mutations and may not have a family history. Physical examination may reveal icterus and splenomegaly. Typical lab findings include mild-to-moderate anemia and markers of ongoing hemolysis including reticulocytosis and increased bilirubin. Elevated LDH and low haptoglobin may not be present because the hemolysis is primarily extravascular—occurring mostly in the spleen. A typical finding in HS is an elevated MCHC.

Hemolytic, aplastic, and megaloblastic crises may occur (1). Hemolytic crises are usually precipitated by a viral illness, are common in children, and are characterized by anemia, jaundice, increased splenomegaly, and reticulocytosis. Aplastic crisis is most commonly associated with parvovirus B19 infection. This virus has a tropism for red cell precursors in the marrow. Giant pronormoblasts are seen in the bone marrow aspirate, and erythropoiesis ceases for 10 to 14 days. The reticulocyte count is typically 0.1% during an aplastic crisis. In patients with severe HS, transfusion is an absolute requirement. Megaloblastic crisis occurs in patients with increased folate demands, like pregnant women, children, and elderly patients. Patients with mild disease who are not known to have HS may first manifest with cholecystitis or aplastic crisis.

Key Diagnostic Dilemma

Peripheral blood smear shows red cells lacking central pallor; many of these cells are small (microspherocytes). A variable degree of polychromasia can be seen. AIHA has the same appearance, and so the workup of HS should include a negative direct antiglobulin test (DAT), also known as Coombs test. The osmotic fragility test reveals increased osmotic fragility either on a fresh or an incubated specimen. Flow cytometric analysis of eosin-5-maleimide binding to erythrocytes reveals reduced binding, reflecting the reduction of Rh-related integral membrane proteins and band 3 in HS diagnosis (1).

Prognosis

Overall, the long-term prognosis for patients with HS is very good with appropriate management. The severity of the condition—mild, moderate, or severe (Table 7.2)—does impact treatment. A major factor contributing to HS mortality is development of

Table 7.2 Classification of Hereditary Spherocytosis				
	Carrier	**Mild**	**Moderate**	**Severe**
Hemoglobin, g/dL	Normal	11 to 15	8 to 12	6 to 8
Reticulocytes, %	<3%	3% to 6%	>6%	>10%
Bilirubin, mg/dL	0 to 1	1 to 2	>2	>2
Peripheral smear	Normal	Mild spherocytosis	Significant spherocytosis	Significant spherocytosis
Osmotic fragility	Normal	Normal to slight increase	Increased	Increased

life-threatening infection from encapsulated organisms in patients who have undergone splenectomy.

Management

Patients with HS typically do well with folic acid supplementation and observation for complications such as cholelithiasis and associated cholecystitis and cholangitis (1). Splenectomy cures or markedly improves the anemia in most HS patients. However, the decision to undergo splenectomy is individualized. Patients with anemia and splenomegaly who are severely symptomatic will benefit from surgery, but post-splenectomy complications, such as increased risk of infection by encapsulated organisms and thrombosis, need to be considered. Partial splenectomy has been done in an effort to improve anemia and preserve the splenic function.

Key Points

1. HS presents with varying degrees of anemia and splenomegaly. The spleen is the primary site of red cell destruction.
2. HS can present at any age and with any severity. The majority of affected individuals have mild or moderate hemolytic anemia.
3. Splenectomy, when indicated effectively, halts hemolysis, although spherocytes may be a persistent finding in the peripheral blood.

HEREDITARY ELLIPTOCYTOSIS AND HEREDITARY PYROPOIKILOCYTOSIS

Introduction

HE is heterogeneous in clinical presentation and severity. Membrane defects in HE and HPP affect the "horizontal" interactions in the membrane skeleton. A common feature of all forms of HE is loss of membrane plasticity, which results in progressive transformation of the cell from discocytes to an elliptocyte or ovalocyte and, in severe cases like HPP, to membrane and RBC fragmentation (1). Variants are described in Table 7.3.

Diagnosis

Most patients with traditional HE are asymptomatic. Occasionally, in homozygotes or compound heterozygotes for one or two molecular defects, more severe hemolytic disease is observed. Approximately 10% of HE patients and all HPP patients have mild-to-moderate anemia with clinical features of pallor, jaundice,

Table 7.3 Hereditary Elliptocytosis Variants

	Genetics	Comments
HE	Autosomal dominant	Smear: Biconcave elliptocytes and in more severe forms, rod-shaped RBCs
Hereditary pyropoikilocytosis	Autosomal recessive: Compound heterozygous or homozygous HE defects	Most severe form of elliptocytosis Defect often in spectrin or protein 4.1 Blood smear often confused with TTP Markedly low MCV (50s) Thermally unstable RBC at 45°C–46°C
Southeast Asian ovalocytosis	Autosomal dominant: genomic mutation in Band 3	Smear: Presence of oval-shaped red cells with one or two transverse ridges or a longitudinal slit on smear Prevalence of 5%–25% in Southeast Asia Rigid RBC membrane Little to no hemolysis

HE, hereditary elliptocytosis; MCV, mean corpuscular volume; RBC, red blood cell; TTP, thrombotic thrombocytopenic purpura.

and gallstones. A markedly low MCV, typically in the range of 50 to 60 fL, may be observed. In HPP, the RBCs are thermally unstable and fragment at lower temperatures compared to RBCs with normal spectrin (1). HPP is characterized by elliptocytosis (Figure 7.3) and a striking poikilocytosis with blebs and fragmentation resulting in a very low MCV—often <50 fL. Southeast Asian ovalocytosis appears to provide some protection against malaria. Most affected individuals experience minimal hemolysis. It has been suggested that the increased rigidity of the membrane could impede the ability of the malarial parasite to effectively invade these red cells, and thereby decrease parasitemia and the clinical severity of malarial infections.

Key Diagnostic Dilemma

Elliptocytes and poikilocytes can be seen on peripheral blood smear in other conditions such as iron deficiency, thalassemia, megaloblastic anemia, myelofibrosis, and myelodysplasia. However, in HE, the percentage of elliptocytes usually exceeds 60%. Additional specialized laboratory investigation may be needed in some cases

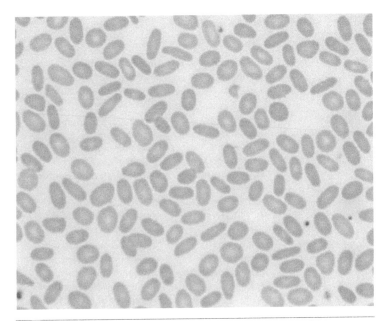

Figure 7.3 Peripheral smear of hereditary elliptocytosis.

to make the diagnosis. This includes separation of solubilized membrane proteins by polyacrylamide gel electrophoresis, which may reveal either an abnormally migrating spectrin or a deficiency or abnormal migration of protein 4.1. An increased fraction of unassembled dimeric spectrin in the extract can be detected by electrophoresis of extracts under non-denaturing conditions.

Prognosis

HE is not common and there is limited information in the medical literature regarding the long-term survival of patients. As in HS, there is nothing to suggest the disease impacts longevity of affected individuals.

Management

Treatment is not necessary for most individuals with common HE. Splenectomy may be of benefit for patients with symptomatic hemolytic anemia.

Key Points

HE is typically mild and may be incidentally recognized when the patient is examined for anemia that is out of proportion to a condition like renal failure or anemia of chronic disease.

OTHER RBC MEMBRANE DISORDERS

Stomatocytosis

Stomatocytes have a wide transverse slit or stoma toward the center of the RBC. A few stomatocytes can be found on the blood smears of healthy individuals or as an artifact. Acquired stomatocytosis can be seen in acute alcoholism and hepatobiliary disease, as well as in malignant neoplasms and cardiovascular disorders.

A very rare autosomal recessive disorder, Rh null, results in loss of the Rh-related protein(s). The Rh null phenotype manifests with stomatocytosis and a chronic hemolytic anemia. These patients can experience complications with transfusions because they are at high risk of producing antibodies against the Rh antigens they lack; hence, they should only receive blood from similarly affected individuals.

HSt is a an autosomal dominant disorder associated with abnormalities in erythrocyte cation channels, resulting in increased RBC Na^+ and overhydration of the cell. Hydrocytosis is marked by stomatocytosis, splenomegaly, and increased RBC osmotic fragility and hemolysis. Xerocytosis is a disorder in which K^+ is lost and the cells are dehydrated. It is marked by osmotic resistance and elevated MCHC. Newborns with these disorders may demonstrate ascites and nonimmune hydrops.

Management

Patients with HSt do not respond to splenectomy and have an increased risk of developing thrombotic events and pulmonary hypertension after splenectomy. Treatment is supportive, and splenectomy should be avoided.

Acanthocytosis

Acanthocytosis, or spur cell anemia, can be inherited or acquired. An acanthocyte typically has a small number of long projections (Figure 7.4). A spur cell is essentially an acanthocyte with one large projection. These cells can be distinguished from echinocytes, which are RBCs with a large number of smaller projections. The echinocyte is often called a burr cell. The autosomal recessive disorder, abetalipoproteinemia, is characterized by the congenital absence of apolipoprotein B in plasma, acanthocytosis, ataxia, and retinitis pigmentosa. Consequently, all plasma lipoproteins containing this apoprotein, as well as plasma triglycerides are nearly absent. Plasma cholesterol and phospholipid levels are markedly reduced. The role of these lipid abnormalities in producing acanthocytes is not well understood. The McCleod phenotype is a rare X-linked disorder in which acanthocytosis is found in association with marked reduction of Kell antigen expression.

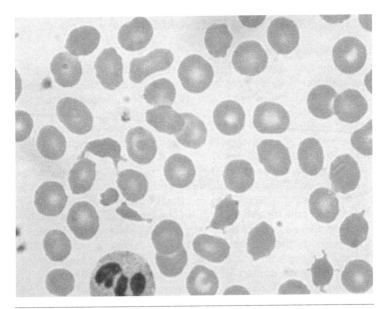

Figure 7.4 Peripheral smear of acanthocytosis, as may occur in liver disease.

Acquired acanthocytosis is associated with advanced or end-stage liver disease. In liver disease, acanthocyte formation is a two-step process involving the transfer of free nonesterified cholesterol from abnormal plasma lipoproteins into the erythrocyte membrane with subsequent remodeling of abnormally shaped erythrocytes by the spleen. Acanthocytes are also seen in patients who have undergone splenectomy or who have disorders such as amyloidosis or celiac disease which result in splenic hypofunction.

RBC ENZYMOPATHIES

Clinical Case 7.2

A 28-year-old man with recently diagnosed HIV/AIDS was started on prophylactic trimethoprim/sulfamethoxazole. He complains of increasing fatigue and dyspnea over a 10-day period. His heart rate is 100/minute, blood pressure (BP) is 89/45 mmHg, and he has new scleral icterus. His Hgb is 6 g/dL, HCT 18%, reticulocyte count 15%, and RPI is 2.5. His LDH is 1,500 and DAT is negative. Peripheral blood smear shows polychromasia with bite and blister RBCs (Figure 7.5).

Diagnosis: Glucose-6 phosphate dehydrogenase (G6PD) deficiency

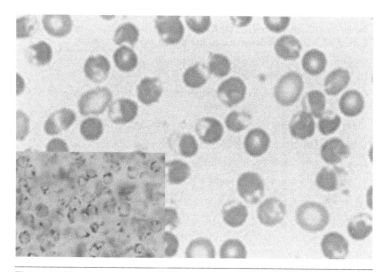

Figure 7.5 Peripheral smear of G6PD deficiency. Blister cells. Inset shows Heinz body stain.

G6PD, glucose-6 phosphate dehydrogenase.

Overview

The glycolytic pathway in RBCs provides adenosine triphosphate (ATP) for the maintenance of RBC membrane and electrolyte balance and 2,3-biphosphoglycerate (2,3-BPG) necessary to modulate the oxygen saturation of Hgb. The hexose monophosphate shunt generates nicotinamide adenine dinucleotide phosphate (reduced form with the H ion) (NADPH) needed to reduce glutathione, so that it can maintain heme iron in the reduced state and prevent oxidant damage to Hb and the RBC membrane. There is also a metabolic pathway for nucleotide salvage which helps to maintain adequate supply of adenine and ATP levels in the RBC.

G6PD DEFICIENCY

Introduction

G6PD deficiency is the most frequently encountered abnormality of RBC metabolism. The *G6PD* gene is on the X chromosome and exhibits extensive polymorphism. Worldwide, over 300 genetic variants of G6PD are described and are categorized according to whether the defect leads to normal activity, moderately deficient activity, or severely deficient activity (Table 7.4), and whether it is associated with hemolytic anemia (2). Most mutations are clinically

Table 7.4 Glucose-6 Phosphate Dehydrogenase Classes to Determine the Extent of Enzyme Deficiency and the Severity of Hemolysis*

Class I	Severely deficient, associated with chronic non-spherocytic hemolytic anemia
Class II	Severely deficient (1%–10% residual activity), associated with acute hemolytic anemia
Class III	Moderately deficient (10%–60% residual activity)
Class IV	Normal activity (60%–150%)
Class V	Increased activity (>150%)

*Class IV and V are of no clinical significance.

silent. G6PD B is the wild-type enzyme. G6PD A+ is a common variant in the African American population, which demonstrates normal enzyme activity. G6PD A– is present in 12% of African American men and 1% of women (Table 7.5) (2). This variant produces an unstable enzyme, which results in moderately reduced enzyme activity in aged RBCs. Other G6PD variants have severely reduced catalytic activity and marked instability or are produced at a decreased rate, rendering both reticulocytes and older cells susceptible to hemolysis. Enzymatic deficiency of this type is seen in Greeks, Italians, Middle Eastern, and Asian populations, as well as Ashkenazi Jews. The common example of this deficiency is the G6PD Mediterranean variant (Table 7.5). G6PD deficiency may protect the carrier during infection with malaria.

Exposure to an oxidant results in depletion of NADPH and oxidation of Hgb and the RBC membrane. Denatured Hgb aggregates form Heinz bodies, which, along with oxidized cell membrane, make the red cells vulnerable to destruction in the spleen. RBCs may also undergo intravascular hemolysis. The degree of hemolysis depends on the type of defect, the level of enzyme activity in the erythrocyte, and the severity of the oxidant challenge. Table 7.6 summarizes the common medications that have been described as G6PD oxidant stressors.

Diagnosis

Initial laboratory tests reveal anemia, hyperbilirubinemia, elevated plasma Hgb, and hemoglobinuria consistent with intravascular hemolysis. Review of the smear will facilitate the diagnosis if key findings are identified: (a) confinement of Hgb to the side of the RBC with the remainder of cell surface being Hgb free (Figure 7.5, blister cell); (b) appearance of bite cells during acute episode; and (c) Heinz bodies revealed with brilliant cresyl blue stain (Figure 7.5, inset).

Table 7.5 Common Glucose-6 Phosphate Dehydrogenase Variants*

Variants	Enzyme Activity/ Class	Ethnicity/Region	Clinical
G6PD B Wild type	Normal catalytic activity Class IV	Caucasians, Asians, and a majority of Blacks	No hemolysis
G6PD A+	Normal catalytic properties	20% to 30% of Blacks from Africa	No hemolysis
Mediterranean	Class II variant Majority of RBCs have grossly deficient enzyme	Greeks, Sephardic Jews, Italians Middle East/ Mediterranean	Hemolysis upon exposure to oxidant Otherwise, no anemia or reticulocytosis
G6PD A−	Class III variant 10% to 15% enzyme activity, but higher in young reticulocytes	African ancestry	Mild-to-moderate hemolysis Sensitivity to primaquine Oldest RBCs undergo hemolysis

*The World Health Organization has classified the different G6PD variants according to the magnitude of the enzyme deficiency and the severity of hemolysis.
G6PD, glucose-6 phosphate dehydrogenase.

The clinical presentation is heterogeneous and linked to the activity level of the enzyme. Patients may experience a chronic hemolytic anemia or have a tendency for acute hemolytic episodes triggered by exogenous agents. Presentations of neonatal jaundice have been reported.

Key Diagnostic Dilemma

Lab values in G6PD deficiency are not unlike those for intravascular hemolysis from other etiologies. Although there is a G6PD enzymatic assay, checking for G6PD activity is not useful during the acute episode. Quantitative G6PD levels should be checked 3 to 4 months (RBC life span) later. Depending on the activity level of the enzyme associated with the patient's variant, the level will be normal during a hemolytic episode due to lysis of the older cells and normal levels in reticulocytes, as can be seen in G6PD A− in

Table 7.6 Glucose-6 Phosphate Dehydrogenase Oxidant Stressors

Acetanilide	Pentaquine
Dapsone	Phenylhydrazine
Dimercaptosuccinic acid	Phenazopyridine
Furazolidone	Primaquine
Glibenclamide	Sulfacetamide
Isobutyl nitrite	Sulfamethoxazole
Methylene blue	Sulfanilamide
Nalidixic acid	Sulfapyridine
Naphthalene	Thiazolesulfone
Niridazole	Toluidine blue
Nitrofurantoin	TNT
Pamaquine	Urate oxidase

TNT, trinitrotoluene.

African Americans (2). A Heinz body stain is more useful during acute hemolysis.

Prognosis

Most patients are asymptomatic and develop problems only when exposed to an oxidative challenge that triggers a hemolytic episode. In newborns, there is an increased risk of neonatal jaundice. The mechanism or risk factors for this observation are not entirely clear. In areas where G6PD deficiency is prevalent, this is probably the most common reason for long-term neurologic consequences in those patients who are not appropriately treated. A fulminant clinical course is a rare complication that may result from acute viral infections (e.g., viral hepatitis A) or oxidant drug exposure. Overall, however, G6PD does not significantly affect life expectancy or quality of life for those affected individuals.

Management

Hemolysis from acute insult is short-lived and rarely requires transfusion. Patients should be advised on how to avoid exposure to oxidant drugs or compounds.

Key Points

1. G6PD deficiency is the most common inherited RBC enzymatic defect, affecting 4 million people worldwide and it is an

important cause of hemolysis in African American men exposed to oxidant drugs.

2. Clinical manifestations include acute hemolytic anemia typically in response to medications.
3. Heinz body stain can be useful in the acute hemolytic episode.
4. Measurement of G6PD activity should be deferred for 3 to 4 months, so that the patient's low baseline level can be recognized.
5. Management of patients with G6PD deficiency depends on the severity of the deficiency and the clinical scenario.

PYRUVATE KINASE DEFICIENCY

Introduction

Pyruvate kinase (PK) deficiency is the most important hemolytic anemia arising from defects in the glycolytic pathway. PK deficiency is rare, with an estimated prevalence of <50 cases per million individuals, primarily of northern European descent (3). Table 7.7 summarizes other rare enzymatic defects of the glycolytic pathway that result in hemolytic anemias.

PK deficiency causes depletion of RBC ATP required for the ATPase-linked sodium–potassium and calcium membrane pumps essential for cation homeostasis, as well as for the maintenance of erythrocyte shape and flexibility. RBC 2,3-BPG content is increased, thus decreasing HbO_2 affinity, which shifts the oxygen saturation curve to the right allowing greater oxygen delivery, thereby compensating for the anemia (3).

PK deficiency is clinically heterogeneous, with presentation ranging from compensated hemolytic anemia to severe anemia. Severity of anemia is usually stable in adulthood, but acute worsening with physiological stress and infections has been noted. Severe cases are common in children and can present with neonatal jaundice or in early childhood with jaundice, splenomegaly, and failure to thrive. Rare cases of hydrops fetalis are reported.

Diagnosis

Labs are consistent with intravascular hemolysis, as previously described. In the most severe cases, marked reticulocytosis, nucleated RBCs, and substantial anisopoikilocytosis can be seen on the peripheral smear (3). Reticulocytes contain residual mitochondria, which offer another source of ATP, thus providing some compensation. The MCV is usually normal or increased. Crenated red cells can be seen on the smear. A marked increase in the reticulocyte

Table 7.7 Enzymatic Defects of Glycolytic Pathway Resulting in Hemolytic Anemia

Enzyme	Role in RBCs	Clinical Manifestations	Neurologic Symptoms	Myopathy	Genetic Transmission
Hexokinase	Embden–Meyerhof pathway	HNSHA, chronic	−	−	AR
Phosphofructokinase	Embden–Meyerhof pathway	HNSHA, chronic (mild)	−	+	AR
Glucosephosphate isomerase	Embden–Meyerhof pathway	HNSHA, chronic	±	−	AR
Triosephosphate isomerase	Embden–Meyerhof pathway	HNSHA, chronic	+	−	AR
Phosphoglycerate kinase	Embden–Meyerhof pathway	HNSHA, chronic	+	+	X-linked

AR, autosomal recessive; HNSHA, hereditary non-spherocytic hemolytic anemia; RBC, red blood cell.

count occurs after splenectomy. Reference laboratories can perform quantitative measurement of the erythrocyte enzyme level necessary to diagnose this condition accurately.

Key Diagnostic Dilemma

As with other hemolytic anemias, review of the smear is critical to identify the etiology of hemolysis. The presence of crenated RBCs can tip the clinician to pursue the enzymatic level for PK. Of note, crenation may also be seen in other clinical conditions such as cirrhosis or diseases associated with abnormalities of RBC membrane lipids.

Prognosis

The disease is clinically heterogeneous, so prognosis varies. People with mild-to-moderate forms of PK deficiency tend to do very well in the long term. People with more severe forms of the disease are symptomatic during early childhood, but tolerate anemia better in adulthood. Severely affected individuals may have complications such as gallstones and stroke (3). As with other diseases in which splenectomy is pursued, splenectomy may predispose the patient to severe infections from pneumococcal or meningococcal bacteria.

Management

Splenectomy can be offered for severe, transfusion-dependent anemia; however, the response is variable and post-op thrombotic complications are noted. Most patients with PK deficiency benefit from splenectomy with an increase in Hgb level of approximately 1 to 3 g/dL (4). Folic acid supplementation is recommended in all patients. Iron overload is a long-term complication, both from multiple transfusions and hyperabsorption, and occasionally requires iron chelation.

Key Points

1. PK deficiency is rare. It can be diagnosed by measuring reduced PK activity in RBCs.
2. For severe disease, RBC transfusions may be necessary. Splenectomy ameliorates transfusion-dependent anemia.

Abnormalities of Nucleotide Salvage Pathway

Three important enzymes in the salvage pathway are pyrimidine 5′ nucleotidase (P5N), adenylate kinase, and adenosine deaminase.

P5N removes pyrimidine nucleotides from RBCs by catalyzing the hydrolysis of uridine monophosphate (UMP) and cytidine monophosphate (CMP), rendering diffusible nucleosides and free phosphates which accumulate and result in insoluble aggregates and coarse basophilic stippling (3). P5N is the enzyme inhibited in lead poisoning. Its clinical presentation is consistent with a variable mild-to-severe hemolytic anemia, jaundice, and splenomegaly.

Deficiency of adenylate kinase (autosomal recessive and associated with psychomotor retardation) or excess of adenosine deaminase (autosomal dominant and associated with immune deficiency) deplete adenine nucleotides and eventually ATP from RBCs, thereby leading to chronic hemolytic anemia (3).

AUTOIMMUNE HEMOLYTIC ANEMIA

Clinical Case 7.3

A 24-year-old woman presented to the emergency department with shortness of breath and fatigue. She was tachycardic and had a temperature of 100.6°F. Her spleen tip was palpable and there was no lymphadenopathy. Her Hgb was 5.5 g/dL with a reticulocyte count of 25%. The white blood cell (WBC) count was increased, and some myelocytes and metamyelocytes were present along with 15 nucleated RBC/100 WBC. Total bilirubin was 2.5 mg/dL with a direct fraction of 0.4 mg/dL. Marked spherocytosis with microspherocytosis and significant polychromatophilia was seen on the peripheral blood smear (Figure 7.6). The DAT was strongly positive for IgG, but negative for C3. Indirect

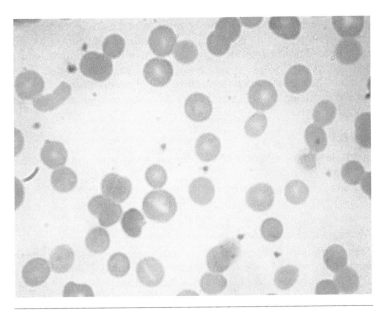

Figure 7.6 Peripheral smear of warm autoimmune hemolytic anemia. Reticulocytosis and spherocytosis in WAIHA.

WAIHA, warm autoimmune hemolytic anemia.

antiglobulin test (IAT) was also positive and reacted to all red cells in the test panel. The RBC eluate was strongly reactive.
   Diagnosis: Warm AIHA

Overview

AIHA is caused by autoantibodies directed against RBC antigens. Incidence rates are approximately one to three per 100,000 cases. AIHA may be idiopathic or associated with lymphoproliferative disorders, autoimmune diseases such as systemic lupus erythematosus (SLE), common variable hypogammaglobulinemia, and certain infections and drugs (5). AIHA can be classified based on the characteristic temperature activity of the responsible antibodies. They can further be classified based on the underlying etiology.

IgG is the typical antibody involved in the pathophysiology of warm AIHA (WAIHA). It shows maximal reactivity at 37°C. Loss of self-tolerance leads to formation of antibodies against the erythrocyte Rh antigen. The etiology of autoimmunity is unclear. Bacterial and viral infections with resultant inflammation have long been implicated in AIHA, with antigen mimicry and increased production of interferon as the possible mechanisms. IgG is not an effective initiator of the classical complement pathway, thus direct complement-mediated hemolysis (aka intravascular) is unusual.

Hemolysis can occur in two different ways:

1. Binding of antibody to Fc receptors on tissue macrophages can result in direct and complete phagocytosis of RBC.
2. Spherocytes generated by partial phagocytosis are sequestered in the splenic cords owing to their limited deformability. They are subsequently phagocytosed by macrophages in the spleen.

The site of RBC removal depends to a great deal on the quantity of antibody coating the RBC. RBCs that are lightly coated with Ig are removed by the spleen and those that are heavily coated are removed by the liver. Phagocytosis of IgG-coated RBC in the spleen is mediated by the Fc receptor of IgG, with FcRIII playing a major role in hemolysis.

IgM is a pentameric structure, which makes it a more effective activator of the complement system. High-titer IgM autoantibodies result in intravascular hemolysis by generating membrane-activating complex (MAC) of the complement pathway. In most cases, the IgM antibodies are at a lower concentration and the complement inhibitor mechanisms counteract the MAC formation. Despite this, there is some deposition of C3b on the RBC membrane. Subsequent interaction with ligand iC3b on liver macrophages leads to immune-mediated RBC hemolysis in the liver.

Diagnosis of AIHA is aided by the use of the DAT (or Coombs), which demonstrates in vivo coating of red cells with IgG or complement (C3) (Figure 7.7). RBCs are washed and then incubated with polyspecific antihuman globulin (AHG) reagent capable of detecting IgG and C3d. The RBCs are washed to remove nonspecific proteins and then the sample is centrifuged to enhance agglutination. If the RBCs agglutinate, the test is considered positive. Interpretation of the DAT results must be made with caution. A positive DAT may be seen in alloimmune hemolysis post-transfusion, as a result of passenger lymphocytes in solid organ transplant recipients, in drug-induced hemolytic anemia, as well as transplacental transfer of antibodies. A negative DAT may be seen when hemolysis is caused by IgA or IgM antibodies, or with low-titer or low-affinity antibodies.

The next step after a positive DAT should include testing for the antibodies to clinically significant RBC antigens and testing the eluate. Elution is done to remove antibody from the RBC. The eluted serum can then be checked for the antibody specificity by

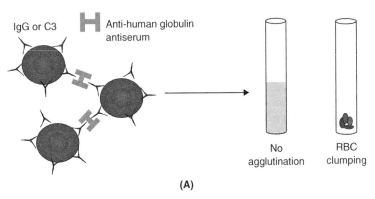

(A)

	IgG subtype	DAT (Coombs)	RBC eluate	Antigen specificity	Hemolysis type
Warm AIHA	IgG mainly	IgG ± C3d	IgG	Mostly Rh	Extravascular
CAD	IgM	C3d	Nonreactive	Mostly anti-I Rarely I or Pr	Intravascular
PCH	IgG	C3d	Nonreactive	P antigen	Intravascular
Mixed type	IgG, IgM	IgG, C3d	IgG		Both

(B)

Figure 7.7 Direct antiglobulin test findings in AIHA

AIHA, autoimmune hemolytic anemia; CAD, cold agglutinin disease; DAT, direct antiglobulin test; PCH, paroxysmal cold hemoglobinuria; RBC, red blood cell.

the IAT or antibody screen. An eluate may have no reaction in drug-induced AIHA.

A diagnosis of immune-mediated destruction of the RBC is supported by RBC surface-bound immunoglobulin and less often by evidence of complement fixation. IgG antibodies bound to red cells require AHG as a cofactor to agglutinate saline-suspended RBC, while IgM antibodies can readily do so without any reagents. The pentameric structure of IgM allows crosslinking, whereas IgG requires AHG to bridge RBCs.

WARM AUTOIMMUNE HEMOLYTIC ANEMIA

Introduction

WAIHA represents 48% to 70% of all AIHA cases and is characterized by autoantibodies (typically IgG) with greatest activity at 37°C. Extravascular hemolysis is the typical mechanism of RBC destruction. Less than half of the cases are idiopathic, with secondary AIHA commonly seen with advanced age. The leading causes of secondary WAIHA are chronic lymphocytic leukemia (CLL), Hodgkin lymphoma, non-Hodgkin lymphoma, and Waldenstrom macroglobulinemia (Table 7.8). Commonly used drugs may elicit hemolysis by (a) altering the antigen on the RBC, thereby resulting in antibodies that cross-react with the unaltered RBC antigen (autoimmune model); (b) directly associating with structures on the RBC to elicit hemolysis (hapten model); or (c) inducing a neoantigen formed by the drug and RBC membrane, which is recognized by the antibody (innocent bystander) (6). A list of culprit drugs is summarized in Table 7.9 (6).

The clinical presentation is highly variable and may present with a waxing and waning course with patients presenting with symptoms secondary to anemia, such as weakness, fatigue, dyspnea, and jaundice. If hepatosplenomegaly and lymphadenopathy are present, an underlying lymphoproliferative disorder may be present.

Diagnosis

Findings of hemolysis include elevated reticulocyte count and indirect bilirubin. Often, the hemolysis is extravascular; but when intravascular hemolysis is present, serum LDH will be elevated and haptoglobin will be low. Rarely, reticulocytopenia may be seen when the antibody also affects the reticulocyte or when there is low folate. The peripheral smear reveals polychromasia and spherocytosis with the presence of microspherocytes (Figure 7.6). As mentioned earlier, DAT is used to confirm the autoimmune nature of observed hemolysis.

Table 7.8 Classification of Antibody-Mediated Red Blood Cell Injury

WAIHA	
Primary	
Secondary	Lymphoproliferative neoplasms Autoimmune disorders Chronic inflammatory disorders Nonlymphoid neoplasms
Drug induced	Hapten model: Penicillin Immune complex model: Quinidine Autoimmune mode: Alpha-methyldopa
CAD	
Idiopathic/primary	
Secondary	Lymphoproliferative Autoimmune Infections (*Mycoplasma*, EBV)
PCH	
Primary	
Secondary	Infections: syphilis

CAD, cold agglutinin disease; EBV, Epstein–Barr virus; PCH, paroxysmal cold hemoglobinuria; RBC, red blood cell; WAIHA, warm autoimmune hemolytic anemia.

Key Diagnostic Dilemma

Spherocytosis is observed in both AIHA and HS; therefore, distinguishing between the two requires additional steps beyond peripheral smear review. The DAT, when positive, can assist in making the diagnosis. Of note, approximately 1% to 10% of AIHAs are DAT negative. This is due to the detection capabilities of the Coombs assay (7). The AHG has the capacity to detect 100 to 500 molecules of IgG or C3 coating RBC; hence, if fewer molecules are present, one can still observe significant hemolysis and a negative DAT. Moreover, the DAT will miss IgA or IgG4, as these are not recognized by the routine assay. A super Coombs test is available at select institutions, and has higher specificity and the ability to detect fewer molecules of IgG or C3 coating the RBC (7).

A common misconception is that the strength of the DAT correlates with the severity of hemolysis. It is important to use the DAT to help to make the diagnosis, but not to anticipate severity of observed hemolysis. Finally, a positive DAT can be seen in patients who are not actively hemolyzing. Between 1:1,000 and 1:14,000 healthy blood donors and from 7% to 8% of hospitalized patients may have a positive DAT (7). Consequently, clinical evaluation

Table 7.9 Drugs Associated With Autoimmune Hemolytic Anemia

Antibiotics	Analgesic and Antipyretics	Chemotherapy	Other
Amoxicillin	Acetaminophen	Carboplatin	Antazoline
Amphotericin B	Aspirin	Cisplatin	Buthiazide
Cefazolin	Diclofenac	Fluorouracil	Carbimazole
Cefotaxime	Dipyrone	Imatinib	Catechin
Cefotetan	Ibuprofen	Methotrexate	Chlorpromazine
Cefoxitin	Methadone	Oxaliplatin	Chlorpropamide
Ceftazidime	Naproxen	Pemetrexed	Cyclofenil
Ceftriaxone	Phenacetin		Cyclosporin
Chloramphenicol	Sulfasalazine		Diethylstilbestrol
Ciprofloxacin	Sulindac		Furosemide
Erythromycin	Tolmetin		Hydrochlorothiazide
Isoniazid			Insulin
Levofloxacin			Nomifensine
Mefloquine			Probenecid
Nafcillin			Radiocontrast medium
p-Aminosalicylic acid			Ranitidine
Penicillin			Tolbutamide
Piperacillin			Triamterene
Pyrimethamine			
Quinidine			
Quinine			
Rifampin			
Stibophen			
Streptomycin			
Temafloxacin			
Tetracycline			
Ticarcillin			
Trimethoprim/ sulfamethoxazole			

including adequate history and laboratory workup is essential in making a diagnosis of AIHA.

Prognosis

WAIHA in children has a good prognosis and is self-limiting. However, if it presents within the first 2 years of life or in the teenage years, the disease can follow a more chronic course, requiring long-term immunosuppression, with serious developmental consequences (8). The reported mortality rate for children with AIHA is approximately 3% to 4% (9). The main causes of death reported are overwhelming sepsis in splenectomized patients, catastrophic bleeding in patients with concurrent immune thrombocytopenic purpura (Evan's syndrome), and complications of underlying malignancy (9).

In adults, first-line therapy with steroids results in 70% to 85% response; however, only one in three cases will achieve long-term remission after discontinuation of steroids (6). Fifty percent of patients require long-term maintenance steroid doses and approximately 30% will require second- or third-line therapies (6). Less than 20% of adults are cured by steroids alone (6).

Management

For patients with an acute onset of disease, AIHA can be life-threatening and the patient should receive blood transfusion. The antibodies typically are directed against blood group antigens Rh complex on all RBCs, except for those who are Rh null. Therefore, crossmatched blood transfusion is not feasible. Phenotypically matched transfusion should suffice in most cases. An extended phenotyping is necessary in patients with prior transfusion history and women with prior pregnancies.

Steroids are the mainstay of treatment in AIHA and should be initiated immediately. The starting dose of prednisone is usually 1 mg/kg/d and is maintained until Hb shows improvement. Prednisone is then slowly tapered over 4 to 8 weeks. Patients are monitored closely during this period with weekly complete blood count (CBC) and reticulocyte count. About 50% patients respond to steroids alone, with only one third of these attaining long-term remission. Addition of rituximab was shown to improve the complete response rates and relapse-free survival. In patients with secondary AIHA, treatment of the underlying etiology is preferred. Second-line treatment:

1. Rituximab: Response rates range from 82% to 87%. It is generally well tolerated, with infusion reactions being the most common issue. Patients should be tested for hepatitis B before treatment with this agent (5).

2. Splenectomy: Overall response rate is approximately 60% to 75%, with higher responses noted in idiopathic AIHA (5).
3. Immunosuppressive agents: Several immunosuppressive agents are available for treatment of relapsed/refractory AIHA (Table 7.10) (5).
4. Intravenous immunoglobulin (IVIG): This has had limited utility in warm AIHA treatment. Case reports show varied response and failure rates.
5. Alemtuzumab: A humanized anti-CD52 monoclonal antibody has been shown to induce responses in patients with AIHA associated with CLL in recent case reports (10).

Key Points

1. The etiology of most cases of WAIHA is unknown. In a minority of cases, an associated disorder may be present, that is, viral infection, autoimmune disorders, lymphoproliferative disorders, common variable immunodeficiency, and drugs.
2. Laboratory findings indicating the presence of hemolysis include elevated levels of indirect bilirubin and LDH, along with reduced levels of haptoglobin. DAT is an important aspect of the diagnosis.
3. Most patients present with acute onset of severe hemolysis and symptomatic anemia requiring emergent treatment, including glucocorticoids and possible transfusions.
4. Relapse rates are high, and second-line treatments include splenectomy, rituximab, and other immunosuppressive modalities.

COLD AGGLUTININ DISEASE

Introduction

Cold agglutinin disease (CAD) is a type of cold AIHA (C-AIHA). It is a rare disorder characterized by hemolytic anemia precipitated by exposure to cold secondary to antibodies directed against polysaccharide antigens (I, i, and Pr) on the surface of RBC. CAD constitutes 16% to 32% of AIHA. Primary CAD is mostly seen in older patients (peak incidence at 70 years) with slight female predilection. Infections such as *Mycoplasma* and low-grade lymphoproliferative disorders such as Waldenstrom macroglobulinemia are the causes of secondary CAD (18). IgM is the culprit in both primary and secondary CAD. Hemolysis occurs when complement is fixed, and C3b-coated RBCs are cleared by macrophages in the spleen and Kupffer cells in the liver. Red cells may also undergo

Table 7.10 Third-Line Immunosuppressive Agents in Autoimmune Hemolytic Anemia

	Initial Dose	Response Rate (%)	Toxicity	Miscellaneous
Azathioprine (11,12)	2 to 4 mg/kg oral once daily	60 to 70	Leukopenia, thrombocytopenia, infections, nausea/vomiting	Given continuously for 6 months and then tapered
Cyclosporine A (12)	2.5 mg/kg oral BID	60	Hypertension, renal insufficiency, rarely MAHA	Monitor CsA levels
Mycophenolate (12, 14, 15)	500 mg oral BID	25 to 70	GI intolerance, myelosuppression	Long-term toxicity not known
Danazol (16,17)	200 mg oral Q6 to 8h	60 to 70	–	A good alternative to splenectomy in elderly
Cyclophosphamide (low dose) (15)	1 to 2 mg/kg/d	40 to 60	Hemorrhagic cystitis, secondary malignancy, infertility	Given concomitantly with prednisone 40 mg/m^2/d
Cyclophosphamide high dose) (12)	50 mg/kg IV days 1 to 4 or 1,000 mg IV weekly × 4	66 to 100	Neutropenic fever, alopecia, nausea/vomiting	Needs mesna and GCSF support

BID, twice a day; GCSF, granulocyte colony-stimulating factor; GI, gastrointestinal; IV, intravenous; MAHA, microangiopathic hemolytic anemia.

direct lysis of RBCs by terminal complement activation. When CAD ensues after *Mycoplasma* infection, the IgM typically reacts with the I antigen on RBC. When Epstein–Barr virus (EBV) is followed by CAD, the antigenic target is i.

Diagnosis

In most cases, patients with CAD present with chronic hemolytic anemia with exacerbations in cold weather. Symptoms include pain or discomfort when swallowing cold foods and Raynaud's phenomenon. A few patients have significant hemoglobinuria (with dark urine) on cold exposure, forcing them to move to warmer climates. Physical examination may reveal acrocyanosis and livedo reticularis, both of which are reversible on rewarming the affected area (18). Rarely, patients develop gangrene of the digits. Splenomegaly is seen infrequently, specifically in secondary CAD associated with lymphoproliferative disorders.

Spurious elevation of MCHC and MCV may be seen in CBCs, owing to agglutination of RBCs (Figure 7.8). DAT is positive for C3b and generally negative for IgG, although up to 25% of patients express a weakly positive IgG. The cold agglutinin titer reflects the

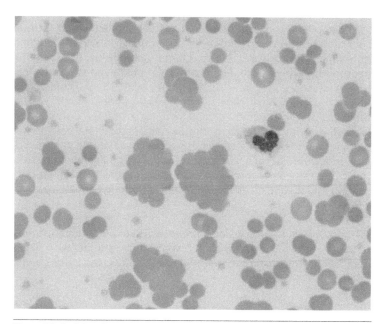

Figure 7.8 Peripheral smear of cold autoimmune hemolytic anemia. Agglutination of RBCs.

RBC, red blood cell.

concentration and avidity of the antibody for its target. The titer is determined by testing serial dilutions of patient serum for their ability to agglutinate RBCs. DAT titers <1:64 are not clinically significant. Most experts consider a titer of 1:512 to be clinically significant and in many cases, for CAD, the titers are >1:2,048 (18). Discerning the thermal amplitude is of greater significance than the antibody titer. It reports the highest temperature at which a cold agglutinin binds the RBC antigen. Most clinically significant cold agglutinins have a thermal amplitude that exceeds 28°C to 30°C.

Evaluation for an underlying disorder in CAD is appropriate in most individuals, especially the elderly. Specific focus should be on infectious, autoimmune, or lymphoproliferative disorders. In the case of lymphoproliferative disease, a serum protein electrophoresis and flow cytometry may reveal a monoclonal protein (IgM κ in >90% of cases) and/or monoclonal B-cell population, respectively.

Key Diagnostic Dilemma

Cold-induced symptoms and hemolytic anemia are characteristics of other diseases and careful evaluation must be undertaken to exclude these entities. Raynaud's and cold symptoms can be associated with autoimmune disorders that are not characterized by a cold agglutinin or with hemolytic anemia. Cryoglobulinemia, for example, is characterized by immune complexes that form in cold temperatures and can cause a number of findings including arthralgias, purpura, skin ulcers, glomerulonephritis, or peripheral neuropathy. While these patients may exhibit Raynaud's and a history of infection, they have no laboratory evidence of a cold agglutinin nor do they have clinical hemolysis. In patients with WAIHA, there are usually no cold-induced symptoms and the Coombs test is positive for IgG rather than complement. Paroxysmal cold hemoglobinuria (PCH) is a C-AIHA that is often associated with a recent viral infection. PCH is associated with IgG which can bind complement, but the cold agglutinin titer is only modestly elevated (i.e., <1:160). The diagnostic test for PCH is the Donath–Landsteiner test.

Prognosis

CAD secondary to *Mycoplasma pneumoniae* or EBV infection tends to be self-limited. CAD associated with lymphoproliferative disorders has prognosis tied to underlying malignancy or autoimmune etiology.

Management

In idiopathic CAD, anemia tends to be mild and chronic; hence, most patients can be observed without treatment. Avoidance of cold temperatures is most helpful. In CAD secondary to infections, no therapy is necessary in most cases. In a minority with significant hemolysis, simple transfusion and as-needed plasmapheresis suffice. In malignancy-associated CAD, treatment of the underlying disease generally controls the CAD.

1. Rituximab: It is the first-line systemic therapy for CAD. Rituximab as a single agent has shown an overall response rate (ORR) of 45% to 54% with a median response duration of approximately 11 months. Complete remissions are uncommon, and 50% to 80% of patients relapse. When used in combination with prednisone, there are more CRs and only a third relapse at 1 year (18,19).

2. Immunosuppressive therapy: Chlorambucil and cyclophosphamide have an estimated ORR of 15% to 45% with a median response duration of 11 months. They are associated with myelotoxicity and require frequent lab monitoring.

3. Plasmapheresis: This tends to be a temporizing procedure as the endogenous antibody production is not affected. This has utility in patients undergoing coronary artery bypass by temporarily decreasing cold agglutinin titers. Plasmapheresis is technically difficult owing to the need to keep the blood warm.

4. Transfusion: Blood needs to be tested at 37°C to minimize the effect of cold agglutinin. When transfusion in necessary, it needs to be done through an in-line blood warmer at 37°C.

Key Points

1. C-AIHA includes CAD and PCH. Cold avoidance can reduce cold-induced symptoms and hemolysis. In cases associated with acute viral infection, the hemolysis may be transient.

2. In cases, such as in CAD, associated with lymphoproliferative processes, it is important to treat the underlying disorder.

PAROXYSMAL COLD HEMOGLOBINURIA

Introduction

PCH was first described by Donath and Landsteiner in 1904 as a syndrome characterized by pain, fever, and hemoglobinuria following cold exposure. It results from a polyclonal IgG antibody (Donath Landsteiner [DL] antibody) directed against the P antigen on the RBC membrane. It may be idiopathic (primary) or secondary to infection (20). When syphilis was more prevalent, PCH was a common association. The DL antibody is a biphasic hemolysin as it sensitizes the RBC in the cold periphery, but only causes hemolysis by activation of complement in the warm core body.

PCH may manifest as chronic hemolysis. It is very rare and should prompt investigation for underlying syphilis. Acute transient hemolysis may occur after an infectious process. The antibody appears 7 to 10 days after the onset of a febrile illness and may persist for 6 to 12 weeks after (20). Hemoglobinuria, jaundice, and pallor occur after exposure to cold. Patients can also present with Raynaud's phenomenon, pallor, and numbness in hands and feet.

Diagnosis
PCH is confirmed by the Donath–Landsteiner test. The patient's serum is incubated with group O RBC expressing P antigen and pooled normal human serum as a source of complement at 4°C for 30 minutes (antibody and early components of the complement are fixed) and then incubated at 37°C for 60 minutes to allow components of complement to be activated (21). The tubes are then centrifuged, and the supernatant is examined for hemolysis. The test is considered positive when there is visible lysis. Hemolysis occurs only if antibody was present and allowed to fix complement at a cooler temperature. Control reaction mixture continuously maintained at 37°C does not exhibit hemolysis.

Key Diagnostic Dilemma
Donath–Landsteiner test is not very sensitive. Normal RBCs are hemolyzed only with difficulty by human complement, especially in patients with PCH of mild-to-moderate severity. A variation of the test includes the use of papain during incubation at 37°C to increase access to the P antigens or utilizing RBCs from a patient with paroxysmal nocturnal hemoglobinuria (PNH), which are much more susceptible to lysis by complement.

As previously mentioned, other clinical entities can also be characterized by cold-induced symptoms and AIHA. These have been previously described, and the differential diagnosis is outlined in section for CAD.

Prognosis
Patients with PCH have a self-limited course. Although the acute presentation may be severe, the long-term outcome is favorable, and most patients make a complete recovery.

Management
Given the transient nature of the disease, supportive care at the time of the attacks is the appropriate approach. Steroids are of limited benefit. When transfusion is needed, both the patient and the blood components must be warmed. In patients with chronic PCH, avoidance of cold is the ideal strategy. Patients with syphilis, when treated, have resolution of the hemolysis in most cases.

Key Points

1. PCH is a type of AIHA in which an antibody binds to P antigen of the RBC in the cold and fixes complement. Upon warming, the antibody dissociates, thereby leading to complement-mediated lyses of RBCs resulting in intravascular hemolysis.
2. Management of acute episode is supportive.

PAROXYSMAL NOCTURNAL HEMOGLOBINURIA

Clinical Case 7.4

A 33-year-old man presents with a history of right upper quadrant (RUQ) pain and elevated transaminases. He has RUQ tenderness and mild jaundice with no splenomegaly. Peripheral blood smear shows normochromic normocytic RBCs. Total and indirect bilirubin values are 3.5 and 0.3 mg/dL, respectively. LDH is 1,500 U/mL with the haptoglobin being <0.4 mg/dL. Prothrombin time (PT), partial thromboplastin time (PTT), and fibrinogen are normal. Urine analysis (UA) shows dark urine with 3+ blood on dipstick, but no RBCs are seen on microscopic study. An abdominal MRI demonstrates thrombosis of the hepatic veins.

Introduction

PNH is an acquired hemolytic disorder with a close relationship to aplastic anemia (AA; see Chapter 4, Acquired Aplastic Anemia and Inherited Bone Marrow Failure Syndromes). It is the result of an acquired somatic mutation of the X-linked gene phosphatidyli-nositol glycan class A (*PIG-A*) that occurs in a hematopoietic stem cell, leading to severe deficiency or absence of *PIG-A*–associated proteins (Figure 7.9A). Because of X-inactivation, women can be affected as often as men. *PIG-A* is responsible for the generation of glycosylphosphoinositol (GPI) linkage that attaches proteins to the exterior of the cell (Figures 7.9B,C) (11). In PNH, two key complement-related proteins are decreased: decay accelerating factor (DAF; CD 55) and membrane inhibitor of reactive lysis (MIRL; CD59) (Figure 7.9C). Their low activity renders the RBCs and other cells vulnerable to complement-induced hemolysis (Figure 7.10). RBC acetylcholinesterase and leukocyte alkaline phosphatase are also decreased.

PNH is thought to occur after an immune attack on the bone marrow stem cells, thereby leading to clonal expansion of PNH clone (Figure 7.11). The mechanism of expansion is unclear, but has been postulated as a possible immune escape or selective advantage of the clone. Acquired AA and PNH are closely related diseases. A small clonal population of PNH cells may be found in two thirds of patients with newly diagnosed AA. Some degree of cytopenias has

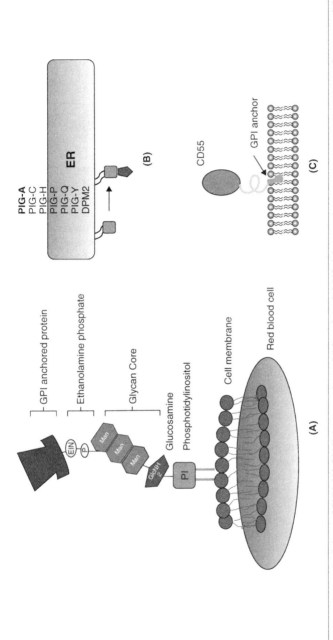

Figure 7.9 Pathophysiology of PNH. (A) GPI-linked protein on RBC surface. **(B)** PIG-A is one of seven subunits involved in the first step of GPI anchor biosynthesis, which takes place in the ER. **(C)** Eventually, the GPI-anchored protein will be transported to the plasma membrane.

ER, endoplasmic reticulum; GPI, glycosylphosphoinositol; PIG-A, phosphatidylinositol glycan class A; PNH, paroxysmal nocturnal hemoglobinuria; RBC, red blood cell.

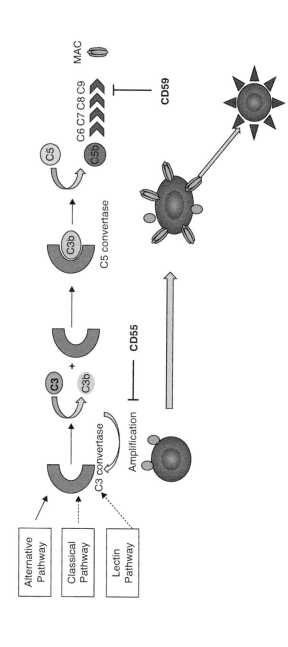

Figure 7.10 Complement-mediated attack. The lectin, classical, and alternative pathways converge at C3 activation. Terminal complement begins with the cleavage of C5 to C5a and C5b, which is triggered by C5 convertase. CD55 inhibits proximal complement activation. CD59 inhibits terminal complement activation. In PNH, CD59 and CD55 are deficient due to lack of the GPI anchor. Intravascular hemolysis caused by MAC predominates.

GPI, glycosylphosphoinositol; MAC, membrane-activating complex; PNH, paroxysmal nocturnal hemoglobinuria.

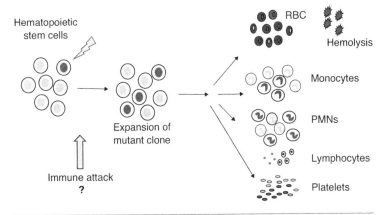

Figure 7.11 Pathogenesis of selective expansion of PNH clone. To cause PNH, the stem cell needs to undergo clonal selection and expansion. The proposed insult is immune attack.

PMNs, polymorphonuclear cells; PNH, paroxysmal nocturnal hemoglobinuria; RBC, red blood cell.

also been described in newly diagnosed PNH patients. In patients with AA, the detection of a PNH clone is a strong evidence for autoimmunity as a cause and predicts response to anti-thymocyte globulin and cyclosporine.

This chapter focuses primarily on the hemolytic anemia management of PNH, with the management of bone marrow failure, including the role of immunosuppressive therapies and hematopoietic stem cell transplantation, presented in Chapter 4, Acquired Aplastic Anemia and Inherited Bone Marrow Failure Syndromes.

Diagnosis

PNH is associated with a wide range of clinical findings, including fatigue, dyspnea, hemoglobinuria, abdominal pain, erectile dysfunction, thrombosis, and bone marrow suppression. In general, the severity of clinical findings is thought to correlate with the size of the PNH clone.

The classical presentation of PNH is that of unexplained hemolytic anemia and associated symptoms, including fatigue, jaundice, and pink urine. Presentations of thrombosis at unusual sites, such as the abdomen (i.e., Budd–Chiari) or cerebrum, have also been described (11). Finally, symptoms consistent with smooth muscle dystonia, such as erectile dysfunction and esophageal spasms, may occur as a result of depletion of nitric oxide (NO) following the release of free Hb into the circulation with the persistent intravascular hemolysis.

Laboratory values are consistent with those of intravascular hemolysis: elevated LDH, low haptoglobin, and the presence of Hgb in serum and urine. Iron deficiency may result from chronic intravascular hemolysis and iron loss via hemoglobinuria and hemosiderinurea. Before the etiology of PNH was discovered, the sucrose hemolysis test and the Ham's test were utilized to detect the fragile RBCs. This has been largely replaced by flow cytometric analysis, which uses fluorescently labeled monoclonal antibodies to detect GPI-linked proteins in patients' peripheral blood. Typical proteins assayed include CD59, CD55, CD14, CD15, CD16, CD24, CD45, and CD64 (11). It is recommended that flow cytometry be performed using at least two target reagents, with each lab using a defined cocktail. The Fluorescent AERolysin (FLAER), a test that utilizes a reagent derived from the bacterial toxin aerolysin and binds directly to the GPI anchor, is also incorporated to confirm diagnosis (Figure 7.12A). Two cell lineages (RBCs and leukocytes) are tested to make the diagnosis, with leukocytes frequently utilized to detect the size of the clone and RBCs used to assess severity of disease (Figures 7.12B,C). Testing of RBC alone is not recommended to evaluate the clone size since PNH cells have a short life span, thereby leading to underestimation of the clone size. It is also not recommended that patients get tested after transfusions since the normal cells will interfere with interpretation of results.

Key Diagnostic Dilemma

The differential diagnosis of PNH includes other hemolytic anemias, other causes of thrombosis in atypical sites, such as myeloproliferative disorders, and other bone marrow failure syndromes, which may coexist with PNH.

Prognosis

PNH is a chronic disease with significant morbidity and mortality. In the pre-anti-complement era, the mean survival for American and Japanese populations was 19.4 versus 32.4 years, respectively (22). However, since the availability of eculizumab, the mortality seems to be similar to age-matched controls (23). This therapy markedly reduces the risk of thrombosis, which has been the leading cause of death, particularly among the American population (22,23). Adverse prognostic factors include age >50 years, severe cytopenias at diagnosis, severe infection, thrombosis, and renal failure (22).

Management

For patients with classic PNH, treatment includes cautious correction of iron deficiency. Rapid correction may result in a wave of

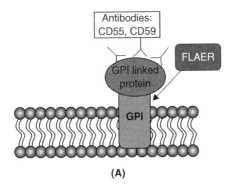

(A)

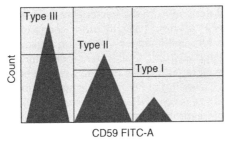

(B)

PNH Types	Clone Size in Granulocytes
Classic PNH	40% to 99%
Acquired aplastic anemia	0% to 10%
MDS	<1%
Healthy individuals	Approximately 0.002

(C)

Figure 7.12 The PNH clone. (A) Diagnosis is made by flow cytometry analysis using antibodies directed against GPI-associated proteins such as CD55 and CD59. FLAER takes advantage of binding of a bacterial protein, aerolysin, to GPI anchor. It is useful for the analysis of WBCs, but not RBCs. **(B)** RBCs are defined by the abundance of GPI-anchored proteins on the surface: PNH Type I cells have normal levels, PNH Type II cells exhibit partial absence, and PNH Type III cells show complete absence. Assessment of RBC population may be useful in determining severity of hemolysis. **(C)** WBCs (monocytes, granulocytes) are the optimal cell type for assessing the PNH clone and determining clinical entity associated with the clone.

FITC-A, fluorescein isothiocyanate; FLAER, fluorescein-labeled aerolysin; GPI, glycosylphosphoinositol; MDS, myelodysplastic syndrome; PNH, paroxysmal nocturnal hemoglobinuria; RBC, red blood cell; WBC, white blood cell.

erythropoiesis followed by a hemolytic crisis. Transfusions may prevent this and may be required to treat anemia. Steroid treatment can reduce hemolysis. Eculizumab, an anti-CD5 antibody, blocks the late phase of complement activation and is an effective, albeit very costly, treatment for patients with PNH who have a transfusion requirement (Figure 7.13A,B) (11,23). Infusions given every 2 weeks reduce or eliminate transfusion needs. Treatment also improves the quality of life and reduces the risk for thrombosis. Eculizumab is associated with increased risk for meningococcal infections and patients should receive vaccination and should also report for antibiotic therapy if they develop fever.

Patients with thrombosis are usually managed with warfarin. Some experts recommend warfarin treatment as prophylaxis in patients with substantial PNH clone size, but no history of thrombosis. Severe PNH is an indication for bone marrow transplantation. Patients with PNH can progress to AA, MDS, or acute leukemia. When AML arises, the PNH defect is no longer present. Conversely, patients with AA who have responded to immunosuppressive therapy need to be periodically assessed for PNH.

Future Directions

Given the excellent results obtained with eculizumab, there has been a great interest to expand the clinical development of second-generation complement modulators. These efforts can be classified into three categories:

1. Inhibitors of the terminal complement effector pathway, targeting C5 and other downstream effectors. As demonstrated by the success of eculizumab, inhibition of the terminal complement effector pathway has been proven as relatively safe and effective (13). Several strategies are under development, aiming to improve the current anti-C5 therapy:

   - Antibody-based C5 inhibitors: ALXN1210, ALXN5500
   - Small interfering anti-C5 RNA: ALNCC5
   - Conversin, a 16 kDa protein of the lipocalin family (from the tick *Ornithodoros moubata*), is capable of binding C5, preventing its cleavage by C5 convertases

2. Inhibitors of early complement activation, targeting C3. Our clinical experience with anti-C5 treatments has demonstrated that inhibition of C5 alone is not enough to prevent all hemolysis, specifically C3-mediated extravascular hemolysis.

   - Compstatin is a 13-residue disulfide bridged peptide that binds to human native C3, as well as its active fragment, C3b. It prevents the cleavage of C3 to C3b and also prevents the incorporation of C3b to form C3/C5 convertases, effectively

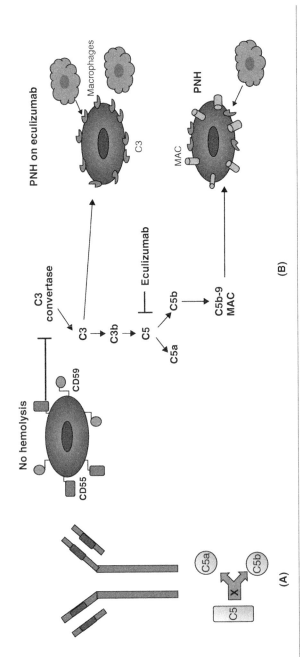

Figure 7.13 Mechanism of action of eculizumab. (A) Eculizumab is a humanized monoclonal antibody with a high affinity for C5, effectively blocking its cleavage. (B) By inhibiting C5 cleavage, eculizumab prevents intravascular hemolysis. Eculizumab does not block extravascular hemolysis due to lack of CD55.

MAC, membrane-activating complex; PNH, paroxysmal nocturnal hemoglobinuria.

abrogating complement activation along the three complement pathways: classical, alternative, and lectin (13).

3. Modulators of initial complement activation upstream of C3:

- Complement factor B (CFB) and complement factor D (CFD) are key molecules upstream of C3 in the alternative pathway. Promising approaches have used small compounds, such as NA-04-WV99 and JD-43-RB65, which prevent the interaction between CFB and CFD.

Key Points

1. PNH results from a somatic mutation in hematopoietic cells resulting in severe deficiency or absence of *PIG-A*–associated proteins.
2. Clinical findings include hemolytic anemia, thrombosis in an atypical location, and other nonspecific symptoms attributable to consequences of hemolysis.
3. In general, the severity is thought to correlate with the size(s) of the PNH clone in untreated patients.
4. Eculizumab has revolutionized the treatment of PNH. New complement inhibitors are in development.

RBC FRAGMENTATION SYNDROMES

Clinical Case 7.5

A 40-year-old woman presents with a BP of 250/160 mmHg and is admitted for management. Heretofore, she has had problems with BP and has been on medications, but she has noticed gradual worsening of her BP. On exam, her skin is taut. Her CBC shows a normal WBC, but she is anemic with an Hgb of 8.5 g/dL, HCT of 25.5, and a platelet count of 75,000. Her creatinine is 2.5 mg/dL and LDH is 800 U/mL. Peripheral blood film shows schistocytes (Figure 7.14), helmet cells, and spherocytes. Platelets are decreased, and many are large. PT, PTT, and fibrinogen are at normal levels.

MAHAs are associated with an array of vascular abnormalities (Box 7.1). Schistocytes, helmet cells, and spherocytes are seen on peripheral blood smear. Two principal disorders that must be considered are TTP and HUS. These are discussed in Chapter 10, Platelet Disorders. Vasculitis, hypertensive crises (especially in scleroderma), and arteriovenous (AV) malformations can be associated with MAHA and mild reduction in platelets. Disseminated intravascular coagulation is complicated by MAHA in 10% to 20% of cases. Microangiopathic hemolytic anemia without thrombocytopenia is a complication of prosthetic heart valvular dysfunction, endocardial repairs, vascular aneurysms, and post-Dacron graft revascularization for peripheral artery disease and extracorporeal circulation

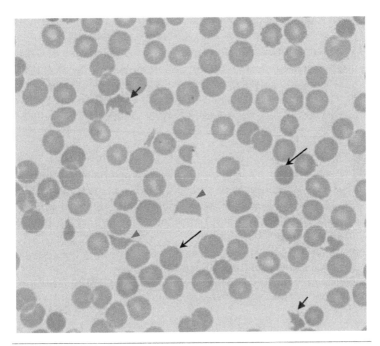

Figure 7.14 Peripheral smear of microangiopathic hemolytic anemia. Noted are several schistocytes (short arrows), spherocytes (long arrows), and helmet cells (red triangles).

devices. Treatment of the underlying condition is the foundation of treatment. Patients with prosthetic valvular dysfunction may do better if cardiac contractility is reduced with beta-blockers. Iron replacement may be necessary for those with significant intravascular hemolysis. Folate supplementation is also recommended as for any hemolytic disorder.

Box 7.1 Causes of Microangiopathic Hemolytic Anemia

Disseminated intravascular coagulation
HELLP syndrome
Thrombotic thrombocytopenic purpura/hemolytic uremic syndrome
Malignancy
Malignant hypertension
Scleroderma renal crisis
Waring Blender syndrome (cardiac valve hemolysis)
Kasabach–Merritt syndrome
Drugs: chemotherapy
Vasculitis (i.e., polyarteritis nodosa, granulomatosis with polyangiitis)

HELLP, hemolysis, elevated liver enzymes, and a low platelet count.

Other Causes of Hemolysis

Infections

Hemolysis is associated with three organisms: malaria (Figure 7.15), *Babesia,* and *Bartonella. Falciparum* malaria is associated with a very high parasite burden, splenic sequestration of infected RBCs, and also intravascular hemolysis. *Babesia* infections also produce hemolysis and are particularly problematic for asplenic individuals. Carion's disease or Arroyo fever is seen in Peru and other areas in South America. *Bartonella* organism attaches to the RBC membrane and causes hemolysis.

Chemical Exposures

Exposure to copper or increased copper levels seen in Wilson's disease can produce hemolysis. Near drowning will induce an osmotic lysis of RBCs as will inadvertent exposure to hypotonic fluid during hemodialysis. Thermal damage due to burns can cause aggregation of spectrin and failure of the RBC cytoskeleton and hemolysis. Membrane blebbing is a feature of these cells in which the lipid bilayer becomes untethered from the inner cytoskeleton.

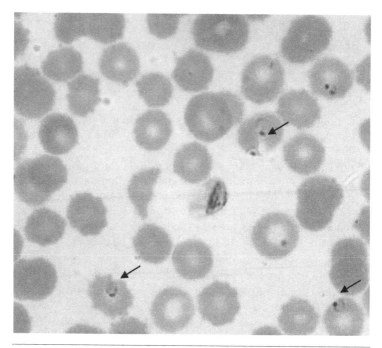

Figure 7.15 Peripheral smear of malaria infection. Noted within RBCs are the *Plasmodium falciparum* rings (arrows).

A similar picture is seen in patients with mutations in spectrin that affect its thermal stability—hereditary pyropoikilocytosis.

Snake envenomation can also cause hemolysis. The bite of the brown recluse spider is associated with a painful skin lesion and hemolysis with spherocytes and weakly positive Coombs due to activation of complement. Perhaps, the most devastating hemolysis with infections is seen with *Clostridium*. *Clostridium perfringens* elaborates a lecithinase with hemolytic properties. Patients may have total destruction of RBCs resulting in circulation of massive amounts of free Hgb and HCT, which is much lower than predicted for the measured Hgb. Serum chemistry studies are also deranged by the massive hemolysis. Patients typically present with gangrenous cholecystitis or gas gangrene of an extremity. Mortality is high despite antibiotics and surgical debridement or amputation.

Hypersplenism

An enlarged spleen is associated with anemia, thrombocytopenia, and leukopenia. Anemia results from sequestration in the enlarged spleen and enhancement of the spleen's normal function which is to cull out damaged RBCs. Hemolysis may not be significant unless there is macrophage activation also as seen with malaria infection.

REFERENCES

1. Gallagher PG. Abnormalities of the erythrocyte membrane. *Pediatr Clin North Am.* 2013;60:1349–1362. doi:10.1016/j.pcl.2013.09.001

2. Cappellini MD, Fiorelli G. Glucose-6-phosphate dehydrogenase deficiency. *Lancet.* 2008;371:64–74. doi:10.1016/S0140-6736(08)60073-2

3. Koralkova P, van Solinge WW, van Wijk R. Rare hereditary red blood cell enzymopathies associated with hemolytic anemia - pathophysiology, clinical aspects, and laboratory diagnosis. *Int J Lab Hematol.* 2014;36:388–397. doi:10.1111/ijlh.12223

4. Haley K. Congenital hemolytic anemia. *Med Clin North Am.* 2017;101:361–374. doi:10.1016/j.mcna.2016.09.008

5. Kalfa TA. Warm antibody autoimmune hemolytic anemia. *Hematology Am Soc Hematol Educ Program.* 2016;2016:690–697.

6. Garraty G. Immune hemolytic anemia associated with drug therapy. *Blood Rev.* 2010;24(4–5):143–150. doi:10.1016/j.blre.2010.06.004

7. Zantek ND, Koepsell SA, Tharp DR, Cohn CS. The direct antiglobulin test: a critical step in the evaluation of hemolysis. *Am J Hematol.* 2012;87:707–709. doi:10.1002/ajh.23218

8. Heisel MA, Ortega JA. Factors influencing prognosis in childhood autoimmune hemolytic anemia. *Am J Pediatr Hematol Oncol.* 1983;5:147–152.

9. Aladjidi N, Leverger G, Leblanc T, et al. New insights into childhood autoimmune hemolytic anemia: a French national observational study of 265 children. *Haematologica.* 2011;96(5):655–663. doi:10.3324/haematol.2010.036053

10. Lundin J, Karlsson C, Celsing F. Alemtuzumab therapy for severe autoimmune hemolysis in a patient with B-cell chronic lymphocytic leukemia. *Med Oncol.* 2006;23:137–139. doi:10.1385/mo:23:1:137

11. Hill A, DeZern AE, Kinoshita T, Brodsky RA. Paroxysmal nocturnal haemoglobinuria. *Nat Rev Dis Primers.* 2017;3:17028. doi:10.1038/nrdp.2017.29

12. Barcellini W. Current treatment strategies in autoimmune hemolytic disorders. *Expert Rev Hematol.* 2015;8(5):681–691. doi:10.1586/17474086.2015.1073105

13. Risitano AM, Marotta S. Therapeutic complement inhibition in complement mediated hemolytic anemias: Past, present and future. *Semin Immunol.* 2016;28:223–240. doi:10.1016/j.smim.2016.05.001

14. Howard J, Hoffbrand AV, Prentice HG, Mehta A. Mycophenolate mofetil for the treatment of refractory auto-immune haemolytic anaemia and auto-immune thrombocytopenia purpura. *Br J Haematol.* 2002;117(3):712–715. doi:10.1046/j.1365-2141.2002.03430.x

15. Zanella A, Barcellini W. Treatment of autoimmune hemolytic anemias. *Haematologica.* 2014;99(10):1547–1554. doi:10.3324/haematol.2014.114561

16. Pignon JM, Poirson E, Rochant H. Danazol in autoimmune haemolytic anaemia. *Br J Haematol.* 1993;83(2):343–345. doi:10.1111/j.1365-2141.1993.tb08293.x

17. Ahn YS, Harrington WJ, Mylvaganam R, et al. Danazol therapy for autoimmune hemolytic anemia. *Ann Intern Med.* 1985;102(3):298–301. doi:10.7326/0003-4819-102-3-298

18. Swiecicki PL, Hegerova LT, Gertz MA. Cold agglutinin disease. *Blood.* 2013;122:1114–1121. doi:10.1182/blood-2013-02-474437

19. Berentsen S, Ulvestad E, Langholm R, et al. Primary chronic cold agglutinin disease: a population based clinical study of 86 patients. *Haematologica.* 2006;91:460–466.

20. Heddle NM. Acute paroxysmal cold hemoglobinuria. *Transfus Med Rev.* 1989;3:219–229. doi:10.1016/S0887-7963(89)70082-1

21. Funato M, Kaneko H, Ozeki M, et al. A positive Donath-Landsteiner test in paroxysmal cold haemoglobinuria. *Eur J Haematol*. 2007;79:462. doi:10.1111/j.1600-0609.2007.00932.x

22. Nishimura J, Kanakura Y, Ware RE, et al. Clinical course and flow cytometric analysis of paroxysmal nocturnal hemoglobinuria in the United States and Japan. *Medicine (Baltimore)*. 2004;83:193–207. doi:10.1097/01.md.0000126763.68170.46

23. Kelly RJ, Hill A, Arnold LM, et al. Long-term treatment with eculizumab in paroxysmal nocturnal hemoglobinuria: sustained efficacy and improved survival. *Blood*. 2011;117:6786–6792. doi:10.1182/blood-2011-02-333997

8 Thalassemia and Hemoglobinopathies

Sumaira Shafi, Iberia Romina Sosa, and Mark Udden

INTRODUCTION

Thalassemias are a heterogeneous group of inherited syndromes characterized by reduced or absent production of the alpha or beta chain of the hemoglobin (Hgb) tetramer (1,2). Adult hemoglobin A (HgbA) is composed of two alpha and two beta chains. In a normal adult, the alpha and beta chains are produced in roughly equal amounts. Mutations or deletions that affect the balance of these globin chains result in the respective thalassemic syndromes. Thalassemia carriers constitute approximately 1.5% of the world population and are seen in all ethnic groups, but it predominantly affects the Mediterranean and the tropical and subtropical regions of Asia and Africa where malaria is or was an endemic. The clinical syndrome is a consequence of decreased Hgb production in the cell and the effects of the excess alpha or beta globin chain on erythropoiesis. This imbalance causes unpaired chains to precipitate, resulting in destruction of red blood cell (RBC) precursors in the bone marrow (ineffective erythropoiesis) and peripheral blood (hemolytic anemia). Decreased Hgb production manifests as hypochromia and microcytosis (1)

While thalassemias are the result of underproduction of a normal globin chain, hemoglobinopathies are structural abnormalities in the globin proteins themselves, which affect the function of the globin tetramer. An important example is a mutation resulting in the replacement of glutamic acid by valine in the sixth amino acid of the beta chain. This results in tactoid formation when Hgb is in the deoxygenated form. This causes deformation and sickling of the RBC—the hallmark of sickle cell disease (3–5). Other Hgb mutations may result in globin with high or low oxygen affinity, RBC instability, and sensitivity to oxidation (6).

During fetal development, there is a switch from fetal Hgb to adult Hgb. Adult alpha genes are expressed in the first trimester, whereas the switch from fetal (gamma) gene expression to the adult beta does not begin until the third trimester and is completed during the first year of life. Problems related to alpha globin, such

225

as thalassemia or hemoglobinopathy, appear at birth. Problems related to beta chain appear in 6- to 12-month-old children (1,3–5).

BETA THALASSEMIA

Clinical Case 8.1

A 30-year-old man is discovered to have anemia as the result of an insurance exam. His Hgb is 11 g/dL with a mean corpuscular volume (MCV) of 68 fL. RBC number is increased. Ferritin is normal, and Hgb electrophoresis shows HgbA$_2$ of 5.6%. His mother has anemia and her parents came to the United States from Sicily.

Introduction

There are two beta globin genes located on each chromosome 11. The beta globin gene is composed of three exons and two introns. A common cause of beta thalassemia is mutations in or near the splice sites, resulting in either reduced expression (β^+) or complete absence (β^0) of the beta globin chain. Numerous other mutations and deletions may also result in a clinical picture of beta thalassemia, thus contributing to the heterogeneity of this disorder (7).

Reduced synthesis of the beta globin subunit results in an excess of alpha chains, which aggregate and denature. The alpha globin precipitates from membrane-bound inclusion bodies which result in oxidative RBC membrane damage in the precursor and mature RBCs leading to apoptosis of the erythroblasts in the bone marrow (ineffective erythropoiesis) and peripheral destruction of the abnormal RBCs by the reticuloendothelial system (extravascular hemolysis). With the reduced oxygen-carrying capacity, there is an increased erythropoietin (EPO) production leading to massive bone marrow expansion and extramedullary hematopoiesis (7). Mouse models of beta thalassemia demonstrate activation of the *JAK2*–STAT5 pathway, which causes proliferation of erythroid progenitors with arrest in differentiation. Decreased hepcidin levels result in iron accumulation (8).

Concomitant alpha thalassemia with beta thalassemia can restore the balance between alpha and beta chain production and result in a milder condition.

Beta Thalassemia Minor

Clinical Case 8.1 describes a typical patient who is heterozygous for a beta thalassemia gene (either β^+ or β^0)—mild anemia with microcytosis and an increase in HgbA$_2$. Patients may have a palpable spleen tip, but are typically asymptomatic. These patients should not take iron unless there is laboratory evidence of iron deficiency. Genetic counseling should be offered. If both prospective parents have beta thalassemia minor, there is a 25% risk that they will have a child affected by beta thalassemia major. Chorionic villous sampling (CVS) can be done to determine if a fetus has beta thalassemia major. In vitro fertilization may be employed to select unaffected embryos for implantation (1,8).

Beta Thalassemia Intermedia

Nearly 10% of beta thalassemia patients have beta thalassemia intermedia. Patients with beta thalassemia intermedia are not transfusion dependent during early childhood. Transfusion dependence may develop later, particularly in third and fourth decades or during periods of erythroid stress (infections, pregnancy). An intermedia phenotype can result through various mechanisms: homozygosity for mild forms of β^+; the concommitant presence of alpha thalassemia, thereby restoring the balance of globin production; or mutations favoring persistence of fetal Hgb production. The clinical picture in these patients tends to be heterogeneous. Clinical features such as declining Hgb, progressive splenomegaly, growth defects, endocrine defects, and frequent hemolytic crises would indicate the need for regular transfusion therapy. Even in the absence of regular transfusions, patients develop iron overload and need regular monitoring (7).

Beta Thalassemia Major

Beta thalassemia major is frequently referred to as Cooley's or Mediterranean anemia. The mutation profile is homozygous or compound heterozygous (HgbE/β thalassemia) resulting in minimal to no beta globin chain production and little to no HgbA. Patients with beta thalassemia major have severe anemia (Hgb <7 g/dL) with substantial ineffective erythropoiesis and transfusion dependence (7).

Diagnosis

Onset of symptoms for beta thalassemia major is at 6 to 12 months of age when fetal Hgb production has fully switched to adult Hgb (1). Patients usually present with fatigue, irritability, growth retardation, and hepatosplenomegaly due to extramedullary hematopoiesis. Extramedullary erythropoiesis may also lead to the development of facial and skeletal changes, as well as the formation of masses which can result in cord compression. Patients may suffer complications of high-output heart failure associated with severe anemia and are likely to develop osteoporosis (1,2,7).

Microcytic, hypochromic anemia with increased reticulocyte count is present in patients with beta thalassemia major. The peripheral smear shows extreme microcytes, target cells, and tear drop cells with fine basophilic stippling (Figure 8.1A,B). Patients who have splenectomies show striking normoblastemia. Hgb electrophoresis shows variably high levels of HgbF and HgbA$_2$ (Table 8.1). Increasingly, a genetic diagnosis is made by looking for characteristic haplotypes or sequencing of the beta globin gene (1).

Late symptoms of thalassemia derive from iron overload which can affect the liver, heart, and the endocrine system. Iron overload is the result of both transfusion and increased gastrointestinal absorption of iron. When iron levels are high and there is liver damage, ferritin may not be a good indicator of body iron stores. Parenchymal iron may be assessed by liver biopsy (1,9). Specialized MRI techniques (MRI*) can also evaluate liver and heart iron content (10).

Key Diagnostic Dilemma

Patients with thalassemia minor are commonly misdiagnosed as having iron deficiency anemia (IDA). Both entities are characterized by microcytosis and hypochromia. As IDA (covered in Chapter 6,

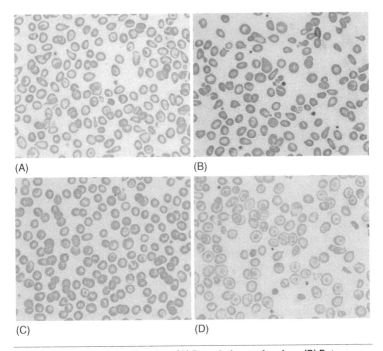

Figure 8.1 Thalassemia disorders. **(A)** Beta thalassemia minor. **(B)** Beta thalassemia intermedia. **(C)** Alpha thalassemia $\alpha^{3.7}/\alpha^{3.7}$. **(D)** Hemoglobin H disease.

Table 8.1 Beta Thalassemia, Overview of Hemoglobin Electrophoresis, Laboratory and Clinical Manifestations

Subtype	Genotype	Hgb Electrophoresis	Clinical Features	Microcytic Anemia	Transfusion Dependence
βThalassemia minor/trait (heterozygotes)	β/β^+ or β/β^0	HgbA$_2$ 3.6% to 7% HgbF up to 5%	Asymptomatic Increased risk for gallstones Mild anemia	Mild	No
βThalassemia intermedia	β^+/β^+	HgbF 10% to 50% HgbA$_2$ >4%	Variable presentation with moderate anemia	Moderate (>7 g/dL)	Transfusion independent
βThalassemia major/Cooley's anemia	β^0/β^0 or β^0/β^+	HgbF up to 95% HgbA$_2$ >5% HgbF 70% to 90% HgbA up to 30%	Severe anemia, skeletal and facial changes, growth retardation, osteoporosis, organ damage from iron overload	Severe (<7 g/dL)	Transfusion dependent

Hgb, hemoglobin.

Hypoproliferative Anemia) is more prevalent, patients with thalassemia minor are often treated with iron supplementation. In mild IDA, however, MCV is rarely below 80 fL, whereas an MCV below 75 fL is common in thalassemia minor. RBC counts are typically high in thalassemia minor, but are suppressed in IDA. The RBC distribution width (RDW) in thalassemia minor is normal, reflecting a homogeneous population, whereas it is elevated in IDA to indicate a heterogeneous RBC population. The peripheral smear shows similar findings to hypochromia and microcytosis. However, target cells prevalent in thalassemia are rare in IDA. Moreover, tear drop cells are typical in thalassemia, but not observed in IDA. Finally, ordering an iron panel should help confirm the diagnosis, as patients with thalassemia minor have normal iron storage parameters or possibly, elevated ferritins. Hgb electrophoresis identifies beta thalassemia carriers, but not alpha thalassemia carriers (1).

Prognosis

The prognosis for beta thalassemia is variable and dependent on the disease phenotype. Survival continues to improve with the advent of iron chelation and hypertransfusion protocols (1,9). Beta thalassemia intermedia has a variable prognosis which depends on the severity of anemia, need for transfusion, and use of iron chelation. In contrast, beta thalassemia minor is a relatively asymptomatic disease that does not limit survival and may never come to medical attention (1).

Untreated beta thalassemia major is fatal in 85% of patients who do not survive to age 5. Cardiovascular complications are the main cause of death either from high-output heart failure or iron overload cardiomyopathy, both of which have improved in recent years with the advent of hypertransfusion protocols and iron chelation therapy, respectively. Survival into the fourth, fifth, or sixth decade is possible now (8). Hematopoietic cell transplantation (HCT), which began in the 1980s, is potentially curative (9).

Management

Thalassemia major patients are transfusion dependent. Patients have significant anemia with Hgb <7 g/dL, features of growth retardation, and skeletal changes if transfusion therapy is not initiated. Hypertransfusion with the goal of attaining Hgb from 9 to 10.5 g/dL is recommended. This suppresses erythropoiesis and gastrointestinal absorption of iron (11). A complete RBC antigen phenotype should be obtained to guide selection of donor units, so that the risk of delayed hemolytic transfusion reaction is reduced (1).

Assessment of iron stores is important in patients with thalassemia. Iron chelation needs to be initiated when the ferritin level is >1,000 ng/mL, liver or cardiac iron concentration exceeds 3 mg iron per gram dry weight, hypertransfusion program is initiated, and/or after transfusion with 20 to 25 units of red cells (1). The options for pharmacologic iron chelation include the oral agents deferasirox and deferiprone and subcutaneous infusion of deferoxamine (Table 8.2). Growth and endocrine defects due to iron deposition in the pituitary, thyroid, and adrenal glands may require consultation with an experienced endocrinologist. Women with beta thalassemia major often require in vitro fertilization to conceive (11). Zinc supplementation may improve bone mineral density in young patients. Compliance with a transfusion program improves the bone strength and reduces fracture risk (11).

Heart failure and cardiac arrhythmias are the main causes of death in patients with beta thalassemia major. Early EKG changes include prolonged PR, first-degree heart block, and premature atrial contractions. Periodic assessment of cardiac iron content by MRI T2* is necessary. Deferiprone is more effective than deferoxamine in reducing cardiac iron load (12).

Splenectomy is considered in patients with large spleens and progressive increase in transfusion requirements or with

Table 8.2 Iron Chelators

	Administration	Pharmacokinetics	Dosing	Side Effects
Deferoxamine	IV or SQ	Half-life 8 to 10 minutes	Nightly 10-12 h continuous SQ infusion of 2 g delivered through battery-driven pump	Local reaction, neurosensory toxicity, visual and auditory impairment, infections with *Yersinia* and mucormycosis
Deferiprone	Oral	Half-life 90 minutes	Every 8 hours	Agranulocytosis, nausea, vomiting, arthropathy, hepatic dysfunction
Deferasirox	Oral	Half-life 12 to 18 hours	Once a day	Elevated serum creatinine, mild GI symptoms, skin rash, well tolerated in general

GI, gastrointestinal; IV, intravenous; SQ, subcutaneous.

worsening cytopenias. Spleen size by itself is not an indicator for splenectomy. Appropriate vaccinations need to be administered prior to surgery. There is an increased risk for thromboembolic disease and sepsis from encapsulated organisms following splenectomy (13).

Stem cell transplant can be offered to children if a human leukocyte antigen (HLA)-matched sibling who is not thalassemic or who is heterozygous is available. When performed early, stem cell transplant is tolerable and can restore normal erythropoiesis. Iron overload can then be managed by phlebotomy (9).

Future Directions

- Hypomethylating agents can increase HgbF production and ameliorate ineffective erythropoiesis (14).
- *JAK2* inhibitors are being investigated for their ability to modulate ineffective erythropoiesis (14).
- Gene therapy has been accomplished with the transfer of a normal beta globin gene into pluripotent hematopoietic stem cell and autotransplantation. An alternative approach is to introduce a deactivating mutation in the promoter of the *BCL11A* gene, which is a key element in the switch from HgbF to HgbA, resulting in increased levels of HgbF (14).

Key Points

- Beta thalassemia is a genetic disorder with reduced synthesis of the beta globin subunit and aggregation of excessive alpha chains, which results in RBC destruction in the bone marrow or spleen.
- Three distinct syndromes include thalassemia major, intermedia, and minor based on the amount of alpha and beta subunits produced as a result of genetic changes.
- Beta thalassemia minor patients are asymptomatic carriers, but need genetic counseling. It is important not to confuse this entity with IDA.
- Beta thalassemia intermedia has a heterogeneous presentation, often not requiring transfusions until later in life or during periods of stress.
- Beta thalassemia major is the most severe form, manifesting during the first year of life, and needs aggressive measures to prevent life-threatening complications.
- Beta thalassemia is characterized by microcytic, hypochromic RBCs with an elevated red cell count and normal RDW. Diagnosis is confirmed by Hgb electrophoresis.

- Early enrollment in hypertransfusion program and iron chelation can prevent long-term complications of beta thalassemia major. Hematopoietic stem cell transplant is potentially curative.

ALPHA THALASSEMIA

Introduction

There are two alpha globin genes (α_2 and α_1) located on each chromosome 16. The α_2 produces more globin than α_1. Deletion of one or more genes results in alpha thalassemia and leads to imbalance in globin chains with an excess of beta chains. Unlike the alpha chain, the beta chains can form relatively stable tetramers β_4 (HgbH). HgbH tetramers primarily affect the mature RBC and not the precursors. Hemolysis is present, but with mild ineffective erythropoiesis. At birth, γ_4 (Hgb Barts) is present. Patients are not as anemic, and erythropoiesis is more effective than that seen with beta thalassemia (2). In African and African American patients, gene deletion may result from a crossover event (unequal genetic exchange) during premeiosis that generates a single gene comprising parts of α_2 and α_1. Homologous recombination between misaligned chromosomes results in a 3.7-kb deletion. Patients with $\alpha\alpha/\alpha^{3.7}$ make up about 30% of the African American population. These patients do not have anemia, but may have borderline MCV. Patients who are homozygous for $\alpha^{3.7}/\alpha^{3.7}$ comprise about 3.5% of the African American population and they may have mild anemia with microcytosis (2). In the Near East and Asia, large deletions of chromosome 16 affect the alpha locus, so that both α_2 and α_1 (--) on chromosome 16 are lost. A typical deletion is found in Southeast Asia (--^{SEA}). In the same population, $\alpha^{3.7}$ with a single functional gene on the chromosome also exists. This can result in situations in which there are two functioning genes (--/$\alpha\alpha$) or only one functioning alpha gene (--/$\alpha^{3.7}$) (2). The former results in microcytosis with mild anemia and the latter results in anemia and what is known as HgbH disease. These patients have a normal life expectancy, but do have anemia and a tendency for iron overload (2).

Parents who share a --/$\alpha\alpha$ genotype may have children who are --/--. A fetus with this genotype is unlikely to survive outside the uterus. The baby's fetal Hgb is mostly γ_4, which has a very high oxygen affinity. Oxygen transport from the placenta is compromised and the infant suffers from hydrops fetalis. Typical pregnancies end in stillbirth, and the mothers develop eclampsia. Intrauterine transfusions may ameliorate this situation (2,15).

There are also non-deletional events that affect the α gene. One of these is a mutation in the stop codon, which results in a longer alpha mRNA that is not efficiently translated. A longer alpha chain is produced (31 additional amino acids) which produces an unstable globin, Hgb Constant Spring, which is common in southern China. When the other chromosome has two gene deletions, HgbH is seen and the anemia can be quite severe (2). Rarely, patients are seen with alpha thalassemia in association with intellectual delay and other developmental abnormalities. One of these involves deletions of the end of chromosome 16 containing the alpha gene loci and other genes responsible for the developmental findings (*ATR-16*). Another is found on a promoter gene on the X chromosome (*ATR-X*). This promoter affects transcription of the alpha gene and other genes, resulting in developmental abnormalities in boys in association with thalassemia. Mutations in *ATR-X* can be acquired in MDS and myeloproliferative neoplasm (MPN) and account for the reports of patients who acquire a thalassemic phenotype as a result of these disorders (2).

Diagnosis

The presence and severity of anemia correlates with the number of functioning globin chains. Alpha thalassemia minor patients experience mild anemia, hypochromia, and microcytosis, which is clinically asymptomatic. The Hgb level is usually >10 g/dL, without overt hemolysis. Patients with HgbH disease have moderate anemia that does not require transfusional support. A retrospective series reports Hgb levels between 8 and 11 g/dL. In some cases, transfusion may be necessary for patients with HgbH during periods of erythropoietic stress (e.g., infection, pregnancy). Complete absence of the alpha gene is not compatible with life. Peripheral smear in Hgb Barts typically shows marked hypochromia and microcytosis, bizarre RBC morphology, and an elevated RBC count (Figure 8.1C,D) (2).

Table 8.3 summarizes the expected Hgb electrophoresis and peripheral smear review findings.

Key Diagnostic Dilemma

As with beta thalassemia minor, alpha thalassemia patients are often misdiagnosed with IDA. However, alpha thalassemia carrier patients exhibit a normal Hgb electrophoresis. While hypochromic microcytic anemia is the hallmark of the thalassemia syndromes, the silent carrier state (most commonly, α-2 thalassemia trait or a-/a-) is often normochromic and the diagnosis is best confirmed by globin gene testing.

Prognosis

Severe alpha thalassemia, characterized by (--/--), with no production of globin chains, leads to intrauterine death due to hydrops fetalis in the absence of intrauterine transfusions. Alpha thalassemia intermedia patients have variable prognosis which depends

Table 8.3 Alpha Thalassemia, Overview of Hemoglobin Electrophoresis, Laboratory and Clinical Manifestations

Phenotype	Genotype	Hgb Electrophoresis	CBC Characteristics	Clinical Characteristics
Silent carrier (α^+-thalassemia trait)	$\alpha\alpha/\alpha-$	Normal	Normal Hgb and MCV	Melanesia and Southeast Asia
αThalassemia minor	$\alpha\alpha/--$ or $\alpha-/\alpha-$	HgbA$_2$ (1.5%–2.5%)	Mild anemia with low MCV	The existence of concomitant unstable alpha chain Hgb variants along with alpha thalassemia trait may result in a lower than expected Hgb (15)
HgbH disease	$\alpha-/--$	HgbH (up to 30%), HgbA$_2$ <4%	Moderate to severe anemia	Skeletal changes, splenomegaly Predominant in Asians and Mediterranean. Rare in Africa
Hydrops fetalis (16)	$--/--$	Hgb Barts (gamma tetramers) No HgbF, HgbA, or HgbA$_2$	Severe anemia with hydrops fetalis	Exclusively in Asians Marked anasarca, hepatosplenomegaly, severe anemia Fatal

CBC, complete blood count; Hgb, hemoglobin; MCV, mean corpuscular volume.

on the severity of anemia, transfusion requirement, and need for iron chelation. Alpha thalassemia minor patients are asymptomatic carriers with no compromised survival and may never come to medical attention (2).

Management

Treatment goals are similar to those for beta thalassemia and are largely dependent on severity of anemia (2).

Key Points

- Alpha thalassemia is a genetic disorder characterized by impaired production of alpha chains from one, two, three, or all four of the alpha globin genes (*HBA1* and *HBA2*), resulting in excess β chains which form tetramers that are unstable and primarily affect mature RBCs; thus, there is little ineffective erythropoiesis.
- Clinical presentations of alpha thalassemia vary based on the number of functioning genes.
- Most of the alpha thalassemia patients exhibit microcytosis, but silent carriers may be normochromic.
- Diagnosis is based on globin gene testing as the Hgb electrophoresis is normal except in HgbH and Hgb Barts when excess tetramers may be visualized.
- Based on the degree of anemia, transfusion and iron chelation are recommended.

HgbE: A THALASSEMIC HEMOGLOBINOPATHY

HgbE is prevalent in Southeast Asians and results from a single nucleotide change in codon 26 of the beta globin gene. HgbE is a "thalassemic hemoglobinopathy." The GAG/AAG substitution activates a cryptic splice site, which if utilized creates an unstable mRNA causing a decreased beta chain synthesis. Transcripts without the abnormal splicing demonstrate the amino acid substitution of lysine for glutamic acid. Individuals with the HgbE trait are asymptomatic with or without mild anemia and variable microcytosis. HgbE-β (β^E/β^0) results in a variable phenotype ranging from thalassemia intermedia to thalassemia major (16).

SICKLE CELL DISEASE

Clinical Case 8.2

A 25-year-old man with HgbSS presents to the hospital for treatment of pain crises. He has developed fever, shortness of breath, and bilateral chest pain.

Pain is described in all extremities, back, and pelvis. Pulse oximetry shows low oxygen saturation on room air with modest improvement while on 4-L oxygen cannula. Chest x-ray shows bilateral infiltrates. His Hgb is 6.5 g/dL and white blood cell (WBC) count is 20,000 with normal differential.

Introduction

HgbS results from a mutation affecting the sixth amino acid of HgbA, resulting in a substitution of glutamic acid by valine. Deoxygenated valine forms a hydrophobic area, which favors gelation of HgbS to form larger polymers or tactoids. These tactoids distort the RBC into a sickle shape. Repetitive deformation of the membrane occurs with reversible sickling as cells are oxygenated in the lung and exposed to hypoxia in the tissues. Ultimately, these cycles of sickling and unsickling lead to permanent red cell membrane damage and an irreversibly sickled RBC—the hallmark of sickle cell disease. In the heterozygous state, reversible sickling occurs with deoxygenation, but does not result in permanent damage to produce irreversible sickle forms in peripheral blood smears which are made with blood exposed to air. In homozygous individuals, sickling results in a hemolytic anemia along with microvascular disease that has long-term effects on organ function and periodic vaso-occlusive disease resulting in pain crises, chest syndrome, and stroke (3–5). Splenic function is affected at an early age, and children typically become functionally asplenic by the age of 6 or 7. The spleen may be affected by vaso-occlusion resulting in splenic sequestration. Neonatal screening programs now identify children with sickle cell disease and allow parents to be educated to bring their children in when they have fever or abdominal pain. This has dramatically reduced death due to pneumococcal infection and unrecognized splenic sequestration. Currently, 90% to 95% of children with sickle cell anemia (SCA) survive to adulthood (17).

Diagnosis

By convention, SCA refers to HbSS. Patients who are compound heterozygotes for HgbS and β^0 have similar presentation and natural history, and are described as having sickle cell disease. HgbSβ^0 is characterized by a slightly higher Hgb and microcytosis. Sickle cell disease also includes HgbSC disease and Sβ^+ thalassemia. These patients have higher Hgb levels and often a milder course. Their spleen persists into adulthood, with the potential for splenic infarction/sequestration in the second or third decade of life (3).

SCA is characterized by chronic hemolysis, usually associated with mild to moderate anemia (hematocrit 20%–30%), reticulocytosis of 3% to 15%, normal MCV, unconjugated hyperbilirubinemia, elevated serum lactate dehydrogenase (LDH), and low serum haptoglobin.

Peripheral blood smear reveals sickled RBCs, polychromasia due to reticulocytosis, and Howell–Jolly bodies due to hyposplenia (Figure 8.2). The RBCs are normochromic, unless there is a concomitant thalassemia or iron deficiency. SICKLEDEX is a quick screening test based on the observation that HgbS is insoluble in concentrated phosphate buffer solutions, whereas HgbA and other Hgb remain in solution. The test is not specific for HgbSS as the trait and other sickling syndromes also give a positive result. Hgb gel electrophoresis constitutes a low-cost method to detect common Hgb variants: HgbA, $HgbA_2$, HgbF, HgbS, and HgbC (3–5). For first-line screening of hemoglobinopathies, gel electrophoresis has been replaced by more sensitive, reliable, and automatable methods such as isoelectric focusing, cation-exchange high-performance chromatography, and capillary electrophoresis (3–5). Prenatal testing can be achieved by chorionic villus sampling at 8 to 10 weeks of gestation. Testing of fetal cells from maternal peripheral blood is now routinely done for chromosomal abnormalities, but studies to validate the reliability of this modality to diagnose SCA are currently underway (17).

Table 8.4 summarizes the expected Hgb electrophoresis and peripheral smear review findings in common sickle hemoglobinopathies.

SCA is characterized by several complications that are covered in the section, Sickle Cell Complications, in this chapter. Specific diagnostic testing for these complications are covered in that section.

Key Diagnostic Dilemma

Performing an Hgb electrophoresis after a blood transfusion makes it difficult to confirm diagnosis since the test reflects the transfused blood. Alkaline pH Hgb electrophoresis does not distinguish Hgb that migrates to the same position, such as $HgbA_2$ and HgbC, making it difficult to identify an HgbSC. In this case, separation of comigrating Hgb can be accomplished at acidic pH (e.g., separation of HgbC from $HgbA_2$).

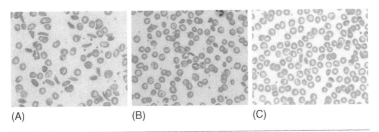

(A)   (B)   (C)

Figure 8.2 Sickle hemoglobinopathies. **(A)** Hemoglobin SS. **(B)** Hemoglobin SC. **(C)** Hemoglobin Sβ thalassemia.

Table 8.4 Common S Hemoglobinopathies—Overview of Hemoglobin Electrophoresis, Laboratory and Clinical Manifestations

Type	Electrophoresis Findings	Clinical Features	Morphology
HgbAS (sickle cell trait)	HgbA and HgbS, HgbA > HgbS	Asymptomatic	No sickling
HgbSS (sickle cell disease)	$HgbA_2$ and HgbS	Moderate anemia	Irreversibly sickled cells
HgbSC	HgbS and HgbC	Mild anemia, less frequent pain, but more frequent ocular and bone complications	Sickling rare + crystalline material called SC poikilocytes
Sickle β^0-thalassemia	HgbS, $HgbA_2$, and HgbF, but no HgbA	Mild to moderate anemia	Irreversibly sickled cells, target cells, and microcytosis
Sickle β^+-thalassemia	HgbS, HgbA and $HgbA_2$, and HgbF	Mild anemia, less pain	Sickling rare

Prognosis

Patients with sickle cell disease (SCD) have increased morbidity and mortality, but the prognosis for SCD has dramatically improved following the institution of comprehensive care that includes newborn screening, immunizations, antibiotics, hydroxyurea, and prevention and treatment of disease complications (e.g., stroke). In areas where comprehensive care is available, the disease has largely shifted from a fatal illness to more chronic disease management. The Dallas Newborn Cohort, which includes 940 patients prospectively enrolled since 1983, showed that acute chest syndrome (ACS) and multiorgan failure have largely replaced bacterial sepsis as the leading causes of death in young patients with SCD. Ninety-five percent of children with SCA now survive to age 16. In contrast, in regions of Africa where newborn screening and access to immunizations and antibiotics is not routine, infections remain the leading cause of death (18).

Two recent studies have demonstrated the benefit of comprehensive care center in the survival of patients with SCA. A 2014 study involving a cohort of adult patients followed at a tertiary care medical center in the United States demonstrated the median survival for HgbSS and HgbSβ⁰ was 58 years and for HgbSC and HgbSβ⁺ was

66 years. In a 2016 study involving 712 patients followed at a tertiary center in the United Kingdom, the median survival for HgbSS and HgbSβ^0 was 67 years. Both studies show that individuals who survive into later adulthood will experience long-term complications, such as renal insufficiency and pulmonary hypertension, which are not often encountered in younger patients (19,20).

Management

Neonatal screening carried out in most states detects affected children while they are still covered by an increased fetal Hgb. Penicillin prophylaxis and early medical assessment of fever or abdominal pain has dramatically reduced mortality due to sepsis and splenic sequestration. Screening for stroke risk by transcranial Doppler and transfusion therapy for at-risk children have decreased the incidence of stroke. The National Heart, Lung, and Blood Institute (NHLBI) guidelines recommend treatment of some form either with hydroxyurea or transfusion for all children. Ideally, care should be coordinated by experienced physicians in a well-organized sickle cell center, as this improves prognosis for this population (19,20).

Early clinical studies established a role for hydroxyurea in increasing HgbF levels. HgbF reduces the concentration of S in the cell, and the presence of the gamma chain in mixed tetramers ($\alpha_2\beta^S\gamma$) inhibits sickling (3–5). Hydroxyurea therapy was shown to be of substantial benefit in the MESH trial in which 150 patients were randomized to hydroxyurea and 150 to placebo. The incidence of pain crises was reduced, and the frequency of chest syndrome decreased by half. Hydroxyurea was well tolerated, and HgbF levels increased substantially in those who were compliant with therapy (21). The BABY HUG trial showed the safety and benefit of hydroxyurea in a pediatric population (22).

Adult care should begin with a smooth transition from pediatric care to adult hematology. Given the chaotic state of healthcare for adults in the United States, this transition has been problematic for many patients with SCA. Hydroxyurea remains the mainstay of treatment. SCA patients who are treated in the community rather than in sickle cell centers are often on subtherapeutic doses of hydroxyurea. Doses should be titrated to near leukopenia to maximize HgbF levels. The NHLBI guidelines are a useful resource for the details of hydroxyurea management (19). Patients with stroke are continued on transfusion indefinitely. Adults have more issues with maintaining access for transfusion. Treatment with iron chelation must continue with careful monitoring of renal and hepatic functions. Management of sickle pain crises requires knowledge of individual needs. Narcotics should be tailored to the individual and based on a treatment plan or contract between the physician and the patient (3–5).

Bone marrow transplantation is an option for a patient with significant morbidity. Results are best in children and adolescents. An adult with SCA has a worse outlook with allogeneic transplants. HLA-matched sibling donors are only available for about 20% of patients. Haploidentical stem cell transplants have been done with some success. A chimeric bone marrow usually results, which is often sufficient to reduce sickling enough to benefit the patient, albeit at the cost of significant immunosuppression (14).

Gene therapy has been the Holy Grail for multiple disorders and has arrived finally for patients with sickle cell disease and beta thalassemia major. Two approaches have been developed. The first which has been tested in pilot studies utilizes a construct containing a modified human HBB$^{BA-T87Q}$ that has a threonine to glycine substitution at amino acid 87 observed in normal HgbF gamma chains. This substitution confers an anti-sickling effect and allows recognition of the novel globin product by Hgb fractionation methods. Stem cells are transduced and then an auto stem cell transplant is carried out. Another approach, still in the laboratory, is the use of Crisper-Caspase 9 technology to insert a downregulating mutation in the promoter for the *BCL11A* gene. The *BCL11A* gene product is a component of the "switch" from gamma gene expression to beta gene expression. In animal models, this results in an increased HgbF up to 50%, which produces a phenotype similar to patients who are heterozygous for S and for the hereditary persistence of fetal Hgb and, as a result, are similar to HgbS trait individuals (14).

L-Glutamine has been introduced as an oral agent that ameliorates the unfavorable redox state of the sickle cell which results in increased oxidation and damage to the red cell membrane. A clinical trial showed a modest improvement in patient outcomes on L-glutamine compared to a placebo control (14).

Inhibition of P-selectin–mediated sickle cell adhesion to endothelium has been achieved with an inhibitory monoclonal antibody, crizanlizumab. A recent clinical trial shows that regular infusions significantly reduce the frequency of pain crises. Both agents were tested in populations that included patients on hydroxyurea therapy presaging an era in which combination therapies are offered to patients to prevent pain crises and slow the progress of sickle vasculopathy (14).

Specific treatment options for sickle cell complications are covered next.

Sickle Cell Complications

Pain crises are the bane of existence for many patients with SCA. Patients vary in the frequency and severity of pain episodes. Some studies show that about 20% of patients have more than two to three crises per year, resulting in visits to emergency department or hospitalization. The remaining 80% of patients have less than one crisis per year reported. Pain can affect the arms, legs, back, and abdomen. Narcotics may be required to control pain. Milder pain can be managed by nonsteroidal anti-inflammatory drugs (NSAIDs) or acetaminophen. Local measures such as hot baths or massage may help. Admission is recommended for patients who have chest pain to observe and evaluate for potential evolution of ACS (3–5).

Stroke occurs in about 5% of patients with HgbSS and about 1% of patients with HgbSC. Stroke is caused by intimal changes and vaso-occlusion in distal internal carotid arteries (ICA) and proximal circle of Willis, including middle cerebral artery (MCA) and anterior cerebral artery (ACA). Transcranial Doppler measurements showing increased flow velocity are predictive of stroke, and most pediatric sickle cell centers employ this as a screen. Patients with high velocities are offered transfusion therapy which effectively reduces stroke occurrence. Strokes in SCA can be infarctive or hemorrhagic. Hemorrhagic stroke is associated with a high mortality. Silent infarction can be found in 18% to 20% of patients who have not had a clinical stroke. Initial management of stroke should include transfusion or exchange transfusion to maximize recovery and long-term transfusion protocols to prevent recurrence. MRI and magnetic resonance angiography (MRA) are effective in the evaluation of stroke. Angiography is more specific for lesions in the central nervous system (CNS) vasculature, but there is risk from exposure to dye which can facilitate sickling. Transfusions should be done before angiography is undertaken. The initial goal of transfusion/exchange should be to keep the percentage of HgbS below 30%. Chronic transfusion requires maintenance of a good access and also careful attention to iron chelation to prevent iron overload. Patients who develop antibodies to red cell antigens or who cannot tolerate transfusion can be switched very slowly to hydroxyurea therapy (3–5).

Splenic sequestration is a complication of sickle vaso-occlusion and occurs between the ages of 1 and 6 in HgbSS children. In adulthood, splenic sequestration is rare and occurs in patients with Hgb SC or Sβ+ because their spleens persist into adulthood. In about one third of these patients, the spleen is palpable. Splenic sequestration and splenic infarction may coexist. Patients present with left upper quadrant (LUQ) pain, decrease in Hgb level of 20% below baseline, and increase in size of the spleen by 2 cm. Patients may develop hypotension requiring emergency transfusions and rarely, splenectomy. A sympathetic left pleural effusion may develop. Treatment is largely supportive with fluid resuscitation, narcotics for pain, and transfusion (3–5).

Aplastic crisis or pure red cell aplasia is a significant problem in SCA. Patients have anemia, shortened RBC life span, and are absolutely dependent on an expanded erythron. Parvovirus B19 is the usual culprit. This virus invades the pronormoblast via interaction with the P antigen, proliferates in the nucleus, and causes cell death. During the infection, the production of RBCs stops and there is reticulocytopenia. If a marrow is done, erythroid hypoplasia is present along with a few giant pronormoblasts with intranuclear inclusions—lantern cells. In typical SCA patients with good immunity, this is a self-limited disease and the management is supportive. Usually, simple transfusions are required. Parvovirus infection can be accompanied by ACS, stroke, nephrotic syndrome, encephalopathy, and myocarditis (3–5).

Infections with encapsulated organisms are a major issue in the care of patients with SCA owing to their lack of splenic function. *Streptococcus pneumoniae* and *Haemophilus influenzae* B are the most common infections. As per the NHLBI guidelines, patients should receive vaccinations for these two organisms as well as for meningococcal disease, hepatitis B, and the annual flu shot. Penicillin prophylaxis is recommended for children until the age of 5—there is a paucity of evidence supporting continuation after that age (3–5).

ACS is a major cause of morbidity and mortality in SCA (clinical case). It is marked by fever, cough, infiltrate on chest x-ray, hypoxemia, and leukocytosis. Patients may have chest pain and dyspnea. There are multiple factors at play in this syndrome: infection, volume overload from overly aggressive attempts to hydrate, fat embolization, reactive airways disease, pulmonary thrombosis, and atelectasis due to poor inspiration while receiving narcotics or due to rib infarction and splinting. The mainstays of treatment are antibiotics, transfusions, oxygen, and use of the incentive spirometer to treat or prevent atelectasis. In a study in which patients routinely underwent bronchoalveloar lavage, an infection was present in about one third—*S. pneumoniae, H. influenzae*, mycoplasma, and chlamydia. Another significant finding was the presence of lipid-laden macrophages consistent with fat embolization originating from bone infarcts. Chest syndrome can occur days after hospitalization for pain crisis—often a severe one with multiple bones involved as a potential source for fat embolization. Management of ACS includes prevention with use of the incentive spirometer in all patients admitted for control of pain. Patients admitted should also have routine monitoring of pO_2. When chest syndrome is recognized, antibiotics, administration of oxygen, and transfusion should be undertaken. Exchange transfusion may be required, especially when the baseline Hgb is above 8 or 9 g/dL and when there is no improvement in oxygenation with more conservative measures (3,4,23).

Pulmonary hypertension is seen in about one third of patients with SCA. Increased pulmonary artery pressure can be estimated from the degree of tricuspid regurgitation on echo Doppler studies of the heart. The increase is usually moderate and seldom reaches the levels seen in idiopathic pulmonary hypertension, and standard echo Doppler estimates are not always substantiated by values obtained during right heart catheterization. High cardiac output appears to be another factor in measurements of pulmonary artery pressure. Nevertheless, this finding is associated with increased mortality in sickle cell disease. Pulmonary hypertension has been correlated with intravascular hemolysis. Free Hgb in the plasma is a powerful scavenger of nitric oxide (NO). NO administration can decrease the pulmonary blood pressure, but is not a practical mode of therapy for patients. Pulmonary hypertension is associated with markers of hemolysis, such as LDH, and also with other complications of sickle cell disease: sickle ulcers and priapism. It is very likely that other phenomena such as red cell interactions with endothelium via adhesion molecules such as P-selectin and increased oxidation are participants in the vasculopathy of SCA and its complications. Consultation with a pulmonologist who has expertise in pulmonary hypertension is helpful. A trial of sildenafil in SCA patients with pulmonary hypertension showed no benefit — patients on the treatment arm had changes in pulmonary artery pressures, but also had increased frequency of pain crises which led to early termination of the study (24). Endothelin blockade, prostacyclin infusion, transfusion therapy, and hydroxyurea are potential treatments for which there are insufficient data (3,23,24).

Nephropathy occurs in patients with SCA. Glomerulopathy with proteinuria responds to treatment with angiotensin-converting enzyme (ACE) inhibitors, which may slow progression of renal disease. Advanced disease can result in the need for hemodialysis (HD) or peritoneal dialysis. HD is sometimes problematic because of an increased incidence of failure of grafts or fistulae created for dialysis access. Renal transplantation has been successful in SCA. EPO must be used with caution in the management of anemia of renal disease in a patient with SCA. The desired Hgb level is the patient's baseline level for his or her SCA. Taking the patient to an Hgb of 10 or higher will result in an increased frequency of crises and access thrombosis. Renal tubular problems also occur in SCA. Renal tubular acidosis, hyperkalemia, and hyperuricemia may be encountered. All adults with SCA have some degree of inability to concentrate the urine, making dehydration an important issue. The management of SCA crises often begins with an effort to rehydrate the patient. Hematuria is also encountered and requires a full workup before assigning blame to sickle cell disease. Renal papillary necrosis is another known complication. Patients also are at risk for pyelonephritis (4,5,25).

Hepatic crises are a serious complication of SCA and can be fulminate and lead to death. Vaso-occlusive disease presents with right upper quadrant (RUQ) pain, hepatic enlargement, and increased levels of transaminases and alkaline phosphatase. The bilirubin level is often strikingly elevated and is a combination of indirect bilirubin from hemolysis and direct reacting bilirubin from hepatic failure. Hgb may also drop precipitously from sequestration of sickle cells in the hepatic sinusoids. Other factors in SCA liver disease include iron overload from frequent transfusions and viral hepatitis. Although most patients with SCA have an elevated bilirubin at baseline, it is usually <5 mg/dL with a low direct reacting fraction. Higher levels of total and indirect bilirubin are seen in patients who also have Gilbert's disease (4,5).

Cholelithiasis is found in 25% to 50% of patients with SCA. Pigment stones from increased bilirubin are typically found. Cholecystitis must be differentiated from abdominal pain associated with a pain crisis. Patients present with RUQ pain and tenderness on palpation during deep inspiration, fever, and elevated bilirubin. About one third of these patients require cholecystectomy after a bout or two of cholecystitis. Laparoscopic cholecystectomy is well tolerated. For general anesthesia, the patients are usually prepared by simple transfusion to an Hgb of 10 g/dL. Exchange transfusion is not necessary, unless the patient has a high Hgb level or when there is a significant history of pulmonary hypertension or other pulmonary disease. If transfusion therapy is omitted, there is an increased risk for pain crises and chest syndrome (4,5,26).

Avascular necrosis (AVN) also affects patients with SCA and most often involves the hips and, less frequently, the humeri. Patients may do well with physical therapy, but hip replacement is often required to maintain mobility without pain. Hip disease may present at a young age in SCA, so most orthopedists delay replacement as long as possible recognizing the relatively short functional durability (about 15 years) of current hip prostheses. Rates of prosthetic hip failure and infection are higher in SCA (4,5).

Retinopathy should be assessed as a part of health maintenance in SCA. Exams are recommended yearly or every other year. Laser treatment of sickle retinopathy is often successful and may prevent progression to glaucoma and loss of eyesight (4,5).

Venous stasis ulcers are a major nuisance for patients with SCA. Treatment is largely supportive, although zinc supplementation may be helpful. The advent of wound care clinics has been a benefit for these patients. Healing is slow even with the best of care. Patients must take ownership of their treatment, which may involve frequent irrigation of the wound and dressing changes (4,5).

Pregnancy in women with sickle cell disease can be managed as a high-risk pregnancy with reasonable chances for successful outcomes. Women should be encouraged to plan their pregnancies. Birth control can be offered and there are a variety of approaches: progesterone ring insertion, progesterone implant or depo injections, and estrogen-containing birth control pills. Before trying to conceive, advice from an experienced obstetrician and/or maternal fetal medicine physician should be sought. Genetic counseling should be offered as part of reproductive planning, and prospective fathers should be tested for sickle trait and beta thalassemia. Hydroxyurea should be stopped, although in some European centers, this practice is not followed and hydroxyurea is continued. There is a paucity of evidence on the teratogenic risk of hydroxyurea, but small studies of women who conceived while on hydroxyurea show no ill effects. During pregnancy, a team-based approach is favored. Based on a study by Koshy et al. (27), the current approach is to offer transfusions when it is apparent that sickle crises are occurring more frequently or with greater severity. Early transfusion therapy is offered to patients carrying twins or if there is a history of prior fetal demise. Pre-eclampsia, intrauterine growth delay, and fetal loss are more common in SCA women. On average, delivery occurs at week 36 to 38. Transfusion beginning early in pregnancy is a consideration, especially for those who were on hydroxyurea before conception. Transfusion therapy at the outset of pregnancy is now being reconsidered. Folic acid supplementation is recommended, but not routine iron supplementation as many women with SCA have normal or increased iron stores. NSAIDs are not used in pregnancy for management of pain (4,5,27).

Emerging Therapies

1. Hypomethylating agents like azacytidine and decitabine can increase HgbF production, which dilutes HgbS, ameliorating the clinical severity of sickle cell disease (14).
2. Gene therapy by beta globin gene correction, insertion of an anti-sickling beta globin gene, use of gamma and delta globin gene, and RNA repair to produce more HgbF are being explored (14).
3. Reduction of the polymerization of HgbS by using compounds like Gardos channel (a calcium-activated potassium channel) inhibitors, Aes-103, and voxelotor (14).

4. Given the success of crizanlizumab, additional inhibitors of selectin binding have been proposed as a therapy for vaso-occlusive events by reducing the interactions between blood cells and the vascular endothelium in individuals with SCD (14).

Key Points

- Sickle Hgb is the result of point mutation in the beta globin chain and is less soluble than normal HgbA.
- SCD constitutes a spectrum of diseases including homozygous SCA, heterozygous sickle cell trait, sickle beta thalassemia, and HgbSC disease.
- SCA patients usually have normocytic anemia with other labs suggesting chronic hemolysis with elevated LDH and reticulocyte count. Hgb electrophoresis confirms the diagnosis.
- SCA results in hemolytic anemia along with microvascular disease that may acutely lead to acute pain crisis, ACS, or ischemic injuries to the heart, brain, and kidneys.
- Spleen may be affected by vaso-occlusion, and affected children may become functionally asplenic by age 5 or 6. This can lead to the risk of infections, especially encapsulated organism, splenic sequestration, and venous thromboembolism.
- Prevention including immunizations and management of chronic complications is the key. Hydroxyurea remains the mainstay of treatment with safety both in adults and children. Hematopoietic stem cell transplant in children and adolescents and transfusion programs are other options. Gene therapy, l-glutamine, and the inhibitory monoclonal antibody, crizanlizumab, have shown some promise in treatment of veno-occlusive crises.
- Transition from a pediatric to an adult hematologist is encouraged. Pregnancy should be contemplated and planned, with experienced maternal fetal medicine obstetricians and a genetic counselor involved in care along with a hematologist.

OTHER SICKLE HEMOGLOBINOPATHIES

Sickle trait affects 7% to 8% of African Americans. It is not associated with increased mortality, except for the rare event of sudden death related to extreme exercise. Individuals with sickle trait may not be able to concentrate their urine, and thus are prone to dehydration and fatal rhabdomyolysis if they exercise without proper attention to fluid intake or ambient humidity. A recent systematic review found strong evidence for an association with proteinuria, chronic kidney disease, venous thromboembolism, and pulmonary embolism.

Moderate strength evidence supported an increased risk for exertional rhabdomyolysis. Data were too weak or lacking to support clinical reports of sickle trait in association with splenic infarction, hematuria, papillary necrosis, or renal medullary carcinoma (4,5).

HgbSC disease is a milder SCA phenotype. Patients have one gene expressing the β S mutation and another with β C. The presence of C Hgb in the RBC favors dehydration by maintaining activation of a K:Cl cotransport activity. Potassium exits the cell taking water with it and the concentration of Hgb increases. The mean corpuscular hemoglobin concentration (MCHC) is usually increased, and the concentration of HgbS reaches that seen in HgbSS. Patients tend to have fewer crises, although there is considerable variability. Problems with the spleen—splenic enlargement, splenic infarction, and sequestration—can occur in young adulthood unlike SCA patients who typically have such problems much earlier and lose splenic function by the end of their first decade. HgbSC patients have more problems with retinopathy and AVN than patients with SCA. Treatment is largely supportive, although there is some evidence for benefit from treatment with hydroxyurea (3,5).

Patients with HgbSβ+ *thalassemia* are very similar to HgbSC patients. They have mild anemia and relatively fewer pain crises and problems with the spleen in adulthood, but may exhibit increased frequency of retinopathy and AVN. HgbSC and Sβ+ patients are frequently misdiagnosed as being sickle trait and are often treated for community-acquired pneumonia or pulmonary embolism without consideration of possible ACS. Although antibiotics and anticoagulation may be helpful, delay or failure to undertake exchange transfusion may result in poor outcomes, including death (3,5).

HgbD is prevalent in northwest Punjab region of India, but may be encountered in other groups. It results from the substitution of glutamine for glutamic acid at the 121st position of the beta chain. Patients with HgbD (both homozygous and heterozygous) disease can be asymptomatic or demonstrate mild anemia. Patients who inherit both HgbD and HgbS exhibit sickling as HgbD promotes Hgb deoxygenation. The diagnosis of HgbAD (D trait) or HgbDD is made by Hgb electrophoresis. HgbS and HgbD have similar electrophoretic mobility on cellulose acetate electrophoresis and isoelectric focusing, but can be differentiated by acid citrate gel electrophoresis or liquid chromatography (23).

NON-SICKLE HEMOGLOBINOPATHIES

Altered Oxygen Affinity

Hgb mutations that stabilize the R state of the Hgb tetramer or destabilize the T state result in a high-oxygen-affinity globin. These can be mutations in the alpha or beta chain, and patients typically have erythrocytosis with autosomal dominant inheritance. EPO levels may be normal, but may also increase dramatically after phlebotomy. Diagnosis is made by measuring the P50, but this requires the ability to perform an oxygenation equilibrium curve, a specialized test performed in limited labs. Variants include Hgb Yakima, Ypsilanti, and Ranier (6).

Unstable Hgbs have mutations that interfere with the secondary, tertiary, or quaternary structure of the globin tetramer. Tetramer instability results in intracellular precipitates, which can be detected by a Heinz body stain similar to the precipitates seen with glucose 6-phosphate dehydrogenase (G6PD) deficiency and oxidant exposure. The isopropanol test is also used to screen for unstable Hgb. Hemolysis occurs and patients have anemia, reticulocytosis, pigmenturia, and splenomegaly (6).

Methemoglobin (Met-Hgb) is an altered state of Hgb in which heme's ferrous (Fe++) iron is oxidized to the ferric (Fe+++) state. Methemoglobinemia can be congenital or acquired. Most cases of hereditary methemoglobinemia are autosomal recessive and are due to homozygous or compound heterozygous deficiency of cytochrome b5 reductase (nicotinamide adenine dinucleotide [NADH] is a cofactor). It is included here because of its association with cyanosis. Treatment, ironically, is with methylene blue, which uses an alternative enzyme NADPH-methemoglobin reductase to redox balance. Another congenital cause of methemoglobinemia is autosomal dominant HgbM (Milwaukee) disease due to mutations in either the alpha or beta or, rarely, gamma globin gene. In most of the mutations, tyrosine is substituted for either proximal or distal histidine in the heme pocket and forms a Fe^{3+}–phenolate complex that resists reduction of Fe^{3+} heme iron to the divalent state. The result is lifelong methemoglobinemia. Administration of methylene blue does not correct this type of congenital methemoglobinemia. There is no effective treatment for the methemoglobinemia seen in this condition, but, in fact, no treatment is required as patients are not symptomatic—they are "more blue than sick" (6,28).

Acquired methemoglobinemia results from increased Met-Hgb formation by various exogenous agents including sulfa-containing medications, nitrates- and nitrites-containing medications, local anesthesia medications, and other chemicals (Table 8.5). A risk factor for acute acquired methemoglobinemia is the asymptomatic heterozygous state for cytochrome b5 reductase deficiency. Presence of abnormal Met-Hgb can be directly analyzed if there is clinical suspicion following the sudden onset of cyanosis with symptoms of hypoxia after administration or ingestion of an agent with oxidative potential. If the patient is symptomatic or if the Met-Hgb level is >20%, specific therapy is urgently indicated. The two

Table 8.5 Agents Associated With Acquired Methemoglobinemia

Acetaminophen	Phenytoin	Nitroprusside
p-Aminosalicylic acid	Chloroquine	Amyl nitrates
Benzocaine	Primaquine	Nitrofurantoin
Bupivacaine	Dapsone	Nitric oxide
Lidocaine	Flutamide	Piperazine
Prilocaine	Metoclopramide	Rifampin
Valproic acid	Nitrates	Sulfonamides

treatments most often employed are methylene blue and ascorbic acid. Methylene blue is relatively contraindicated when the patient has G6PD deficiency (28).

Key Points

- Patients with congenital methemoglobinemia have lifelong cyanosis and are generally asymptomatic.
- Patients with acquired methemoglobinemia display symptoms at Met-Hgb levels >20%, such as headache, fatigue, lethargy, and shortness of breath. At Met-Hgb levels >30% to 40%, respiratory depression, seizures, and altered consciousness may occur.
- The presence of Met-Hgb is suspected when there is clinical cyanosis in the presence of normal PaO_2. Blood is found to be chocolate colored.
- In congenital cases, avoidance of aniline derivatives and nitrates is recommended.
- In acquired cases, in which the patient is asymptomatic and Met-Hgb levels are <20%, removal of the offending agent is enough. If the patient is symptomatic, the levels are higher, and the patient does not have G6PD deficiency (covered in Chapter 7, Approach to Hemolytic Anemias), then use of IV methylene blue is recommended.

REFERENCES

1. Olivieri NF. The beta-thalassemias. *N Engl J Med.* 1999;341:99–109. doi:10.1056/NEJM199907083410207
2. Harteveld CL, Higgs DR. Alpha-thalassaemia. *Orphanet J Rare Dis.* 2010;5:13. doi:10.1186/1750-1172-5-13
3. Rees DC, Williams TN, Gladwin MT. Sickle-cell disease. *Lancet.* 2010;376:2018–2031. doi:10.1016/S0140-6736(10)61029-X

4. Rodgers GP. Overview of pathophysiology and rationale for treatment of sickle cell anemia. *Semin Hematol*. 1997;34:2–7.

5. Ballas SK, Kesen MR, Goldberg MF, et al. Beyond the definitions of the phenotypic complications of sickle cell disease: an update on management. *Sci World J*. 2012;2012:1–55. doi:10.1100/2012/949535

6. Nagel R. Unstable hemoglobins; hemoglobins with altered O2 affinity. In: Steinberg M, Forget B, Higgs D, eds. *Disorders of Hemoglobin Genetics, Pathophysiology, Clinical Management*. Cambridge: Cambridge University Press, 1999.

7. Nienhuis AW, Nathan DG. Pathophysiology and clinical manifestations of the beta-thalassemias. *Cold Spring Harb Perspect Med*. 2012;2:a011726. doi:10.1101/cshperspect.a011726

8. Gardenghi S, Ramos P, Marongiu MF, et al. Hepcidin as a therapeutic tool to limit iron overload and improve anemia in beta-thalassemic mice. *J Clin Invest*. 2010;120:4466–4477. doi:10.1172/JCI41717

9. Caocci G, Orofino MG, Vacca A, et al. Long-term survival of beta thalassemia major patients treated with hematopoietic stem cell transplantation compared with survival with conventional treatment. *Am J Hematol*. 2017;92:1303–1310. doi:10.1002/ajh.24898

10. St Pierre TG, El-Beshlawy A, Elalfy M, et al. Multicenter validation of spin-density projection-assisted R2-MRI for the noninvasive measurement of liver iron concentration. *Magn Reson Med*. 2014;71:2215–2223. doi:10.1002/mrm.24854

11. Cazzola M, Borgna-Pignatti C, Locatelli F, et al. A moderate transfusion regimen may reduce iron loading in beta-thalassemia major without producing excessive expansion of erythropoiesis. *Transfusion*. 1997;37:135–140. doi:10.1046/j.1537-2995.1997 .37297203514.x

12. Pennell DJ, Udelson JE, Arai AE, et al. Cardiovascular function and treatment in beta-thalassemia major: a consensus statement from the American Heart Association. *Circulation*. 2013;128:281–308. doi:10.1161/CIR.0b013e31829b2be6

13. Taher AT, Musallam KM, Cappellini MD, Weatherall DJ. Optimal management of beta thalassaemia intermedia. *Br J Haematol*. 2011;152:512–523. doi:10.1111/j.1365-2141.2010.08486.x

14. Gardner RV. Sickle cell disease: advances in treatment. *Ochsner J*. 2018;18:377–389. doi:10.31486/toj.18.0076

15. Carr S, Rubin L, Dixon D, et al. Intrauterine therapy for homozygous alpha-thalassemia. *Obstet Gynecol*. 1995;85:876–879. doi:10.1016/0029-7844(94)00334-A

16. Fucharoen S, Weatherall DJ. The hemoglobin E thalassemias. *Cold Spring Harb Perspect Med.* 2012;2:a011734. doi:10.1101/cshperspect.a011734

17. Almeida AM, Henthorn JS, Davies SC. Neonatal screening for haemoglobinopathies: the results of a 10-year programme in an English Health Region. *Br J Haematol.* 2001;112:32–35. doi:10.1046/j.1365-2141.2001.02512.x

18. Quinn CT, Lee NJ, Shull EP, et al. Prediction of adverse outcomes in children with sickle cell anemia: a study of the Dallas Newborn Cohort. *Blood.* 2008;111:544–548. doi:10.1182/blood-2007-07-100719

19. Elmariah H, Garrett ME, De Castro LM, et al. Factors associated with survival in a contemporary adult sickle cell disease cohort. *Am J Hematol.* 2014;89:530–535. doi:10.1002/ajh.23683

20. Gardner K, Douiri A, Drasar E, et al. Survival in adults with sickle cell disease in a high-income setting. *Blood.* 2016;128:1436–1438. doi:10.1182/blood-2016-05-716910

21. Steinberg MH, McCarthy WF, Castro O, et al. The risks and benefits of long-term use of hydroxyurea in sickle cell anemia: a 17.5 year follow-up. *Am J Hematol.* 2010;85:403–408. doi:10.1002/ajh.21699

22. Wang WC, Ware RE, Miller ST, et al. Hydroxycarbamide in very young children with sickle-cell anaemia: a multicentre, randomised, controlled trial (BABY HUG). *Lancet.* 2011;377:1663–1672. doi:10.1016/S0140-6736(11)60355-3

23. Schnee J, Aulehla-Scholz C, Eigel A, Horst J. Hb D Los Angeles (D-Punjab) and Hb Presbyterian: analysis of the defect at the DNA level. *Hum Genet.* 1990;84:365–367. doi:10.1007/BF00196236

24. Klings ES, Machado RF, Barst RJ, et al. An official American Thoracic Society clinical practice guideline: diagnosis, risk stratification, and management of pulmonary hypertension of sickle cell disease. *Am J Respir Crit Care Med.* 2014;189:727–740. doi:10.1164/rccm.201401-0065ST

25. Drawz P, Ayyappan S, Nouraie M, et al. Kidney disease among patients with sickle cell disease, hemoglobin SS and SC. *Clin J Am Soc Nephrol.* 2016;11:207–215. doi:10.2215/CJN.03940415

26. Vichinsky EP, Haberkern CM, Neumayr L, et al. A comparison of conservative and aggressive transfusion regimens in the perioperative management of sickle cell disease. *N Engl J Med.* 1995;333:206–213. doi:10.1056/NEJM199507273330402

27. Koshy M, Burd L, Wallace D, et al. Prophylactic red-cell transfusions in pregnant patients with sickle cell disease. A randomized cooperative study. *N Engl J Med.* 1988;319:1447–1452. doi:10.1056/NEJM198812013192204

28. Cortazzo JA, Lichtman AD. Methemoglobinemia: a review and recommendations for management. *J Cardiothorac Vasc Anesth.* 2014;28:1043–1047. doi:10.1053/j.jvca.2013.02.005

9

Iron Metabolism Disorders and Porphyria

Kirtan D. Nautiyal and Martha Pritchett Mims

HEREDITARY HEMOCHROMATOSIS

Clinical Case 9.1

A 49-year-old Caucasian male presents for a routine evaluation by his primary care provider. He complains of mild fatigue and pain in the small joints of his hands. Exam is unremarkable. Initial laboratory evaluation shows a normal complete blood count, but the aspartate transaminase (AST) and alanine transaminase (ALT) are elevated above the upper limit of normal. An ultrasound of the liver is ordered, which shows normal echotexture and no biliary ductal dilatation. He denies alcohol abuse. Further labs demonstrate ferritin of 700 mcg/mL (elevated), and an iron panel, demonstrating a transferrin saturation of 70%. Genetic testing identifies homozygous C282Y mutations in the HFE gene. The patient is initiated on a regular phlebotomy program removing 500 mL of whole blood weekly. After several months, his ferritin and transaminases normalize. He is pleased that his fatigue is improved along with his laboratory abnormalities; however, his hands continue to cause him pain.

Introduction

Hereditary hemochromatosis (HH) is a genetically heterogeneous, autosomal recessive disorder characterized by inappropriately increased absorption of dietary iron, which may result in oxidative damage to the heart, liver, and other essential organs. Multiple genetic mutations can lead to this clinical phenotype, but the most prevalent is the C282Y substitution in the *HFE* gene, seen in one out of 10 individuals of Northern European descent. However, there is great phenotypic variability among patients with these mutations, and additional genetic and environmental factors are important in determining whether clinical iron overload develops. In addition, the initial clinical manifestations of the disease are subtle and non-specific, further complicating the diagnostic process (1).

HH results from hepcidin deficiency. Hepcidin binds to the transmembrane iron transporter ferroportin and facilitates its internalization and degradation. Absence or dysfunction of hepcidin results in increased expression of ferroportin in the macrophages and at the basolateral surface of intestinal epithelial cells, permitting increases in the level of serum iron. Low levels of hepcidin might be secondary to mutations of the *HFE* or *TfR2* genes (adult hemochromatosis) or the *HJV* or *HAMP* genes (juvenile hemochromatosis). Rarely, gain-of-function mutations in the genes coding for ferroportin render it insensitive to regulation by hepcidin and result in the same clinical phenotype (2).

Primary HH must always be distinguished from secondary iron overload due to repeated blood transfusions or ineffective erythropoiesis (as observed in thalassemia, sideroblastic anemia, and myelodysplastic syndrome), as the subsequent workup and treatment of these conditions varies greatly. In general, the same principles of iron chelation (Table 9.1) apply to patients with secondary iron overload.

Diagnosis

Due to more frequent testing of the liver function and iron levels in the primary care setting and greater awareness of the disease among healthcare providers, HH is rarely diagnosed with the classic triad of cirrhosis, diabetes, and increased skin pigmentation observed in advanced disease. Rather, in its early stages, HH manifests in middle age with nonspecific symptoms such as chronic fatigue, decreased libido, and arthralgias at the second and third metacarpophalangeal joints (Box 9.1). Men typically present in their 40s, while women are usually not diagnosed until their 50s due to the temporizing effects of iron loss through menstruation and pregnancy.

Early lab abnormalities may include mildly elevated serum transaminases and an increased serum ferritin. However, serum ferritin alone is not a reliable, specific marker of iron overload, especially as it is affected by alcohol intake and the presence of chronic inflammatory conditions. Thus, individuals found to have an elevated serum ferritin (>200 mcg/L in males and >150 mcg/L in females) should have a measurement of transferrin saturation, as it is a more sensitive and specific marker for early iron overload. Persistent fasting transferrin saturation above 45% should prompt genetic evaluation, which includes *HFE* gene mutation analysis for the C282Y substitution and the less-common *H63D* mutation. In the presence of iron overload as defined herein, the identification of a C282Y/C282Y homozygote is diagnostic of HH. While the C282Y/H63D compound heterozygote can also result in the HH phenotype, the clinical significance of C282Y/wild-type and H63D/wild-type heterozygotes or H63D/H63D homozygotes is much less clear (Figure 9.1). Other causes of secondary iron overload should be considered in these individuals. Following the diagnosis of HH,

Table 9.1 Pros and Cons of Available Iron Chelating Agents

Iron Chelating Agent	Pros	Cons
Deferoxamine	Can be used when renal clearance is as low as 10 mL/min No dose changes for hepatic impairment Can be used in children aged 3 and older	Must be given IV, IM, or SQ Can cause the following: • Rash • GI symptoms (nausea, vomiting, abdominal pain, diarrhea) • Pain at the injection site • Cataracts and other ophthalmic problems • Hearing loss and tinnitus • Renal failure • Allergic reactions
Deferasirox	Oral agent Approved for children aged 2 or older	Can cause the following: • Rash • Acute renal failure and death, not to be used if eGFR is <40 mL/min/1.73 m² • Liver injury requiring frequent measurement of serum transaminases and bilirubin • Hearing loss • GI hemorrhage, especially in older patients • Marrow suppression • Changes in vision
Deferiprone	Oral agent No dose changes required for hepatic or renal impairment	• Can cause the following: • Agranulocytosis • Rash • Nausea, vomiting, abdominal pain, diarrhea • Arthralgias • Elevated liver enzymes • Zinc deficiency

eGFR, estimated glomerular filtration rate; GI, gastrointestinal; IM, intramuscular; IV, intravenous; SQ, subcutaneous.

all first-degree adult relatives of the affected patient should also be counseled on their risk of developing the disease and screened with measurement of their iron levels and a *HFE* genetic mutation analysis (2).

Only a fraction of patients with serum iron overload and an *HFE* mutation will develop clinically apparent end-organ damage. Patients with HH and a serum ferritin <1,000 mcg/L should be

Box 9.1 Signs and Symptoms of Hereditary Hemochromatosis

- Chronic fatigue
- Decreased libido
- Arthralgias (most prominent at the second and third metacarpopha-langeal joints)
- Skin hyperpigmentation
- Impaired glucose tolerance
- Hepatomegaly
- Cardiac dysfunction

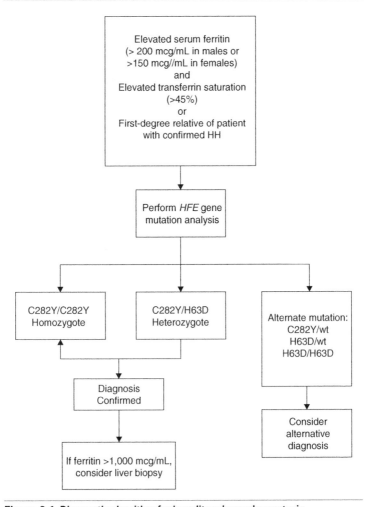

Figure 9.1 Diagnostic algorithm for hereditary hemochromatosis.

HH, hereditary hemochromatosis

screened for diabetes, with no further organ-specific investigations unless laboratory abnormalities or clinical symptoms dictate. In contrast, those with a serum ferritin >1,000 mcg/L should undergo liver biopsy to assess for the presence or absence of cirrhosis. Liver biopsy provides prognostic as well as diagnostic information.

Diagnostic Dilemma

Elevated ferritin is relatively common among hospitalized patients with other medical issues, thus screening is best done in the outpatient setting if possible. In young patients with suspected iron overload, one should also consider the rarer iron metabolism disorders.

Management

Experts agree that a therapeutic phlebotomy program is the cornerstone of treatment for HH (3). Phlebotomy is maximally effective before the onset of end-organ damage such as diabetes or cirrhosis, but some disease features such as joint pain and fatigue can be reversed with aggressive treatment. In the absence of large, randomized controlled trials, the guidelines for the initiation and endpoints of treatment are based on expert opinion.

The consensus for any patient with HH is to begin phlebotomy when serum ferritin exceeds the upper limit of normal. Hemoglobin should be checked prior to every phlebotomy and ferritin checked monthly while still abnormal. A unit (500 mL) of whole blood can be removed once or twice a week until the target ferritin is reached (50–100 mcg/L) while maintaining hemoglobin in an acceptable range (11–12 g/dL). Phlebotomy is usually stopped in pregnant women due to gestational anemia and the loss of iron associated with fetal development and delivery. Also deserving of special consideration are elderly patients, many of whom require less-frequent phlebotomy as they age.

In patients intolerant of phlebotomy, providers may consider initiating iron chelation therapy. Though there are no randomized trials comparing its efficacy to that of regular phlebotomy, chelation has proven very effective in the treatment of secondary iron overload. Deferoxamine, the oldest, has the most available clinical data but requires regular infusions, which dampen compliance. The oral chelators, deferasirox and deferiprone, are more easily taken, but have their own side effect profiles, which must be discussed with patients prior to starting therapy.

As noted, disease features such as fatigue and skin pigmentation can improve quickly with treatment. Joint pain is also improved in many patients, though a significant population does not see any change in their arthralgias and some may even have a transient increase in symptoms during phlebotomy. Diabetes is not reversible, though there are reports of decreased insulin requirements and less-labile blood sugars following iron chelation or phlebotomy. While regression of liver fibrosis can occur with aggressive phlebotomy, cirrhosis cannot be reversed once it has begun. Hepatocellular carcinoma is a dreaded complication of excess iron deposition in the liver with an estimated 20-fold higher risk than the general population. Cardiac changes may improve with phlebotomy if not too advanced at the time of discovery (4).

Prognosis

In 1996, the outcomes of 251 patients diagnosed with HH in Germany between 1947 and 1991 were published. The survival of the overall cohort was reduced compared to matched controls; however, the group of patients diagnosed in the last decade of the study (when more aggressive phlebotomy practices were taking hold) and without cirrhosis or diabetes enjoyed normal survival.

More recently, a larger French cohort of 1,085 C282Y homozygotes was followed for a median of 8.3 years. While those patients with serum ferritin >2,000 mcg/mL had a significant increase in liver-related mortality, specifically related to hepatocellular carcinoma, the rate of mortality in the overall patient cohort did not differ from the general population.

Thus, if identified early and treated appropriately prior to the development of end-organ damage, it appears that patients with HH can live a normal life span (5).

Future Directions

The management of HH remains largely based on expert opinion. Both the threshold for starting therapy and its eventual endpoint as determined by serum ferritin levels are topics of ongoing debate. Additional trials are needed to better define these values.

Liver MRI can estimate the hepatic iron load and determine the presence or absence of cirrhosis. Whether MRI can supplant the traditional use of liver biopsy to provide this prognostic information after the diagnosis of HH is also a matter for further investigation.

Key Points

- HH is a genetically heterogeneous, autosomal recessive disorder characterized by increased, inappropriate absorption of dietary iron, resulting in oxidative damage to the heart, liver, and other essential organs.
- Diagnosis is made on the basis of increased iron stores as evidenced by elevated serum ferritin and transferrin saturation and the subsequent identification of an underlying genetic mutation.

- Therapeutic phlebotomy is the cornerstone of effective treatment.
- With routine phlebotomy reducing ferritin levels to normal, affected patients can live a normal, healthy life span.

THE PORPHYRIAS

Clinical Case 9.2

A 25-year-old female presents to the emergency department with recurrent epigastric abdominal pain. She has had three such visits over the last 6 months. The pain is crampy and associated with nausea and vomiting. She complains of feeling tired and "foggy." Her examination, including a neurologic evaluation, is non-focal. Laboratory values including a complete blood count and comprehensive metabolic panel are within normal limits Urine pregnancy test is negative. A CT of the abdomen and pelvis with intravenous (IV) contrast is unremarkable. Due to intractable pain, the patient is admitted for further evaluation. The day following admission, the patient has a tonic–clonic seizure.

The patient's physician learns that she had been started on oral contraceptives from her primary care provider a few months before. Given that all prior workup is unrevealing, acute intermittent porphyria (AIP) is suspected. A random urine assay for porphobilinogen is sent. The patient is continued on opioid analgesics and started on D10 at a rate of 100 mL/hour with some improvement in her symptoms. Several days later, her urine porphobilinogen returns at 20 times the upper limit of normal. She is started on IV hemin at a daily dose of 3 mg/kg. Her contraceptives are discontinued. Her symptoms resolve over the next few days, and she is discharged.

Introduction

Heme is a coordination complex consisting of a single iron molecule bound to a porphyrin ring. Heme is a required cofactor not only for hemoglobin in the erythrocytes, but also for myoglobin in the muscle cells and cytochromes in the liver. The porphyrias are a group of inherited disorders resulting from defects in heme biosynthesis. They are distinguished based on which of the seven enzymes in this biosynthetic pathway are affected, with varying clinical features depending on which toxic precursors accumulate as a result (6).

To aid providers, several classification schemes have been proposed to group porphyrias with similar features. One such schema separates porphyrias based on where the toxic metabolites are overproduced and where the clinical symptoms are seen (Figure 9.2):

Acute hepatic porphyrias: Defective heme synthesis in the liver and symptoms mainly in the nervous system

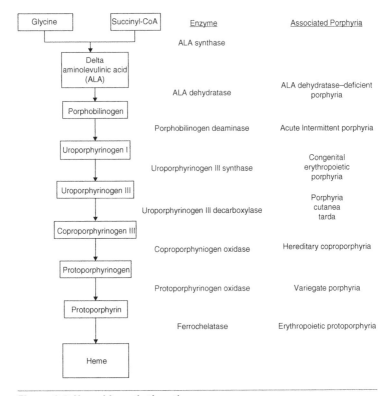

Figure 9.2 Heme biosynthetic pathway.

- AIP
- Hereditary coproporphyria (HCP)
- Variegate porphyria (VP)
- Delta aminolevulinic acid (ALA) dehydratase–deficient porphyria

Erythropoietic photocutaneous porphyrias: Defective heme synthesis in erythrocytes and mainly cutaneous symptoms

- Congenital erythropoietic porphyria (CEP)
- Erythropoietic protoporphyria (EPP), and its recently recognized X-linked form, XLP

Hepatic photocutaneous porphyria: Defective heme synthesis in the liver and mainly cutaneous symptoms

- Porphyria cutanea tarda (PCT)

Diagnosis

The clinical presentation of the various porphyrias varies subtly. The most commonly seen porphyria in the acute setting is AIP, while the most prevalent porphyria in the general population is PCT (7).

Acute Intermittent Porphyria

AIP results from a heterozygous deficiency in porphobilinogen deaminase, the third enzyme in the heme biosynthetic pathway. Only about 10% of patients with a predisposing mutation will present with an acute attack, highlighting the important role of environmental triggers such as medications (cataloged in official databases such as the one maintained by the American Porphyria Foundation—www.porphyriafoundation.com/drug-database). The most important medications acting as exacerbating factors include many antiseizure medications including phenytoin, barbiturates, and some anesthetics. It is generally thought that benzodiazepines are safe. Fasting, tobacco, drug or alcohol use, acute infection, and stress can also trigger attacks. Most acute attacks occur in young women of reproductive age due to the use of oral contraceptives, the progesterone surge seen at the beginning of a menstrual cycle, or the onset of pregnancy.

An attack typically presents with progressive fatigue, severe abdominal pain, nausea, vomiting, tachycardia, hypertension, and neuropsychiatric signs including difficulty concentrating and proximal muscle weakness (Box 9.2). Initial laboratory evaluation may reveal transaminitis and hyponatremia. If misdiagnosed on presentation, as is common, muscle weakness may progress in a fashion similar to that seen in Guillain–Barre syndrome and neurologic dysfunction may progress to frank seizure activity.

The diagnosis depends on clinical suspicion, which is often not prompted by the nonspecific symptoms outlined in Box 9.2. Random urine porphobilinogen concentration is sensitive for the diagnosis of AIP. Collected urine should be protected from light; otherwise, the porphobilinogen will polymerize and darken in color, possibly causing a false negative on testing. Unfortunately, this

---

Box 9.2 Signs and Symptoms of Acute Intermittent Porphyria

- Acute abdominal pain
- Nausea and vomiting
- Dysautonomia (tachycardia, hypertension, sweating)
- Polyneuropathy
- Psychiatric disturbances
- Fatigue
- Seizure

test is typically sent out to a reference laboratory and may have an extended turnaround time, resulting in further delays in care. If a rarer acute hepatic porphyria such as VP or HCP is suspected, additional tests may be required. Serum plasma porphyrin fluorescence emission testing can help differentiate VP and AIP, as each will respond to a characteristic wavelength of light on this assay. Fecal porphyrin testing can differentiate HCP and AIP, as a high level of coproporphyrinogen III is seen only in the former. Direct sequencing of the underlying porphobilinogen deaminase gene is the most sensitive and specific test for AIP and can be obtained if there is still doubt about the diagnosis following the recommended testing.

Porphyria Cutanea Tarda

With the exception of EPP, the cutaneous porphyrias present in adulthood with fragile skin, slow healing, bullae, hyperpigmentation, and facial hypertrichosis. PCT, the most prevalent, is caused by reduced activity of uroporphyrinogen decarboxylase, the fifth enzyme in the heme biosynthesis pathway. Only 10% to 20% cases are familial, caused by an autosomal dominant mutation in the gene encoding for this enzyme. Most cases are instead sporadic, resulting from a combination of susceptibility factors, including iron overload from HH, alcohol abuse, hepatitis C or HIV infection, estrogen use, and certain chemical exposures.

PCT is diagnosed with a random urine or serum porphyrin profile showing a predominance of uroporphyrin and heptacarboxyporphyrin. In some cases, VP and HCP can have symptoms that mimic those of PCT. As in the workup of AIP, measurement of fecal porphyrins and serum porphyrin fluorescence emission testing can distinguish these overlap syndromes.

Erythropoietic Protoporphyria

EPP, due to a partial deficiency of ferrochelatase, presents in childhood with photosensitivity resulting in burning, itching, and erythema on exposure to sunlight. With repeated episodes, patients may suffer hyperkeratosis and lichenification of affected skin.

Patients are diagnosed by measurement of serum protoporphyrin levels. EPP can be distinguished from the related condition XLP by measurement of zinc protoporphyrin, which is elevated in the latter and not in the former. Rarely, EPP can have a late onset in adulthood; measurement of erythrocyte porphyrin levels can differentiate it from PCT.

Diagnostic Dilemmas

Diagnosis of an acute porphyria between attacks can be quite difficult as the levels of the porphyrin precursors may be normal. Comprehensive testing may be required for such patients and may require genetic testing and referral to an expert.

Management

Acute Intermittent Porphyria

Upon diagnosis of AIP, any offending medications should be discontinued immediately. In addition to analgesia (opiates are safe) and antiemetics, the patient should be started on a dextrose-containing IV fluid such as D10. The administration of glucose can downregulate the activity of ALA synthase, the first enzyme in the heme biosynthetic pathway, and may be enough to end mild attacks (those without seizures or significant neuropathy). Patients with more severe symptoms should also receive IV hemin at a dose of 3 to 4 mg/kg daily, which provides additional negative feedback on the activity of ALA synthase. In a Finnish series of 51 attacks in 22 patients, hemin at a dose of 3 mg/kg was started within 4 days in 96% of the reported cases. All patients responded. The mean duration of symptomatic pain was 2.5 ± 0.97 days, and in 90% of the attacks, the total hospitalization time was 7 days or less (8).

Prophylactic scheduled hemin infusions may be considered for patients with frequent attacks despite correction of possible inciting factors. For those patients with attacks refractory to hemin, liver transplantation represents a therapy of last resort.

Complications of hemin therapy include phlebitis in small-bore IV lines, platelet aggregation, prolonged prothrombin time, and iron overload with repeated infusions. Reconstituting the powdered hemin preparation with albumin rather than water has been shown to reduce the incidence of phlebitis.

Porphyria Cutanea Tarda

The management of PCT, on the other hand, is mainly preventive. Patients should avoid bright sunlight and practice good skin care. Avoidance of environmental triggers such as alcohol should be advised. Patients with underlying HH should start on a program of regular phlebotomy. Those with underlying hepatitis C or HIV infections should receive antiviral treatment, though the correlation between viral response and resolution of cutaneous symptoms is not clear. For persistent cutaneous symptoms, twice weekly chloroquine (100 mg) or hydroxychloroquine (125 mg) can be prescribed, as these drugs complex with excess uroporphyrin and promote its release from the liver. As the levels of uroporphyrin fall, the drugs can be tapered off.

Erythropoietic Protoporphyria

EPP is also managed preventively. Patients must avoid the sun and may even suffer skin damage with certain indoor lights. While there is some evidence for the use of beta carotene to limit sun damage, most patients do not see any benefit. Case reports support the use of activated charcoal and colestipol to facilitate excretion of protoporphyrins.

Prognosis

Older literature reported mortality rates nearing 25% during an acute attack of AIP. Though a severe attack may still be fatal, with greater availability of hemin and a deeper understanding of which drug triggers must be avoided in the hospital, this outlook has been steadily improving.

Nonetheless, a 2014 report on the clinical experience of 108 patients with AIP makes it clear that the disease can still cause significant chronic complications, mainly due to delays in establishing the diagnosis. In this cohort, 43% suffered from persistent peripheral neuropathy, 43% from hypertension, and 29% from chronic kidney disease. The prevalence of hypertension, psychiatric illness, and seizure disorder were greater in these patients, compared to age- and gender-matched controls. Due to their frequent presentations with abdominal pain, many patients had undergone abdominal surgeries—13% with an appendectomy and 15% with a cholecystectomy. Though not seen in this group, patients with AIP are at higher risk for hepatocellular carcinoma even in the absence of cirrhosis due to the accumulation of mutagenic porphyrins in the liver tissue (7).

With appropriate measures, PCT improves in the vast majority of patients, though it can recur with worsening iron overload in those patients with underlying HH or re-exposure to known environmental triggers.

Due to the lack of effective treatments, EPP is difficult to manage, and most patients suffer from chronic pain and skin changes that markedly affect their quality of life.

Future Directions

A recent phase 1 clinical trial explored the efficacy of a novel gene therapy in the treatment of AIP (9). In the study, investigators administered a recombinant viral vector containing a functioning copy of the porphobilinogen synthase gene. The treatment was safe at the doses tested. Though there was no appreciable change in the levels of porphobilinogen or ALA, there was a trend toward fewer hospitalizations and two patients were able to discontinue regular hemin therapy. Another experimental approach utilizes small interfering RNA (siRNA) to directly disrupt the synthesis of ALA synthase. In a phase 1 trial, injection of the RNA resulted in reduced expression of ALA synthase with minor side effects. These therapies may represent an alternative to liver transplant in patients who are refractory to hemin infusions.

Afemelanotide is an analog of α-melanocyte stimulating hormone which darkens the skin tone and prevents phototoxicity in patients with EPP. A recent phase 3 randomized controlled trial demonstrated an increased duration of sun exposure without pain and improved quality of life in these patients. Though approved for use in Europe, it is still pending evaluation by the U.S. Food and Drug Administration (10).

Key Points

- The porphyrias are a group of inherited disorders resulting from defects in heme biosynthesis. They are distinguished by which of the seven enzymes in this biosynthetic pathway are affected, with varying clinical features depending on which toxic precursors accumulate as a result.
- AIP is a relapsing, remitting condition resulting from a deficiency of porphobilinogen synthase. Though there are effective treatments, the diagnosis is often delayed for years due to nonspecific symptoms. Chronic complications can result.
- PCT is a chronic condition typically associated with underlying susceptibility factors like HH and hepatitis C virus (HCV) infection. Skin symptoms usually improve with treatment of the precipitating factor.
- EPP is a pediatric-onset condition associated with marked phototoxicity. Treatment is largely supportive.

REFERENCES

1. Bacon BR, Adams PC, Kowdley KV, et al. Diagnosis and management of hemochromatosis: 2011 Practice guideline by the American Association for the Study of Liver Diseases. *Hepatology*. 2011;54:328–343. doi:10.1002/hep.24330
2. Powell LW, Seckington RC, Deugnier Y. Haemochromatosis. *Lancet*. 2016;388:706–716. doi:10.1016/S0140-6736(15)01315-X
3. Adams PC, Barton JC. How I treat hemochromatosis. *Blood*. 2012;116:317–325. doi:10.1182/blood-2010-01-261875
4. Bardou-Jacquet E, Morcet J, Manet G, et al. Decreased cardiovascular and extrahepatic cancer-related mortality in treated patients with mild HFE hemochromatosis. *J Hepatol*. 2014;62:682–689. doi:10.1016/j.jhep.2014.10.025
5. Niederau C, Fischer R, Pürschel A, et al. Long-term survival in patients with hereditary hemochromatosis. *Gastroenterology*. 1996;110:1107–1119. doi:10.1053/gast.1996.v110.pm8613000

6. Bissell DM, Anderson KE, Bonkovsky HL. Porphyria. *N Engl J Med*. 2017;377:862–872. doi:10.1056/NEJMra1608634

7. Bonkovsky HL, Maddukuri VC, Yazici C, et al. Acute porphyrias in the USA: features of 108 subjects from porphyria consortium. *Am J Med*. 2014;127:1233–1241. doi:10.1016/j.amjmed.2014.06.036

8. Tenhunen R, Mustajoki P. Acute porphyria: treatment with heme. *Semin Liver Dis*. 1998;18:53–55. doi:10.1055/s-2007-1007140

9. D'Avola D, López-Franco E, Sangro B, et al. Phase I open label liver-directed gene therapy clinical trial for acute intermittent porphyria. *J Hepatol*. 2016;65:777–783. doi:10.1016/j.jhep.2016.05.012

10. Langendonk JG, Balwani M, Anderson KE, et al. Afamelanotide for erythropoietic protoporphyria. *N Engl J Med*. 2015;373:48–59. doi:10.1056/NEJMoa1411481

10 Platelet Disorders

Hyojeong Han and Sarah E. Sartain

INTRODUCTION

Platelets are small, discoid-shaped anucleate cells derived from megakaryocytes in the bone marrow (1). They range in size from 2 to 4 µm and circulate in the peripheral blood for 7 to 10 days before being removed by macrophages (1). Platelets function not only in thrombosis and primary hemostasis (Figure 10.1), but also in more complex processes including blood vessel repair, inflammation, immunity, and tumor growth/metastasis (1). In primary hemostasis, platelets adhere to the exposed subendothelial collagen at the site of blood vessel injury by interacting with von Willebrand factor (VWF) via glycoprotein Ib (GPIb) on the platelet surface (1). Adhered platelets recruit more platelets to form the platelet plug (1). Platelet disorders (Figure 10.2) are complex and extensive. Therefore, the evaluation of a patient for a platelet disorder should be approached systematically beginning with a detailed history, paying specific attention to ethnicity, consanguinity, family history, bleeding history, and associated medical complications consistent with some of the inherited platelet disorders (2). Initial evaluation for platelet disorders should include complete blood count (CBC) with peripheral smear (2). Additional evaluation can be performed based on history, CBC, and peripheral smear findings (2). In this chapter, we review the evaluation and management of platelet disorders.

INHERITED PLATELET DISORDERS

Disorders with Low Platelet Count (Thrombocytopenia)

Wiskott–Aldrich syndrome (WAS)

Clinical Case 10.1

A mother delivered a newborn baby boy at 38 weeks of gestation via C-section. She had routine prenatal care and a negative infectious workup during pregnancy; family history was only notable for diabetes in the maternal grandmother. Approximately 36 hours after birth, the baby was admitted to the

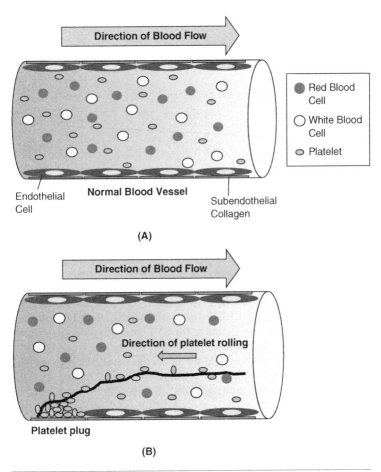

Figure 10.1 Illustration of a normal blood vessel and primary hemostasis. (A) In a normal blood vessel, endothelial cells are intact and subendothelial collagen is not exposed. (B) Upon endothelial cell injury, ULVWF is released and platelets interact with VWF via glycoprotein Ib on the platelet surface. Platelets then roll along ULVWF until they adhere to the exposed subendothelial collagen. Adhered platelets recruit more platelets to form the platelet plug, resulting in primary hemostasis.

ULVWF, ultra large von Willebrand factor; VWF, von Willebrand factor.

neonatal intensive care unit for fever. Infectious workup revealed a urinary tract infection, and antibiotics were initiated. Platelet count was 65 × 10⁹/L and this decreased during admission. The infant required a platelet transfusion for a platelet count <20 × 10⁹/L. Thrombocytopenia was attributed to the urinary tract infection, and after completing a 14-day course of antibiotics,

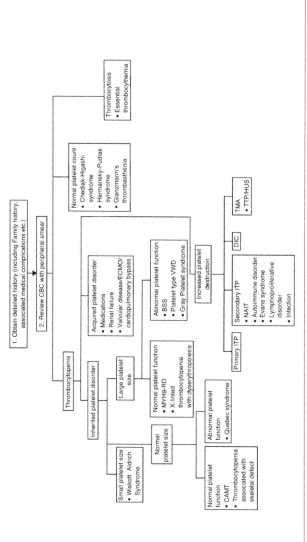

Figure 10.2 Diagnostic algorithm for platelet disorders.

BSS, Bernard–Soulier syndrome; CAMT, congenital amegakaryocytic thrombocytopenia; CBC, complete blood count; DIC, disseminated intravascular coagulation; ECMO, extracorporeal membrane oxygenation; HUS, hemolytic uremic syndrome; ITP, immune thrombocytopenia; MYH9-RD, MYH9-related disorders; NAIT, neonatal alloimmune thrombocytopenia; TMA, thrombotic microangiopathies; TTP, thrombotic thrombocytopenic purpura; VWD, von Willebrand disease.

the infant was discharged home. In the next 3 months, the infant had multiple respiratory tract infections requiring hospitalization, and ongoing thrombocytopenia (platelet count ranging from 6 × 10⁹ to 15 × 10⁹/L). He required red blood cell and platelet transfusions for hematochezia, melena, and petechiae.

Given the frequent infections, bleeding, and persistent thrombocytopenia, his pediatrician was suspicious for WAS. Genetic testing was consistent with WAS, and the baby boy was referred to the allergy/immunology and bone marrow transplant services for further management.

Introduction

WAS is an X-linked recessive disorder with the classic triad of microthrombocytopenia, eczema, and immunodeficiency (3). The incidence of WAS in the United States and Canada is approximately 1:250,000 male births (3). In this complex inherited disorder, the *WAS* gene encodes for WAS protein (WASp), responsible for actin polymerization required for numerous cellular functions (i.e., cell structural changes, division, endomitotic processes, migration, and chemotaxis) (3). Consequently, presenting symptoms can be variable. One should have high suspicion for WAS in a male infant who presents with a history of frequent infection and thrombocytopenia.

Clinical Presentation

WAS generally presents within the year of life with the classic triad of thrombocytopenia, eczema, and immune deficiency (3). WAS patients can also develop autoimmunity and malignancy (3). Approximately 70% of WAS patients are diagnosed with autoimmunity which includes autoimmune cytopenias (i.e., hemolytic anemia, neutropenia), arthritis, vasculitis, inflammatory bowel disease, and immune-mediated renal disease (3). Moreover, WAS patients with autoimmune disease have increased risk for malignancy (3). The prevalence of malignancy in WAS patients is 13% to 22%, with the average onset at age 9 (3). Patients typically present with lymphomas (predominantly non-Hodgkin type and often Epstein–Barr virus [EBV] induced), but can also present with lymphoblastic leukemias, myelodysplasia, myeloproliferative disorders, and other non-lymphoreticular malignancies (i.e., seminoma, testicular carcinoma, glioma, neuroma, Kaposi sarcoma) (3). Table 10.1 summarizes the clinical presentation of WAS (3).

Diagnosis

Diagnostic evaluation of WAS includes the following (3):

- *CBC:* Thrombocytopenia
- *Peripheral blood smear.* Confirms thrombocytopenia, with small platelet size. Mean platelet volume ranges between 3.5 and 5 fL (normal platelet volume 6–10 fL)

Table 10.1 Clinical Presentation of Wiskott–Aldrich Syndrome

Clinical Manifestation	Symptoms
Thrombocytopenia	• Most common presenting symptom; present at birth • Spontaneous and/or posttraumatic bleeding • Ranges from petechiae to severe hematomas • Possible life-threatening intracerebral or intestinal hemorrhage
Immunodeficiency	Increased infection risk by bacterial, viral, and fungal organisms, including opportunistic organisms • Bacterial infection: Otitis media, sinusitis, abscess, enterocolitis, urinary tract infection, meningitis, sepsis • Viral infection: Varicella, herpes simplex virus, Epstein–Barr virus, cytomegalovirus, human papillomavirus • Opportunistic infection: Candidiasis, extensive molluscum contagiosum, aspergillosis, *Pneumocystis jiroveci* pneumonia
Autoimmunity	• Autoimmune cytopenias (i.e., hemolytic anemia, neutropenia, thrombocytopenia) • Arthritis, vasculitis • Inflammatory bowel disease • Immune-mediated renal disease (i.e., IgA nephropathy, Henoch–Schonlein purpura)
Atopy	• Affects over 80% of WAS patients • Eczematous rash, tends to develop during first year of life • Allergic rhinitis, asthma • Food allergy
Malignancy	• Lymphomas: predominantly non-Hodgkin lymphoma type and often Epstein–Barr virus induced • Lymphoblastic leukemia • Myelodysplasia, myeloproliferative disorders • Non-lymphoreticular malignancies (i.e., seminoma, testicular carcinoma, glioma, neuroma, Kaposi sarcoma)

WAS, Wiskott–Aldrich Syndrome.

• *T- and B-cell subsets*:
  ○ Abnormalities in T-cell numbers and function
  ○ Decrease in memory B cells

- *Flow cytometry analysis of lymphocyte subpopulation*:
  - Low CD8 T-cell counts
  - Reduced numbers of B lymphocytes
  - Lower proportions of memory B cells in adult WAS patients
- *Immunoglobulin level*:
  - Low level of IgM and isohemagglutinins
  - Elevated IgA level
  - Normal IgG level
  - Responses to unconjugated pneumococcal antigens are typically defective
- *WASp expression in peripheral blood leukocytes*:
  - Abnormal or lacking
  - WASp expression interpretation is not straightforward; WAS diagnosis must be confirmed by genetic analysis
- *Genetic analysis of WAS gene*:
  - Definitive diagnosis and essential
  - Determines specific mutation in WAS gene

Management

Curative treatment of WAS is allogeneic hematopoietic stem cell transplant (HSCT) (3). HSCT outcomes in WAS have improved significantly, with current literature reporting approximately 90% survival at 5 years and approximately 75% to 80% survival at 8 to 10 years after HSCT (3). Overall outcomes are variable depending on the age at transplant, severity of the disease, and type of donor (3). Umbilical cord blood and mismatched related donor transplants are associated with lower overall survival, and transplant at older age is associated with worse overall survival (3). Even if HSCT is successful, patients can have post-HSCT complications, the most common of which is autoimmunity (3). Up to 55% of transplanted WAS patients develop autoimmune manifestations such as autoantibody-mediated cytopenias (3). Given the severity of the post-HSCT–related complications, HSCT is often reserved for patients with the severe WAS phenotype; for those with a mild phenotype, the decision to transplant is made case by case.

Supportive Management

Close monitoring and supportive measures (listed in Table 10.2) are indicated in WAS patients (3). Prophylactic transfusions to maintain platelet counts within a determined range is not recommended to avoid development of anti-human leukocyte antigen

Table 10.2 Supportive Management of Wiskott–Aldrich Syndrome Patients

Clinical Manifestation	Supportive Management
Thrombocytopenia	Prevent bleeding complications: • Precautions against falls • Use of protective devices such as bicycle helmet • Avoidance of high-contact, high-risk sports Active bleeding: • Use of antifibrinolytic agents • Platelet transfusions • Any other blood product as needed
Immunodeficiency	Prompt treatment of infection Prophylaxis: • Decision to use antibacterial, antiviral, and/or antifungal prophylaxis depends on the frequency, severity, and type of infection
Autoimmunity	Combination of immunosuppressive agents such as high-dose corticosteroids, IVIg, rituximab, cyclophosphamide, azathioprine, vincristine
Atopy	Treat eczema, allergic rhinitis, asthma, and food allergy similar to general population

IVIg, intravenous immune globulin.

(anti-HLA) antibodies, reduce transfusion efficacy in case of emergency, and improve the chance for successful engraftment post-HSCT (3).

Emerging Treatments

Unfortunately, <20% of WAS patients have human leukocyte antigen (HLA)-identical family donors available for HSCT, and mismatched donor HSCT confers increased morbidity and mortality (3). Gene therapy studies are being conducted in the United States and Europe with a goal of transplanting autologous hematopoietic stem cells transduced with the gene encoding normal WASp (3). Benefits include decreased risks of graft rejection and graft versus host disease (GVHD) (3). Limitations of gene therapy include: (a) risk of insertional oncogenesis by viral vector; (b) continued thrombocytopenia; (c) lack of long-term data and follow-up assessing the functional reconstitution of humoral immunity; and (d) lack of long-term outcome and safety data (3). Close follow-up of patients receiving gene therapy is needed to understand the long-term outcomes.

MYH9-RELATED DISORDERS

Clinical Case 10.2

A 6-year-old boy with history of frequent epistaxis presented to his pediatrician's office with an acute febrile illness. The CBC demonstrated a platelet count of 7 × 10⁹/L. The child was initially diagnosed with immune thrombocytopenia (ITP) and CBC was monitored closely. He continued to have thrombocytopenia and frequent, self-resolving nosebleeds. Upon further investigation, family history revealed frequent epistaxis in his brother, mother, and maternal uncle. Prothrombin time (PT), partial thromboplastin time (PTT), fibrinogen level, and von Willebrand panel were normal. Peripheral blood smear showed large platelets and neutrophils with prominent Dohle bodies. MYH9 gene analysis revealed an MYH9 gene mutation.

Introduction

May–Hegglin anomaly, Sebastian syndrome, Fechtner syndrome, and Epstein syndrome are autosomal dominant thrombocytopenia disorders initially thought to be distinct syndromes (4). However, it is now recognized that there are no distinguishing features among the disorders, and all are characterized by mutation of the *MYH9* gene (4). Clinical presentation varies not only within families carrying the same mutation, but also in the individual patient during his or her lifetime (4). Therefore, May–Hegglin anomaly, Sebastian syndrome, Fechtner syndrome, and Epstein syndrome are now grouped under the single heading of "MYH9-related disorders" (MYH9-RD) (4). The *MYH9* gene encodes non-muscle myosin IIA heavy chain, which is part of the contractile cytoskeleton of megakaryocytes, platelets, and neutrophils. Bone marrow megakaryopoiesis is ineffective in these patients (4).

Clinical Presentation

As seen in Figure 10.2, MYH9-RD presents with macrothrombocytopenia (Figure 10.3) (4). Platelets can be as large as red blood cells. Bleeding tendency due to thrombocytopenia varies from patient to patient and can range from easy bruising to mucosal bleeding (i.e., epistaxis, gum bleeding) and/or menorrhagia (4). Some patients have spontaneous bleeding episodes requiring platelet or red blood cell transfusion; life-threatening spontaneous or postpartum hemorrhage has rarely been reported (4). Patients with less-severe thrombocytopenia are usually asymptomatic and low platelet count is incidentally discovered when CBC is obtained for an unrelated clinical problem (4).

Organ involvement in MYH9-RD is presented in Table 10.3 (4).

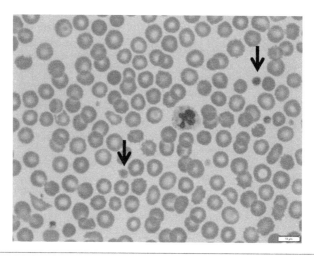

Figure 10.3 Peripheral blood smear of a patient with May–Hegglin anomaly. Platelets (black arrows) are as large as red blood cells.

Source: Courtesy of Dr. M. Tarek Elghetany, Department of Pathology and Immunology and Pediatrics, Texas Children's Hospital/Baylor College of Medicine.

Diagnosis

Definitive diagnosis of MYH9-RD is made by identifying a mutation within the *MYH9* gene by genetic analysis (4). Additional evaluation to help guide the diagnosis of MYH9-RD follow (4):

1. *CBC* showing thrombocytopenia with abnormally large platelets. Platelets are often as large as red blood cells, and automated blood cell counters can recognize platelets as red blood cells

2. *Peripheral smear* showing decreased platelet count with large platelets. Neutrophil inclusion bodies (Dohle-like bodies) are often seen in the cytoplasm

3. Normal *platelet aggregation test*

4. Presence of *comorbidities* such as sensorineural hearing loss, cataracts, glomerulonephritis

5. *Bone marrow biopsy* is not required for diagnosis

Identification of the mutation in the *MYH9* gene is important for prognosis because some mutations are associated with higher incidence of kidney damage, deafness, or isolated thrombocytopenia (4).

Table 10.3 Clinical Presentation of MYH9-Related Disorders

Organ System	Clinical Presentation
Bone marrow	• Leukocyte inclusion bodies seen at birth • Thrombocytopenia • Platelet counts between 20×10^9 and 130×10^9/L • Bleeding symptoms including easy bruising, menorrhagia, epistaxis, gum bleeding
Kidney	• Kidney damage occurs in approximately 30% of patients • Variable presentation in members of the same family • Presents with proteinuria, with or without microscopic hematuria • Approximately 70% of patients with proteinuria develop renal failure within a few years • Once the renal function is altered, progression to renal failure requiring dialysis or kidney transplant is rapid
Eye	• Approximately 16% of patients develop cataracts • Mean age of onset: 23 years
Ear	• Approximately 60% of patients develop progressive hearing loss, usually bilateral sensorineural defect • Onset ranges from the first to sixth decade of life

Management

Current management of MYH9-RD is supportive (Table 10.4) (4). Thrombocytopenia increases the risk of bleeding; therefore, prevention of bleeding (e.g., fall precautions, avoiding contact sports, avoiding medications that can impair platelet function) is important (4). Prophylactic platelet transfusion to maintain the platelet count in a determined range is not recommended due to risk of alloimmunization and subsequent refractoriness to platelet transfusion (4). MYH9-RD patients should receive platelet transfusions for active bleeding that cannot be managed by local measures (4). Hearing loss is progressive and there is no cure at this time; moreover, there is no report of a successful cochlear implant in an MYH9-RD patient (4). The current recommendation is to avoid hazardous noise and ototoxic drugs (4).

Once MYH9-RD patients develop proteinuria, about 70% rapidly progress to renal failure (4). There are reports of using angiotensin receptor blocker (ARB) or angiotensin-converting enzyme (ACE) inhibitors to slow the progression of renal disease, but the study sample size is too small to conclude if these drugs are effective in preventing or delaying renal failure (4).

Table 10.4 Current Management of MYH9-Related Disorders

Clinical Manifestation	Management
Thrombocytopenia	• Avoid medications that impair platelet function • Regular dental care and good oral hygiene to avoid gum bleeding • Hormonal contraceptives to prevent menorrhagia For surgery: • There is no safe platelet count to prevent bleeding • Major surgery or invasive procedure: Recommend maintaining platelet count $>50 \times 10^9$/L
Hearing loss	• Avoid hazardous noise • Avoid ototoxic drugs
Cataracts	• Regular eye exam
Renal disease	• Avoid nephrotoxic drugs • Dialysis or kidney transplant may be required

Emerging Treatment

Use of eltrombopag (oral nonpeptide agonist of the thrombopoietin [TPO] receptor) is an emerging strategy to improve thrombocytopenia in patients with MYH9-RD (4). One clinical trial showed 12 MYH9-RD patients with platelet counts $<50 \times 10^9$/L at baseline had improved platelet count after 3 to 6 weeks, along with improvement in bleeding symptoms (4). There is no information on the safety of long-term use of eltrombopag, specifically in regard to bone marrow fibrosis.

X-LINKED THROMBOCYTOPENIA WITH DYSERYTHROPOIESIS

Introduction

X-linked thrombocytopenia with dyserythropoiesis is an inherited platelet disorder with a mutation in the *GATA1* gene (5). *GATA1* is a transcription factor that plays a role in both erythroid and megakaryocytic differentiation of hematopoietic progenitors (5). Patients present with thrombocytopenia and anemia, which can range from mild to severe (5). Thrombocytopenia presents in infancy with easy bruising and/or mucosal bleeding (5). Anemia can range from minimal (mild dyserythropoiesis) to severe (hydrops fetalis requiring in utero transfusion) (5). In extreme circumstances, patients may have severe hemorrhage and/or require lifelong red blood cell transfusions (5). Some patients show improvement in anemia and risk of bleeding with age (5).

Diagnosis

CBC demonstrates anemia and thrombocytopenia; platelets are large with decreased granular content, and red blood cells can vary in size (5). Due to the complexity and heterogeneity of the disease, diagnosis may be challenging. Initial presentation is similar to WAS without the associated immunodeficiency; therefore, WAS should be ruled out when evaluating a patient with suspected X-linked thrombocytopenia with dyserythropoiesis (5). Evaluation should include CBC, peripheral blood smear, and bone marrow aspirate and biopsy to confirm that anemia and thrombocytopenia are due to ineffective hematopoiesis (5). Bone marrow evaluation demonstrates small, dysplastic megakaryocytes with signs of incomplete maturation, dyserythropoiesis, and hypocellularity of erythroid and granulocytic lineages (5). Megakaryocyte number may be increased or decreased (5). Definitive diagnosis of X-linked thrombocytopenia with dyserythropoiesis is by detection of a *GATA1* gene mutation (5).

Management

Supportive measures for patients with X-linked thrombocytopenia with dyserythropoiesis include (5):

- Periodic CBC
- Platelet transfusion for bleeding symptoms (i.e., epistaxis not controlled with local measures, gingival bleeding, or gastrointestinal [GI] bleeding)
- Red blood cell transfusion for symptomatic anemia
  - If patients require repeated red blood cell transfusions, they should be monitored for iron overload
- Avoidance of medications that impair platelet function (i.e., aspirin, nonsteroidal anti-inflammatory drugs [NSAIDs])
- Avoidance of activities with high risk of trauma

For patients with severe symptoms, curative bone marrow transplant can be considered (5).

BERNARD–SOULIER SYNDROME

Introduction

Bernard–Soulier syndrome (BSS) is an autosomal recessive disorder affecting the platelet function, size, and number (1). Functionally, platelets cannot adhere to the subendothelium or VWF due to a defect in the platelet glycoprotein complex GPIb/IX/V (1,6).

Clinical Presentation

Patients with BSS typically present with easy bruising, epistaxis, gum bleeding, and cutaneous bleeding (e.g., menorrhagia) (6). The severity of bleeding varies among patients (1,6). In severe cases, patients may have joint bleeding and/or intracranial hemorrhage (7). Though BSS is an autosomal recessive disorder, heterozygous patients usually present with bleeding tendency, albeit milder in nature (6).

Diagnosis

CBC often shows thrombocytopenia with platelet counts between 30×10^9 and 200×10^9/L (1). Platelets are large and platelet aggregation studies are normal to physiological agonists such as epinephrine, adenosine diphosphate (ADP), collagen, and arachidonic acid (6). However, addition of ristocetin to platelet function studies produces defective platelet aggregation (1,6). BSS is confirmed with either genetic testing demonstrating a mutation in *GP1BA*, *GP1BB*, and/or *GP9* genes or by flow cytometry to assess GPIb-IX-V expression on the platelet surface (6).

Management

BSS patients need to be educated on the measures to prevent bleeding complications, including avoidance of medications that impair platelet function and avoidance of risk-taking behavior that could lead to even minor trauma (1,6). Platelet transfusions should be conserved for uncontrolled bleeding to avoid development of alloimmunization (6). If a patient experiences moderate to major bleeding symptoms, activated factor VIIa (FVIIa) can be used to reduce bleeding times (6). Desmopressin may shorten bleeding episodes for some patients (6).

Emerging Treatment

Clinical trials utilizing gene therapy are ongoing as potentially curative therapy for BSS (1).

PLATELET-TYPE VON WILLEBRAND DISEASE

Introduction

Platelet-type von Willebrand disease (VWD) is a rare autosomal dominant disorder with a similar phenotype as type 2B VWD (7,8). While both diseases result in enhanced binding of platelets to VWF, there are differences in the mechanism of disease (7). In platelet-type VWD, there is a gain-of-function mutation in the glyco-protein 1BA (*GP1BA*) gene responsible for encoding glycoprotein 1b alpha (Gp1bα), a subunit of the platelet receptor responsible for platelet–VWF interaction. In type 2B VWD, there is a gain-of-function mutation in the A1 domain of VWF, the site where platelets bind to VWF (7,8). In both disorders, enhanced VWF and platelet interaction leads to increased platelet clumping and enhanced clearance of platelets and high-molecular-weight VWF multimers (7). To differentiate between type 2B VWD and platelet-type VWD, DNA analysis is required (7,8).

Clinical Presentation

Clinical presentation of platelet-type VWD is similar to type 2B VWD (8). Patients present with mild-to-moderate mucocutaneous bleed-ing symptoms such as frequent and severe epistaxis and excessive bleeding following tooth extraction, tonsillectomy, or other surgi-cal procedures (7,8). There is thrombocytopenia with large platelet size/volume (7).

Diagnosis

Once there is suspicion for type 2B VWD, it is important to obtain DNA analysis to distinguish between platelet-type VWD and type 2B VWD for management purposes (7). Initial evaluation for both disorders will show the following (7,8):

- CBC: Thrombocytopenia with elevated mean platelet volume (MPV)
- Peripheral blood smear: Decreased platelet count with large platelet size; sometimes platelet clumping is observed, which is caused by spontaneous binding of circulating VWF to platelets
- VWF multimer assay: Shows decreased amount of high-molec-ular-weight VWF multimers

To definitively diagnose platelet-type VWD, demonstration of a mutation in the *GP1BA* gene is required (8).

Management

Treatment of platelet-type VWD is different from type 2B VWD. Factor VIII/VWF replacement therapy or agents that increase the release of endogenous VWF (such as DDAVP [1-desamino-8-d-ar-ginine vasopressin]) are used in type 2B VWD for management or prevention of bleeding (8). The use of these agents in platelet-type VWD is prohibited, as they will exacerbate the condition by causing further decreases in the platelet count (8). Management of bleeding symptoms or prevention of bleeding from surgical procedures in patients with platelet-type VWD requires platelet transfusions or, if possible, low-dose factor VIII/VWF concentrates (VWF:RCo of approximately 40–47 µ/dL) to increase the hemostatic activity to a limit that does not induce a drop in the platelet count (8). Platelet transfusion is usually sufficient to achieve hemostasis (8).

CONGENITAL AMEGAKARYOCYTIC THROMBOCYTOPENIA

Introduction

Congenital amegakaryocytic thrombocytopenia (CAMT) is an auto-somal recessive bleeding disorder with a severe bleeding phenotype (9). CAMT is caused by mutations in the TPO receptor gene (*c-Mpl*) expressed on megakaryoctyes, leading to absent or diminished pro-duction of platelets (9). Interestingly, CAMT is also regarded as an inherited bone marrow failure syndrome because CAMT patients progress to trilineage bone marrow failure (9). The clinical course of the disease varies depending on the type of mutation in *c-Mpl* (9).

Clinical Presentation

CAMT patients present with symptomatic thrombocytopenia early in life (usually at birth), which includes easy bruising, petechiae, and mucosal bleeding (9). CBC shows platelet counts of <50 × 10^9/L (9). The clinical course of the disorder depends on the type of mutation (9):

1. *Type I mutation*: Premature stop codon or frameshift in *c-Mpl* resulting in complete elimination of receptor signaling. Patients with the Type I mutation have persistent thrombocytopenia and rapid progression to trilineage bone marrow failure. The mean age onset of trilineage bone marrow failure is 1 year and 11 months.

2. *Type II mutation*: Splicing defect or amino acid substitution on the *c-Mpl* gene. These patients have transient modest improve-ments in platelet counts during the first year of life with delayed onset of marrow failure (mean age of onset 5 years).

Diagnosis

CBC usually shows platelet counts of <50 × 10^9/L. Peripheral blood smear shows low platelet count with normally sized platelets (9). If bone marrow aspiration and biopsy is performed, pathology shows marked megakaryocytic hypoplasia (9). The CBC should be monitored closely because CAMT patients often develop pancyto-penia, with onset varying depending on the type of mutation (9). If

Table 10.5 Differential Diagnosis for Thrombocytopenia in Infancy

Prenatal etiologies	• Preeclampsia • Placental insufficiency • Intrauterine growth retardation
Infectious etiologies	• TORCH • Sepsis
Immune etiology	NAIT
Inherited disorder	• Fanconi anemia • Thrombocytopenia with absent radii • Congenital amegakaryocytic thrombocytopenia with radioulnar synostosis • Dyskeratosis congenital

NAIT, neonatal alloimmune thrombocytopenia;
TORCH, toxoplasmosis, rubella cytomegalovirus, herpes simplex, and HIV.

plasma TPO levels can be obtained, they are elevated, often 10-fold or more above the normal range (9). Mutation analysis of the *c-Mpl* gene confirms the diagnosis of CAMT (9). Because thrombocytopenia usually presents at birth, other causes of thrombocytopenia in infancy should be excluded during the workup (Table 10.5) (9).

Management

Currently, the only definitive treatment available for CAMT patients is HSCT (9). Matched related donor transplantation is preferred because outcomes are less favorable for patients without a matched related donor due to delayed engraftment, graft rejection, GVHD, and regimen-related toxicity (9). While awaiting HSCT, patients will require the following (9):

1. Platelet transfusions and other therapies such as antifibrinolytic agents when bleeding symptoms develop
2. Red blood cell transfusions once anemia develops
3. Antibiotics for febrile neutropenia

Because CAMT patients do not have the *c-Mpl* receptor on megakaryocytes, TPO receptor agonists are not useful and thrombocytopenia does not improve with immunoglobulins, corticosteroids, or splenectomy (9).

THROMBOCYTOPENIA-ASSOCIATED SKELETAL DEFECTS

Thrombocytopenia-associated skeletal defects are presented in Table 10.6.

Table 10.6 Summary of Thrombocytopenia Associated With Skeletal Defects

TAR	
Presentation	At birth: • Bilateral absent radii with presence of thumb • Thrombocytopenia (platelet count between 10 and 100×10^9/L) ○ Thrombocytopenia usually resolves over the first year of life • Elevated plasma TPO level • Possible other non-skeletal abnormalities – gastroenteritis, renal malformations, cardiac defects, and so forth
Diagnosis	• Typical bilateral radii abnormalities • No associated mutations identified
Management	• Multisystem evaluation ○ To assess non-skeletal abnormalities • Referral to orthopedic surgery service ○ Management of skeletal abnormalities • Referral to other subspecialties depending on the presence of non-skeletal abnormalities • Platelet transfusion for management of bleeding or prior to surgical procedures • Even after resolution of thrombocytopenia, long-term monitoring for late recurrence of thrombocytopenia
ATRUS	
Presentation	• Radioulnar synostosis • Other skeletal defects: ○ Clinodactyly ○ Syndactyly ○ Hip dysplasia • Severe normocytic thrombocytopenia • Easy bruising and bleeding • Sensorineural hearing loss
Diagnosis	CBC: Severe thrombocytopenia with normal mean platelet volume Bone marrow biopsy/aspirate: Absent megakaryocytes Genetic testing: Mutation of *HOXA11*
Management	• Referral to orthopedic surgery • Platelet transfusion for management of bleeding or prior to surgery • Red blood cell transfusion for symptomatic anemia • Hematopoietic stem cell transplant to correct thrombocytopenia and bleeding symptoms

(*continued*)

Table 10.6 Summary of Thrombocytopenia Associated With Skeletal Defects (*continued*)

DiGeorge Syndrome/VCFS	

Presentation	• Macrothrombocytopenia
	• 22q11 mutation associated comorbidities:
	  ○ Cardiac abnormalities
	  ○ Cleft palate
	  ○ Thymic aplasia
	  ○ Mental retardation
	  ○ Immune deficiency

Diagnosis	• Hemizygous loss of allele of *GP1BB* located at 22q11
Management	• Multidisciplinary approach to manage comorbidities

ATRUS, amegakaryocytic thrombocytopenia with radioulnar synostosis; CBC, complete blood count; TAR, thrombocytopenia with absent radii; TPO, thrombopoietin; VCFS, velocardiofacial syndrome.

Source: From Carubbi C, Masselli E, Nouvenne A, et al. Laboratory diagnostics of inherited platelet disorders. *Clin Chem Lab Med.* 2014;52(8):1091–1106. doi:10.1515/cclm-2014-0131; Geddis AE. Congenital amegakaryocytic thrombocytopenia and thrombocytopenia with absent radii. *Hematol Oncol Clin North Am.* 2009;23(2):321–331. doi:10.1016/j.hoc.2009.01.012; Thompson A, Woodruff K, Feig S, et al. Congenital thrombocytopenia and radio-ulnar synostosis: a new familial syndrome. *Brit J Haematol.* 2001;113(4):866–870. doi:10.1046/j.1365-2141.2001.02834.x

Thrombocytopenia-associated skeletal defects include:

1. Thrombocytopenia with absent radii (TAR)
2. Amegakaryocytic thrombocytopenia with radioulnar synostosis (ATRUS)
3. DiGeorge syndrome/velocardiofacial syndrome (VCFS)

These disorders have skeletal defects and other associated medical complications along with thrombocytopenia (7,9). Therefore, these patients require a multidisciplinary approach to management/treatment.

Thrombocytopenia With Absent Radii

TAR is inherited in either an autosomal recessive or autosomal dominant pattern with variable penetrance (9). At this time, no associated mutations have been identified (9). Patients are born with bilateral radial aplasia with the presence of thumbs (9). Platelet counts range between 10 and 100 × 10^9/L and peripheral blood smear shows normal platelet size (9). TPO level is elevated (9). TAR patients can have non-skeletal abnormalities that include gastroenteritis, renal malformations, and cardiac defects (9). Therefore, when a child is born with absent radii, a multisystem evaluation should be undertaken (9). Generally, over the first year of life, platelet count and bleeding symptoms improve (9). Management for patients with TAR includes (9):

- Referral to orthopedic service for management of absent radii
- Referral to other subspecialties as needed based on the presence of non-skeletal abnormalities
- Management of bleeding symptoms or prevention of bleeding during surgical procedures with platelet transfusions

Even after resolution of thrombocytopenia, patients with TAR need to be monitored for late recurrence of thrombocytopenia or leukemia, as there are reports of patients with TAR developing acute myeloid or lymphoid leukemias (9).

Amegakaryocytic Thrombocytopenia With Radioulnar Synostosis

ATRUS is inherited in an autosomal dominant pattern (7). ATRUS is associated with a mutation in the Homeobox gene *HOXA11*, which plays a central role in skeletal development and hematopoiesis (7). Patients present with thrombocytopenia and absent bone marrow megakaryocytes (10). Associated symptoms include (7,10):

- Aplastic anemia
- Skeletal abnormalities:
  - Radioulnar synostosis: Proximal fusion of the radius and ulna causing limited pronation and supination of the forearm
  - Clinodactyly
  - Syndactyly
  - Hip dysplasia
- Sensorineural hearing loss

A few ATRUS patients have developed hypoplastic anemia and pancytopenia (10). Due to severity of thrombocytopenia and bleeding complications, patients often undergo HSCT (10). Other than stem cell transplant, patients require frequent platelet transfusions and red cell transfusions if anemia is present and referral to orthopedic surgery for management of skeletal abnormalities (9,10).

DiGeorge Syndrome/VCFS

DiGeorge syndrome/VCFS has an autosomal dominant inheritance pattern (7). Patients usually have hemizygous loss of the allele of *GP1BB* located at 22q11 (7). Because *GP1BB* is one of the three genes defective in BSS, patients can exhibit macrothrombocytopenia with mild bleeding symptoms (7). Mutations in 22q11 also exhibit anomalies including cardiac abnormalities, cleft palate, thymic aplasia, mental retardation, and immune deficiency (7). These patients also require a multidisciplinary team approach, given multiple comorbidities associated with the 22q11 mutation.

GRAY PLATELET SYNDROME

Gray platelet syndrome (GPS) is a rare inherited platelet disorder notable for thrombocytopenia, large platelet size, and agranular platelets present on peripheral blood smear (7). Platelets appear gray due to reduced or absent alpha (α-) granules (7). The syndrome can be inherited in a recessive or dominant pattern, and defects are seen in more than one gene (7). Diagnostic evaluation is notable for (7):

1. CBC: Thrombocytopenia
2. Peripheral blood smear: Abnormally large, agranular, gray platelets
3. Platelet aggregation assay: Collagen-induced platelet aggregation is reduced; response to ristocetin is normal or slightly impaired, but never absent. However, the platelet aggregation assay is not always helpful due to variability in results in GPS patients.

QUEBEC SYNDROME

Quebec syndrome, as the name suggests, is confined to French Canadians and inherited in an autosomal dominant pattern (7). These patients have tandem duplication in the *PLAU* gene, resulting in overexpression and storage of urokinase plasminogen activator by platelets leading to increased fibrinolysis (7). As a result, patients present with thrombocytopenia with delayed bleeding tendency (7). Platelet aggregometry shows decreased aggregation in response to epinephrine, but these findings are not specific to Quebec syndrome (7). Definitive diagnosis is made by genetic testing for *PLAU* duplication using polymerase chain reaction (PCR) and Southern blotting techniques (7).

Key Points

- WAS is an X-linked recessive disorder with the classic triad of microthrombocytopenia, eczema, and immunodeficiency.
- Curative treatment of WAS is HSCT.
- MYH9-RD are autosomal dominant disorders with ineffective megakaryopoiesis.
- Unlike WAS, MYH9-RD presents with macrothrombocytopenia.
- X-linked thrombocytopenia with dyserythropoiesis patients present with thrombocytopenia and anemia. Because the initial

presentation is similar to WAS, WAS should be ruled out when evaluating a patient with suspected X-linked thrombocytopenia with dyserythropoiesis.

- BSS is an autosomal recessive disorder affecting the platelet function, size, and number. Patients present with macrothrombocytopenia with defective platelet aggregation to ristocetin.

- Platelet-type VWD is an autosomal dominant disorder with similar presentation as type 2B VWD; however, platelet-type VWD has a gain-of-function mutation in the *GP1BA* gene, resulting in enhanced binding of platelets to VWF.

- To differentiate between type 2B VWD and platelet-type VWD, DNA analysis is required.

- CAMT is an autosomal recessive disorder with a severe bleeding phenotype due to absent or diminished production of platelets. Definitive treatment is HSCT.

- Thrombocytopenia-associated skeletal defects have other associated medical complications along with thrombocytopenia; therefore, these patients require a multidisciplinary approach to management.

DISORDERS WITH A NORMAL PLATELET COUNT

Chediak–Higashi Syndrome
Introduction

Chediak–Higashi syndrome (CHS) is an autosomal recessive disorder with severe immunodeficiency, frequent bacterial infection, variable albinism, progressive neurologic dysfunction, and bleeding tendency (11). These patients have a normal platelet count, but prolonged bleeding time due to abnormal platelet function (11).

Clinical Presentation

Patients with CHS present with partial albinism, recurrent pyogenic infection, and easy bruising and mucosal bleeding due to defective platelets (11). The disorder progresses to an "accelerated phase," where lymphocytes and macrophages infiltrate into major organs of the body (11). Finally, in the third to fifth decade of life, patients develop progressive neurologic dysfunction exhibited by weakness, ataxia, sensory deficits, and progressive neurodegeneration (11).

Diagnosis

Patients are diagnosed with CHS by the presence of large, peroxidase-positive, cytoplasmic granules in both hematopoietic and non-hematopoietic cells (7). Other evaluation reveals the following (7,11):

- CBC:
  - Neutropenia
  - Normal platelet size and count
    - Reduced number of dense granules
- Prolonged bleeding time
- Other clinical findings:
  - Oculocutaneous albinism
  - Recurrent infection

Management

Because of recurrent bacterial infection, patients should be started on prophylactic antibiotics (11). HSCT can cure the hematologic and immunologic complications – neutropenia, platelet dysfunction, immune deficiency, and the "accelerated phase" – but cannot prevent progressive neurologic deficits (11).

HERMANSKY–PUDLAK SYNDROME

Introduction

Hermansky–Pudlak syndrome (HPS) is a rare autosomal recessive disease of subcellular organelles present in many tissues including melanosomes, lysosomes, and platelet-dense granules (7). There are 10 known subtypes of HPS (12).

Clinical Presentations

Patients present with variable hypopigmentation of the hair, skin, and irides, and exhibit easy bruising or bleeding that is often mild (12). Certain subtypes of HPS cause progressive pulmonary fibrosis (12). These patients initially present with dyspnea and pulmonary function testing that indicates restrictive lung disease (12). Ultimately, high-resolution CT of the chest will show reticular opacities, thickened interlobular septa, and ground glass infiltrates consistent with pulmonary fibrosis (12). Patients who develop pulmonary fibrosis face mortality in the fourth to fifth decade of life (12). Some patients have granulomatous colitis, which resembles Crohn's disease and most often involves the colon (12).

Diagnosis

There should be suspicion for HPS in patients with oculocutaneous albinism, along with a history of easy bruising or bleeding (12). HPS patients have a normal platelet count, but a prolonged bleeding time (7). When platelets are closely examined via electron microscopy, delta granules are reduced in number (12). Genetic testing is

> **Box 10.1 Diagnostic Criteria for Hermansky–Pudlak Syndrome**
>
> Tyrosinase-positive oculocutaneous albinism
> - Absent brown/black pigment from hair, eyes, and skin
>
> Bleeding disorder due to platelet dysfunction
> - Symptoms can be mild to severe
>
> Absent delta granules on platelet electron microscopy

recommended to determine the specific subtype of HPS because each subtype has a specific phenotype requiring close follow-up/monitoring (12). Box 10.1 summarizes the diagnostic criteria for HPS (7,12).

Management

Current management of HPS (Table 10.7) is limited, but includes proper protection from the sun, controlling bleeding topically with thrombin and Gelfoam, avoiding NSAIDs and/or aspirin, and possible platelet transfusion in the setting of trauma (12). Ongoing research aims to understand the molecular bases of HPS to provide better treatment for this disorder (12).

Table 10.7 Management of Hermansky–Pudlak Syndrome

Albinism	Protection from sun to prevent skin cancers
Bleeding complications	• Avoid anticoagulant or antiplatelet agents such as aspirin, NSAIDs, warfarin • Prophylactic IV DDAVP for procedures • Control local bleeding topically with thrombin and Gelfoam • Platelet transfusion in the setting of trauma
Granulomatous colitis	Treatment similar to Crohn's colitis: • Anti-inflammatory agents • Immunosuppressants • Infliximab (anti-tumor necrosis factor)

Pulmonary fibrosis	• No known specific therapies
	• Referral for lung transplant evaluation
	• Referral to pulmonary rehabilitation program
	• Immunizations:
	  ○ Yearly influenza vaccine
	  ○ Pneumococcal polysaccharide vaccinations (PPSV23)
	  ○ Pneumococcal conjugate vaccine (PCV13) for patients >65 years old

DDAVP, 1-desamino-8-d-arginine vasopressin; NSAIDs, nonsteroidal anti-inflammatory drugs.

GLANZMANN'S THROMBASTHENIA

Clinical Case 10.3

A 7-year-old girl was referred to Hematology for history of excessive bruising, described as spontaneously occurring large bruises or development of hematomas in the setting of trauma. She also had spontaneous gum bleeding at least once a week. An extensive bleeding evaluation including von Willebrand panel, CBC, PT/PTT, fibrinogen level, and hemoglobin profile was normal. Platelet aggregometry showed absent platelet aggregation to both ADP and collagen. Genetic testing revealed a mutation consistent with Glanzmann's thrombasthenia.

Introduction

Glanzmann's thrombasthenia is a rare autosomal recessive disorder with a functional defect in platelet glycoprotein (GP)IIb/IIIa (αIIbβ3 integrin), which is responsible for platelet binding to proteins such as fibrinogen, VWF, and fibronectin (7). Patients present with mucocutaneous bleeding – purpura, epistaxis, gingival hemorrhage, and menorrhagia (7). The disorder is divided into type I and type II based on GPIIb/IIIa deficiency (1):

- Type I: Severely deficient in GPIIb/IIIa complexes along with absent fibrinogen in the alpha-granules of platelets; clot retraction is absent.
- Type II: Approximately 5% to 25% of platelets have normal GPIIb/IIIa complexes and fibrinogen is present in the alpha-granules of platelets; clot retraction is present, but decreased.

Approximately 78% of the patients belong to Type I subgroup and approximately 14% belong to Type II subgroup (1). Remaining patients display qualitative defects in GPIIb/IIIa (1). Heterozygous individuals are asymptomatic because 50% of the normal amount of GPIIb/IIIa is sufficient for platelet aggregation (7).

Clinical Presentation

Bleeding symptoms can occur soon after birth with a variable clinical presentation ranging from bruising only to severe and potentially fatal hemorrhages (1). Review of the Glanzmann's thrombasthenia registry, a prospective, observational, international registry that enrolled 218 patients, revealed that the first bleeding symptoms occurred at a median age of 1 year (mean 5.6 years) (13). Bleeding episodes were mostly mucocutaneous—bruising, purpura, epistaxis, gingival and other oral bleeding, menorrhagia, and GI bleeding—and less frequently related to hemarthrosis or intracranial hemorrhage (13). Bleeding complications were observed frequently after trauma and surgical procedures (13). Appropriate precaution to prevent bleeding must be discussed with the patient and patient's family to avoid bleeding-related morbidity and mortality.

Diagnosis

Individuals with Glanzmann's thrombasthenia have a normal platelet count and morphology on CBC and peripheral blood smear (1). Platelet function assays are abnormal with prolonged PFA-100 closure time; with platelet aggregometry, platelets do not aggregate to agonists such as ADP, collagen, thrombin, and adrenaline, but do aggregate in the presence of ristocetin (7). Flow cytometry detecting the presence of GPIIb (CD41) and GPIIIa (CD61) proteins on the surface of platelets shows diminished or absent GPIIb/IIIa complexes on platelets for Type I and Type II subgroups (1,7). For the qualitative disorders, platelet aggregation is necessary because flow cytometry shows normal quantities of GPIIb/IIIa (1). Definitive diagnostic testing is confirmed by detection of a genetic mutation in the *ITGA2B* or *ITGB3* gene encoding for GPIIb and GPIIIa, respectively (7,13) (Table 10.8).

Management

Management consists of controlling bleeding symptoms. For patients with menorrhagia, oral contraceptive pills (OCPs) and

Table 10.8 Diagnosis of Glanzmann's Thrombasthenia

Platelet aggregation assay	• Absent aggregation in the presence of ADP, collagen, thrombin, and adrenaline • Aggregation in the presence of ristocetin
PFA-100 assay	Prolonged closure time
Flow cytometry (detection of GPIIb and GPIIIa on the surface of platelets)	• Type I: 0% to 5% of platelets with GPIIb/IIIa complexes • Type II: 5% to 20% of platelets with GPIIb/IIIa complexes • Variant/qualitative: >20% of platelets with GPIIb/IIIa complexes
Genetic testing	Detect genetic mutation in *ITGA2B* or *ITGB3* gene

ADP, adenosine diphosphate; GP, glycoprotein.

Source: From Krishnegowda M, Rajashekaraiah V. Platelet disorders: an overview. *Blood Coagulation Fibrinolysis.* 2015;26(5):479. doi:10.1097/01. mbc.0000469521.23628.2d; Carubbi C, Masselli E, Nouvenne A, et al. Laboratory diagnostics of inherited platelet disorders. *Clin Chem Lab Med.* 2014;52(8):1091–1106. doi:10.1515/cclm-2014-0131; Poon M-C, Minno G, d' Oiron R, Zotz R. New insights into the treatment of Glanzmann Thrombasthenia. *Transfus Med Rev.* 2016;30(2):92–99. doi:10.1016/j. tmrv.2016.01.001

antifibrinolytic agents are recommended. Minor bleeding can usually be managed with topical agents, while moderate to severe bleeding may require a combination of antifibrinolytic agents, platelet transfusions, or recombinant factor VIIa (rFVIIa) (13). Platelet transfusions should be reserved for severe bleeding episodes because repeated transfusion can lead to development of GPIIb/IIIa antibodies to donor platelets, inhibiting GPIIb/IIIa function (13). Thus, rFVIIa product is preferred over platelet transfusion to achieve hemostasis (13). To prevent postsurgical bleeding, patients can receive a combination of antifibrinolytic agents and rFVIIa (13). HSCT is considered in patients with severe and recurrent bleeding, but because of posttransplant-related complications, other therapeutic options are being pursued (13). One option is gene therapy, which has the potential to cure Glanzmann's thrombasthenia, but remains experimental (13).

Key Points

- CHS patients have a normal platelet count, but have abnormal platelet function resulting in prolonged bleeding time.
- HPS should be considered in patients with oculocutaneous albinism and history of easy bruising or bleeding.
- Glanzmann's thrombasthenia is a rare autosomal recessive disorder with a functional defect in platelet GPIIb/IIIa, resulting in mucocutaneous bleeding.

DISORDERS OF INCREASED PLATELET DESTRUCTION

Primary ITP
Clinical Case 10.4

A previously healthy 2-year-old boy presented to the emergency department with diffuse petechiae and bruises for 2 days. Four weeks earlier, he had been diagnosed with a upper respiratory tract viral infection, which had since resolved. He was otherwise well appearing and active with no gum bleeding or blood in the urine or stool. Family history was unremarkable, and the boy had no allergies and was not taking any medications. Vital signs were normal; physical exam was notable for diffuse petechiae with scattered bruises. Oral exam was normal. Platelet count was $5 \times 10^9/L$; hemoglobin, white blood cell count, liver enzymes, and electrolytes (including BUN/creatinine) were within normal range.

Introduction

ITP is an acquired, immune-mediated disorder resulting in destruction of circulating platelets (14). The incidence, management, and treatment of ITP vary between children and adults.

Pediatrics

Clinical Presentation

Pediatric ITP affects four to six out of 100,000 children per year and presents with bruising, petechiae, and mucosal bleeding (15). Serious and/or life-threatening bleeding (such as intracranial hemorrhage) can occur, but is uncommon (15). In fact, the rate of new serious bleeding in the first 28 days of diagnosis of ITP is only about 0.6% (15). Moreover, the platelet count does not correlate with the severity of bleeding. Platelet counts generally improve over time, but 5% to 10% of children with ITP will develop severe, chronic, and/or refractory disease (15).

Diagnosis

Primary ITP is a diagnosis of exclusion; other causes of thrombocytopenia should be ruled out because there is no specific test or evaluation to diagnose primary ITP. Obtaining a detailed history and physical exam are important in excluding other causes of thrombocytopenia (14). CBC and peripheral blood smear are the initial laboratory tests of choice (14). In the past, bone marrow examination was recommended for initial evaluation, but the 2011 American Society of Hematology (ASH) evidence-based practice guideline for ITP no longer considers bone marrow examination to be necessary for diagnosis (14). ITP is divided into the following categories based on the length of disease (14):

- Acute ITP: Onset of thrombocytopenia up to 3 months
- Persistent ITP: 3 to 12 months after diagnosis
- Chronic ITP: Platelet count $<100 \times 10^9$/L for longer than 12 months
- Refractory ITP: ITP that does not respond to, or relapses after, splenectomy

Management

Despite parental anxiety, the 2011 ASH guideline recommends observation alone in children with ITP who have no "wet" bleeding (mucosal bleeding, including wet purpura), regardless of platelet count (14). Skin bruising and petechiae are not considered criteria for treatment (14). The decision to start therapy is based on severity of the associated bleeding, reliability of the family for close follow-up, and potential loss or gain of quality of life (14). Once the decision is made to start therapy, initial therapy recommendations include (14):

- Single dose of intravenous immunoglobulin (IVIg)
- Short course of corticosteroids

IVIg is chosen over corticosteroids if a more rapid increase in platelet count is desired (14). Anti-D immunoglobulin (anti-D) therapy can also be used as first-line therapy, but it carries a black box warning by the U.S. Food and Drug administration (FDA) for rare but serious and potentially life-threatening intravascular hemolysis (14). However, anti-D is an effective first-line therapy for Rh-positive, nonsplenectomized children without anemia or evidence of autoimmune hemolysis (14,15).

For children who do not respond to first-line therapy and have persistent severe bleeding symptoms, and/or have chronic ITP, secondary ITP should be ruled out (see the section "Secondary ITP" for more information) (15). Therapy options for children with ongoing bleeding despite first-line therapy and/or chronic ITP include (14–16):

- *Rituximab*: Rituximab depletes B cells by binding to CD20 antigen surface markers and removes autoreactive B-cell clones. There are no randomized trials for rituximab therapy in children with ITP, but in four cohort studies and 10 case reports, there is evidence that children with chronic ITP have an overall response rate of 61%. Late relapses are possible after achieving remission with rituximab; therefore, long-term follow-up is necessary.

- *High-dose dexamethasone:* There are limited studies on high-dose dexamethasone therapy in children and adolescents with chronic or persistent ITP. However, adult ITP clinical trials demonstrated patients treated with high-dose dexamethasone (dose of 0.6 mg/kg/d × 4 days every 4 weeks for one to three cycles) had better complete response rate when compared to standard prednisone therapy of 1 mg/kg/d for 2 weeks. Therefore, the 2011 evidence-based practice guidelines for ITP suggest high-dose dexamethasone may be considered for children with significant ongoing bleeding despite treatment with IVIg or conventional doses of corticosteroids; or as an alternative to splenectomy or in children who do not respond favorably to splenectomy.

- *TPO receptor agonists*: TPO agonists bind to TPO receptors on megakaryocytes, leading to increased platelet production. There are two TPO receptor agonists (romiplostim and eltrombopag) approved for treatment of chronic ITP in adults, and there are ongoing studies on the use of TPO receptor agonists in children with ITP.

- *Immunosuppressive agents*: Agents such as azathioprine, cyclophosphamide, cyclosporine, sirolimus, or mycophenolate can be used in chronic ITP, but there is limited evidence for their efficacy in children.

- *Splenectomy*: Approximately 85% of patients undergoing splenectomy have an immediate platelet count improvement and about 70% to 80% have a sustained response. However, splenectomy is an irreversible procedure, placing young children at risk for complications, including infection. Therefore, if the decision is made to perform splenectomy, children should be vaccinated against all encapsulated organisms 2 weeks before surgery and receive booster immunizations every 5 years. Prophylactic penicillin or an equivalent antibiotic should be prescribed to children <5 years old and to older children for at least 2 years after surgery to prevent infection.

Adults

Clinical Presentation

The incidence of primary ITP in adults is 3.3/100,000 adults per year with a prevalence of 9.5/100,000 (16). In younger adults, ITP prevalence is higher in women, but for the elderly (age >65 years), the prevalence of ITP in men and women is equal (16). The pathophysiology of ITP is similar between adults and children, but management is different because most children have self-limited disease, while in adults ITP is often a chronic disorder.

Diagnosis

Primary ITP in adults is a diagnosis of exclusion. Thus, other causes of thrombocytopenia should be ruled out. Obtaining a detailed history and physical exam are important (14). The 2011 ASH guideline for ITP recommends obtaining additional laboratory tests including HIV, hepatitis C, CBC and peripheral blood smear; bone marrow evaluation is not necessary for diagnosis (14).

Management/Treatment

First-line treatment for adults with primary ITP is administered for platelet counts <30 × 10^9/L and includes the following (14,16):

- Corticosteroids: Prednisone 1 mg/kg/d for 2 to 4 weeks has been the standard first-line treatment. However, one randomized clinical trial showed patients treated with high-dose dexamethasone as a pulse had better complete response rate (platelet count ≥150 × 10^9/L) when compared to standard prednisone therapy of 1 mg/kg/d for 2 weeks. The reported dexamethasone dose for the clinical trial was 40 mg daily (or 0.6 mg/kg/d) for 4 days, with courses repeated monthly based on platelet count.
- IVIg: Recommended initial dose is 1 g/kg. If the patient does not respond to the initial dose, a higher dose may be considered.
- Anti-D: Anti-D carries a black box warning by the FDA for rare, but serious and potentially life-threatening intravascular hemolysis. Anti-D is an effective first-line therapy for Rh-positive, nonsplenectomized patients without anemia or evidence of autoimmune hemolysis and should be considered in appropriate patients.

If a more rapid increase in platelet count is required, IVIg and corticosteroids can be combined (14). For patients who are unresponsive to, or relapse after initial corticosteroid therapy, splenectomy is recommended as per the ASH guideline for ITP (14). Most recently, fewer patients are undergoing splenectomy due to risk of infection, thrombosis, and immediate postoperative complications (16). Despite the risk, the 5-year response rates of splenectomy are 60% to 70% (15–17).

In adults with ITP who do not respond to first-line therapy and/or have persistent bleeding symptoms, secondary ITP should be ruled out (14,17). Once patients are confirmed to have refractory primary ITP, management depends on the platelet count and bleeding symptoms. If a patient has platelet counts of 30 × 10^9/L or greater and is mostly asymptomatic, he or she may be observed without treatment (17). However, if a patient has platelet counts below 30 × 10^9/L and experiences bleeding symptoms or diminished health-related quality of life, treatment is recommended (17). Cuker et al. divided refractory ITP treatments into three tiers based on efficacy, safety, and quality of evidence (17). Tier 1 treatments have a relatively favorable therapeutic index and are supported by good evidence (17). Tier 2 treatments are frequently prescribed in combination with a Tier 1 or another Tier 2 drug with different mechanisms of action (e.g., using an agent that boosts platelet production in combination with a drug that interferes with platelet clearance) (17). Tier 3 treatments are characterized by low response rates and/or high toxicity (17). Therefore, Tier 3 treatments are considered only for severely refractory patients with a history of serious or life-threatening bleeding (17). If a patient is unable to maintain a hemostatic platelet count with Tier 1 treatment, the provider should encourage the patient to participate in a clinical trial (17). If there is no appropriate clinical trial available, treatments in Tier 2 or 3 should be considered (17).

The three tier-based treatment system is summarized in Table 10.9 (17).

Key Points

- Primary ITP is a diagnosis of exclusion; therefore, other causes of thrombocytopenia should be ruled out.
- Management and treatment of primary ITP differ between children and adults.

Secondary ITP
Secondary ITP is thrombocytopenia due to an underlying disorder, including autoimmune and lymphoproliferative disorders and

Table 10.9 Three Tiers of Treatment Options for Refractory Immune Thrombocytopenia

Tier 1	Low-dose corticosteroids	Outcome: Rarely sustains hemostatic platelet counts at very low maintenance doses of prednisone (≤5 mg/d) Side effects: • Long-term treatment generally well tolerated • Cumulative toxicities: Weight gain, diabetes mellitus, hypertension, decreased bone mineral density, cataract formation
	Rituximab	Outcome: • Meta-analysis (19 studies) showed 63% of patients achieved platelet count >50 × 10^9/L with median duration of response of 11 months • Long-term observational study showed response rate (platelet count >50 × 10^9/L) at 5 years was 21% for adults and 25% for children • Platelet responses are similar in splenectomized and nonsplenectomized patients • Reported dose: 375 mg/m² once per week ×4 weeks Side effects: • Infusion reaction • Serum sickness • Prolonged immune suppression (low immunoglobulin level) • Risk for viral reactivation – screen for hepatitis B before administering Outcome: **Romiplostim**
	TRAs	• Reduced bleeding and improved health-related quality of life • Randomized, placebo-controlled trial of 63 splenectomized adult patients: Overall response (platelet count ≥50 × 10^9/L at any time during the study) was 79%

(continued)

Table 10.9 Three Tiers of Treatment Options for Refractory Immune Thrombocytopenia (*continued*)

		• Given once per week as subcutaneous injection
		• Dose: start at 1 mcg/kg/wk and increase by 1 mcg/kg each week (maximum dose 10 mcg/kg/wk) until the platelet count shows ≥50 × 10⁹/L
		Eltrombopag
		• Phase 3 trial: Platelet count was ≥50 × 10⁹/L for at least 6 weeks of the last 8 weeks in 51% of splenectomized patients on eltrombopag
		• PETIT trials: 36%–40% of children on eltrombopag maintained a platelet count ≥50 × 10⁹/L
		• FDA approved for children aged 1 year and older with chronic ITP
		• Pill taken once per day
		• Reported dose: Start at 50 mg/d (or 25 mg/d for East Asian ancestry, liver impairment, or age 1–5 years) and increase (maximum 75 mg/d) until the platelet count is ≥50 × 10⁹/L
		Side effects:
		• Bone marrow reticulin observed
		• Possible rebound thrombocytopenia when TRAs are discontinued
		• Hepatotoxicity may occur with eltrombopag; monitor liver function tests for patients on eltrombopag
		Outcome:
Tier 2	VAs	**Vincristine, vinblastine**
		• Evidence drawn mostly from studies conducted in 1970s to 1980s
		• Poor durability of response
		• Not a good option for long-term remission
		Side effects:

(*continued*)

Table 10.9 Three Tiers of Treatment Options for Refractory Immune Thrombocytopenia (*continued*)

Dapsone	Outcome: • No randomized clinical trials • Based on prospective and retrospective cohort studies • Overall response rates between 40% and 75% Side effects: • Methemoglobinemia • Agranulocytosis, aplastic anemia • Hypersensitivity • Gastrointestinal complications • Hemolysis in patients with G6PD deficiency
Danazol	Outcome: • Variable response rate (10%–70% depending on the study) • Better response rate when patients are on therapy for a prolonged period • Danazol is more likely to elicit response in patients who respond well to corticosteroids Side effects • Hepatotoxicity • Virilizing effect on women
Cyclophosphamide	Used infrequently due to limited data and potential for serious long-term sequelae – malignancy and infertility

(*continued*)

Table 10.9 Three Tiers of Treatment Options for Refractory Immune Thrombocytopenia (*continued*)

	Antimetabolites	Outcome: **Azathioprine, 6-mercaptopurine** • Azathiorpine: Overall response rate of 64% in one adult study • Side effects: Myelosuppression, hepatotoxicity, pancreatitis **MMF** • Overall response rate: 50%–60% • Side effects: Headache and gastrointestinal symptoms
	Cyclosporine A	Outcome: • Response rate was 50%–60% in the largest study of 20 patients; however, the rate of discontinuation of therapy due to side effects was 30% • A study of 14 children demonstrated a response rate of approximately 30% • Requires regular monitoring of blood pressure, renal function, and drug levels Side effects: • Hypertension • Nephrotoxicity
Tier 3	• ATRA • Autologous HSCT • Colchicine • Interferon α • Plasma exchange	• Consider Tier 3 if suitable clinical trial is not available • Patients with serious bleeding who do not respond to or are ineligible for Tier 1 and Tier 2 treatment options • Low response rates and/or high toxicity

ATRA, all-trans retinoic acid; FDA, U.S. Food and Drug Administration; HSCT, hematopoietic stem cell transplant; ITP, immune thrombocytopenia; MMF, mycophenolate mofetil; TRAs, thrombopoietin receptor agonists; VAs, vinca alkaloids.

infection, to name a few. Treatment for secondary ITP involves controlling or treating the underlying condition. In this section, we discuss the common causes of secondary ITP.

Neonatal Alloimmune Thrombocytopenia

Neonatal alloimmune thrombocytopenia (NAIT) is a severe thrombocytopenia in an otherwise well-appearing newborn (18). The incidence of NAIT is 0.5 to 1/1,000 live births (18). Initial presenting symptoms include severe bruising, diffuse petechiae, intracranial hemorrhage, or death after delivery (18). Platelet counts are usually $<50 \times 10^9$/L in the newborn, while maternal platelet count is in the normal range (18). NAIT is due to placental transfer of maternal IgG antibodies against paternally inherited fetal human platelet alloantigens (HPA) (18). Thrombocytopenia usually resolves within the first 2 weeks of life (18). Testing maternal serum for HPA antibodies, as well as genotyping HPA of both parents to document HPA incompatibility are important measures for determining the risk of NAIT in future pregnancies (18). Immediate treatment for very severe thrombocytopenia (platelet count $<30 \times 10^9$/L) is platelet transfusion (18). Random donor platelet transfusion will elevate the platelet count and reduce the chance of bleeding, even though the platelet products are not compatible with maternal antibody (18). In addition, IVIg can be given to prolong the survival of the transfused platelets and lessen the overall period of thrombocytopenia (18). Moderately severe thrombocytopenia (platelet count 30×10^9–50×10^9/L) without obvious bleeding can be managed with IVIg treatment alone (18).

Autoimmune Disorders

Systemic Lupus Erythematosus (SLE)

Approximately 20% to 25% of patients with SLE develop moderate-to-severe thrombocytopenia (19). The etiology of thrombocytopenia is multifactorial and includes (19):

1. Antiplatelet glycoprotein antibodies
2. Immune complexes of diverse composition
3. Antiphospholipid antibodies (APLA)
4. Vasculitis
5. Thrombotic microangiopathy
6. Hemophagocytosis
7. Autoantibodies to the *c-Mpl* receptor (TPO receptor) and/or megakaryocytes
8. Bone marrow stromal changes

Antiphospholipid Syndrome

Approximately 25% of patients with antiphospholipid syndrome (APS) develop mild-to-moderate thrombocytopenia as non-thrombotic manifestation of APS (19).

Thyroid Disease

Individuals with hyperthyroidism usually have mild-to-moderate thrombocytopenia because platelet survival is reduced (19). However, platelet counts return to normal once patients achieve a euthyroid state (19). For individuals with hypothyroidism, mild thrombocytopenia can occur most likely due to impaired production (19). Once appropriate hormone replacement therapy is started, platelet counts return to normal (19).

Evans Syndrome

Evans syndrome presents as immune hemolytic anemia, ITP, and occasionally immune neutropenia (19). Involvement of two or three hematopoietic cell antibodies can be associated with complex immunodeficiency (19). Over 50% of children and some adults with Evans syndrome have autoimmune lymphoproliferative syndrome (ALPS) (19). ALPS is a chronic accumulation of nonmalignant lymphocytes leading to lymphadenopathy and splenomegaly (19). Laboratory evaluation of T-cell subsets shows >1% CD3+, CD4–, CD8– (double-negative) T cells (19). ITP and Evans syndrome also occur in approximately 10% to 15% of patients with common variable hypogammaglobulinemia (19). Therefore, when an individual presents with hemolytic anemia and ITP, ALPS and common variable hypogammaglobulinemia should be on the differential diagnosis as there are implications of long-term management (19).

Lymphoproliferative Disorders

ITP can also present in patients with chronic lymphocytic leukemia (CLL), CD8 T lymphocyte large granular lymphocytic leukemia (LGL), and Hodgkin disease (19).

Infection

Human Immunodeficiency Virus

Thrombocytopenia is seen throughout the different stages of HIV infection (19). In the initial stage, patients develop thrombocytopenia due to an immune component similar to primary ITP (19). As the disease progresses, the platelet count decreases due to ineffective hematopoiesis from megakaryocyte infection or marrow infiltration (19). Thrombocytopenia can also develop due to underlying opportunistic infections, malignancy, medications (i.e., interferon and antiviral agents), and less frequently, thrombotic microangiopathy (19).

Hepatitis C Virus

Hepatitis C virus (HCV) infection is also associated with ITP likely due to the following (19):

- Binding of HCV to platelets followed by development of anti-HCV antibody to the platelet membrane
- Circulating antiviral immune complexes
- Infection of megakaryocytes
- Bone marrow suppression due to HCV or interferon therapy

Posttransfusion Purpura

Posttransfusion purpura (PTP) is a rare, but dramatic cause of ITP. PTP is typically seen in individuals who received multiple transfusions and presents with hemorrhage and sudden-onset thrombocytopenia up to 7 days after blood product transfusion containing platelet antigens (19). PTP occurs in approximately 1% of Caucasians who are homozygous for the HPA1b allele on GPIIIa, resulting in development of anti-HPA1a antibodies (19). Interestingly, PTP is not seen in women who delivered child(ren) with NAIT because these women have circulating anti-HPA1a antibodies from prior exposure to paternally inherited fetal HPA1a (19). Standard therapy is IVIg to prevent bleeding (19). HPA1a-negative patients diagnosed with PTP who require transfusions should receive blood products from an HPA1a-negative donor. Alternatively, washed packed RBCs may also work as they theoretically remove HPA1a-positive platelets.

HEPARIN-INDUCED THROMBOCYTOPENIA

Introduction

Heparin-induced thrombocytopenia (HIT) is a life-threatening immune complication that occurs after exposure to unfractionated heparin (UFH) or, less commonly, to low-molecular-weight heparin (LMWH) (20). HIT occurs when platelet-activating antibodies bind to platelet factor 4 (PF4)/heparin (H) complexes, resulting in immune-mediated thrombocytopenia and a hypercoagulable state (20). Approximately 33% to 50% of HIT cases are complicated by thrombosis—venous or arterial thrombosis—which can be limb- or life-threatening (21). Early recognition of HIT is crucial to prevent these associated complications.

Unfortunately, HIT is a challenging clinical diagnosis. Hospitals are using UFH or LMWH increasingly for thromboprophylaxis in hospitalized patients, leading to overdiagnosis and treatment of HIT (20). However, HIT occurs only in <0.1% to 5% of heparin-exposed patients, and the incidence varies by drug- and/or patient-related

Table 10.10 Risk Factors Associated With Heparin-Induced Thrombocytopenia

Drug-Related Risk Factors	Patient-Related Risk Factors	Other Risk Factors
UFH: incidence of HIT is 10-fold higher compared to LMWH	HIT exceedingly rare in children	Duration of therapy: ≥6 days of therapy increases the risk of HIT
Fondaparinux: Rarely associated with HIT	HIT exceedingly rare in obstetric patients	Source of heparin: Bovine source increases the risk of HIT compared to porcine source
	Surgical patients are at greater risk of HIT compared to patients receiving heparin for medical indications	

HIT, heparin-induced thrombocytopenia; LMWH, low-molecular-weight heparin; UFH, unfractionated heparin.

risk factors (Table 10.10) (20). Furthermore, the gold standard diagnostic testing for HIT takes a long time to give a result, and HIT immunoassays, even though quick to generate results, are associated with poor specificity (20). Therefore, clinical and laboratory evaluations are required to diagnose HIT.

Clinical Presentation

Patients with HIT usually present with a decline in platelet counts and/or new thrombotic complications after exposure to UFH or LMWH (20). Platelet decline is observed 5 to 14 days after heparin exposure, but for patients who were exposed to heparin in the past 100 days, the drop in platelet count can occur within a median of 10.5 hours (20). This rapid drop in platelet count is because HIT antibodies can circulate in the body for up to 100 days after an episode of HIT (20). Sometimes thrombocytopenia is the only manifestation, which is known as isolated HIT (20). However, because thromboembolic complications occur in approximately 17% to 53% of patients who present with isolated HIT, patients should be evaluated for thrombosis with upper and lower extremity Doppler ultrasounds (20). Both venous and arterial thrombotic events occur, but the most common location is in a lower extremity vein (20).

Diagnosis

Diagnosis of HIT requires clinical assessment and laboratory evaluation (Figure 10.4) (20). The initial step is recognizing the decline in

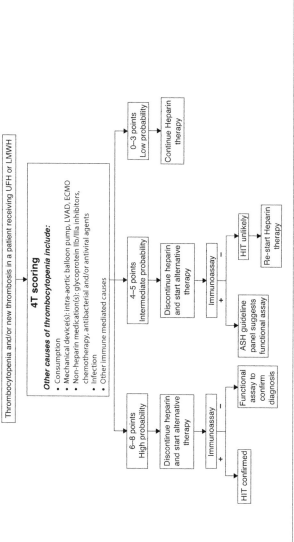

Figure 10.4 HIT diagnosis algorithms. Refer to Table 10.12 for 4T scoring.

ASH, American Society of Hematology; ECMO, extracorporeal membrane oxygenation; HIT, heparin-induced thrombocytopenia; LMWH, low-molecular-weight heparin; LVAD, left ventricular assist device; UFH, unfractionated heparin.

Source: Modified from Lee G, Arepally G. Heparin-induced thrombocytopenia. *Ash Educ Program Book.* 2013;2013(1):668–674. doi:10.1182/asheducation-2013.1.668

Table 10.11 Other Causes of Thrombocytopenia

Consumption	Infection Disseminated intravascular coagulopathy Splenomegaly/hepatomegaly Thrombotic microangiopathy
Poor bone marrow production	Aplastic anemia Malignancy Myelodysplasia
Destruction	Mechanical devices: • Intra-aortic balloon pump • LVAD • ECMO Immune mediated: • ITP • Lupus • Anti-phospholipid antibody syndrome Non-heparin medications: • Glycoprotein IIb/IIIa inhibitors • Antibacterial and antiviral agents • Chemotherapeutic agents • Nonsteroidal anti-inflammatory drugs

ECMO, extracorporeal membrane oxygenation; ITP, immune thrombocytopenia; LVAD, left ventricular assist device.

platelet count in the setting of heparin therapy. Unfortunately, some patients on heparin therapy are also critically ill and thrombocytopenia may be due to other etiologies such as infection, non-heparin medications, or mechanical devices (Table 10.11) (20). Therefore, other causes of thrombocytopenia should be evaluated. When patients present with thrombosis in rare and unusual sites—adrenal vein thrombosis, cerebral vein thrombosis, skin necrosis, and venous limb gangrene—clinicians should have a high suspicion for HIT (20).

The ASH guidelines recommend using the 4Ts scoring system (Table 10.12), which has been validated in numerous studies for excluding HIT (20,21). When the 4Ts scoring system reveals low probability (0–3 points) of HIT, no further evaluation is recommended. However, when the 4Ts scoring system reveals intermediate (4–5 points) or high (6–8 points) probability, further laboratory evaluation is recommended.

The gold standard test for HIT is the functional serotonin release assay (SRA) (21). This test uses platelets from normal donors labeled with radioactive serotonin (20). The platelets are incubated with the patient's plasma in the presence of buffer or various doses of heparin (20). If HIT antibodies are present in the patient's plasma,

Table 10.12 The 4Ts Scoring System for Diagnosis of Heparin-Induced Thrombocytopenia

4Ts	Condition	Points
Thrombocytopenia	Platelet count falls >50% and nadir ≤20,000/mm^3	2
	Platelet count falls 30% to 50% or nadir 10 to 19,000/mm^3	1
	Platelet count falls <30% or nadir <10,000/mm^3	0
Timing of platelet count fall	Between days 5 and 10 or ≤1 day if prior heparin exposure within the last 30 days	2
	Consistent with fall between 5 and 10 days but unclear, onset after day 10, or fall ≤1 day with prior heparin exposure within 30 to 100 days	1
	Platelet count falls <4 days without recent heparin exposure	0
Thrombosis or other sequelae	Confirmed new thrombosis, skin necrosis, or acute systemic reaction after IV unfractionated heparin bolus	2
	Progressive or recurrent thrombosis, non-necrotizing skin lesions, or suspected thrombosis, not proven	1
	None	0
Other causes of thrombocytopenia	None apparent	2
	Possible	1
	Definite	0

Note: Interpretation: 0 to 3 points, low probability; 4 to 5 points, intermediate probability; 6 to 8 points, high probability.

Source: From Lee G, Arepally G. Heparin-induced thrombocytopenia. *Ash Educ Program Book.* 2013;2013(1):668–674. doi:10.1182/asheducation-2013.1.668

platelets are activated and they release radioactive serotonin (20). The test has high specificity (>95%), but is not readily available and samples may have to be sent to outside performing laboratories (20). Other tests that can easily be utilized are immunoassays (Table 10.13), but they have poor specificity compared to functional assays (20,22). In certain circumstances, both the immunoassay and functional assay are utilized to assist in the diagnosis of HIT (20).

Table 10.13 Immunoassays for Heparin-Induced Thrombocytopenia Diagnosis

Antibody Specificity	Types of Immunoassay	Assay Description
Polyspecific (IgG, IgA, IgM)	ELISA, PaGIA, CLIA	• Use immobilized PF4/H complexes on microtiter plates or gel particles to identify antigen-specific antibodies in plasma or serum • Widely available • Rapid turnaround time • Sensitivity >99% • Poor specificity (30%–70%) due to their detection of nonpathogenic antibodies caused by exposure to UFH or LMWH
IgG specific	ELISA, CLIA	• Detect IgG antibodies that elicit platelet activation • Improved specificity which also means slightly lower sensitivity • Some patients with true HIT may have a negative IgG assay and need to rely on the polyspecific assay

CLIA, chemiluminescent immunoassay; ELISA, enzyme-linked immunosorbent assay; H, heparin; HIT, heparin-induced thrombocytopenia; IgA, immunoglobulin A; IgG, immunoglobulin G; IgM, Immunoglobulin M; LMWH, low-molecular-weight heparin; PaGIA, particle gel immunoassay; PF4, platelet factor 4; UFH, unfractionated heparin.

Management

If patients have a low probability 4Ts score, they do not need further testing and heparin therapy should be continued (20). For patients with an intermediate or high probability 4Ts score, heparin therapy should be discontinued and an alternative anticoagulant should be started (20). Available alternative anticoagulants include argatroban, bivalirudin, danaparoid, fondaparinux, and direct oral anticoagulants (DOACs). An alternative anticoagulant is chosen based on availability, cost, route of administration, patient's organ function (e.g., kidney function, liver function, bleeding risk), and experience of the clinician (Table 10.14) (21). However, argatroban or bivalirudin are preferred in patients with increased bleeding risk, or potential need for urgent procedures because of their shorter half-life (21). DOACs' safety and dosing for acute HIT is not well established, thus the authors recommend caution or alternative options in the acute setting of thrombocytopenia.

Table 10.14 Treatment Options for Heparin-Induced Thrombocytopenia

Drug	Mechanism of Action	Route of Administration	Elimination Route	Half-Life	Dosing	Laboratory Monitoring	Notes
Argatroban	DTI	IV	Hepatic	50 minutes	No bolus Infusion: 2 µg/kg/min Hepatic (bilirubin >1.5 mg/dL): 0.5 to 1.2 µg/kg/min	APTT 1.5 to 3× baseline	Can be used in pregnancy
Bivalirudin	DTI	IV	Enzymatic	20 to 30 minutes	No bolus Infusion: 0.15 mg/kg/hr	APTT 1.5 to 2.5× baseline	For renal or liver dysfunction, dose reduction may be necessary
Danaparoid	Indirect FXa inhibitor	IV	Renal	24 hours	Bolus: <60 kg: 1,500 U 60 to 75 kg: 2,250 U 75 to 90 kg: 3,000 U >90 kg: 3,750 U Initial infusion: 400 U/hr × 4 hours, then 300 U/hr × 4 hours Maintenance infusion: 200 U/hr Renal dysfunction: 150 U/hr	Danaparoid-specific anti-Xa activity (goal: 0.5–0.8 U/mL)	Not available in the United States Can be used in pregnancy or when breastfeeding

(continued)

Table 10.14 Treatment Options for Heparin-Induced Thrombocytopenia (*continued*)

Drug	Mechanism of Action	Route of Administration	Elimination Route	Half-Life	Dosing	Laboratory Monitoring	Notes
Fondaparinux	Indirect FXa inhibitor	SC	Renal	17 to 21 hours	<50 kg: 5 mg qdaily 50 to 100 kg: 7.5 mg qdaily >100 kg: 10 mg qdaily	None	Not approved for treatment of acute HIT Can be used in pregnancy
Apixaban	Direct FXa inhibitor	PO	Primarily hepatic	8 to 12 hours	HIT with thrombosis: 10 mg PO twice daily × 7 days, then 5 mg PO twice daily HIT without thrombosis: 5 mg PO twice daily until platelet recovery	None	Not approved for treatment of acute HIT Dosing recommendations extrapolated from VTE recommendations
Dabigatran	DTI	PO	Renal	12 to 17 hours	HIT with thrombosis: 150 mg PO twice daily after 5 days of non-heparin parenteral anticoagulation HIT without thrombosis: 150 mg twice daily until platelet recovery	None	Not approved for treatment of acute HIT Dosing recommendations extrapolated from VTE recommendations

(*continued*)

Table 10.14 Treatment Options for Heparin-Induced Thrombocytopenia (*continued*)

Drug	Mechanism of Action	Route of Administration	Elimination Route	Half-Life	Dosing	Laboratory Monitoring	Notes
Rivaroxaban	Direct FXa inhibitor	PO	Renal	5 to 9 hours	HIT with thrombosis: 15 mg twice daily ×3 weeks, then 20 mg once daily HIT without thrombosis: 15 mg twice daily until platelet recovery	None	Not approved for treatment of acute HIT Dosing recommendations extrapolated from VTE recommendations

APTT, activated partial thromboplastin time; DTI, direct thrombin inhibitor; FXa, factor Xa; HIT, heparin-induced thrombocytopenia; IV, intravenous; PO, per os; SC, subcutaneous; VTE, venous thromboembolism.

Patients with laboratory-confirmed diagnosis of isolated HIT should have a Doppler ultrasound of the upper and lower extremities to look for subclinical thrombosis because the presence of clot(s) would alter the duration of anticoagulant therapy (20). Patients should remain on an alternative anticoagulant until the platelet counts are back to baseline (20). At that point, patients can be initiated on warfarin therapy and continued on anticoagulation therapy for the following duration (20):

- For patients with isolated HIT, up to 4 weeks of anticoagulation
- For patients with thrombosis, 3 months of anticoagulation

For patients with refractory or progressive thromboses despite being on an alternative anticoagulant, plasmapheresis should be considered to reduce antibody burden (20).

Key Points
- HIT is a life-threatening complication that occurs after exposure to UFH or LMWH.
- HIT can be complicated by venous or arterial thrombosis, which can be life-threatening. Therefore, early recognition of HIT is crucial to prevent complications.

DISSEMINATED INTRAVASCULAR COAGULATION

Introduction
Disseminated intravascular coagulation (DIC) is an extreme form of coagulation activation due to an underlying process – trauma, crush injuries, central nervous system (CNS) injuries, heat stroke, burns, hemolytic transfusion reactions, cancer, cardiac arrest, fat embolism, aortic aneurysm, giant hemangiomas, infection, obstetric conditions (placental abruption, placenta previa, retained dead fetus), and so forth (23,24). In these cases, cell injury and/or death results in initiation of massive ongoing activation of coagulation, which can exhaust coagulation factors and platelets, resulting in severe bleeding complications (23,24).

Diagnosis
Diagnosis of DIC is mainly clinical, with a few available laboratory tests that can aid in the diagnosis (23–25). Classic DIC presents with prolonged PT and PTT, thrombocytopenia, and increased markers of fibrin formation and/or degradation (24). Platelet count is usually <100 × 10^9/L, and about 10% to 15% of patients with DIC have platelet counts of <50 × 10^9/L (25). These latter patients have a fourfold to fivefold higher risk of bleeding compared to patients

with higher platelet counts (24). Monitoring the platelet count is important because a recent study has shown that sustained thrombocytopenia for >4 days after ICU admission, or a drop in platelet count >50% during the ICU course, is related to a fourfold to sixfold increase in mortality (25).

Management

Because DIC occurs due to an underlying process, treatment of DIC involves treatment of the underlying condition (23,24). Supportive care is provided concurrently, which includes the following (23,24):

- Transfuse platelets in actively bleeding patients with low platelet counts.
- Transfuse fresh frozen plasma (FFP) or fibrinogen in actively bleeding patients with prolonged PT/PTT or hypofibrinogenemia.
- Consider LMWH therapy if thrombosis develops.

THROMBOTIC MICROANGIOPATHY SYNDROMES

Thrombotic thrombocytopenic purpura (TTP) and hemolytic uremic syndrome (HUS) are part of "thrombotic microangiopathy syndromes" (21). Clinical features of thrombotic microangiopathy syndrome include microangiopathic hemolytic anemia, thrombocytopenia, and organ injury (26). There are nine disorders classified under the thrombotic microangiopathy syndromes, but in this chapter, we will discuss TTP and HUS (26).

Thrombotic Thrombocytopenic Purpura
Clinical Case 10.5

A 20-year-old woman presented to the emergency department with 5 days of fever, fatigue, petechiae, and an episode of syncope. She had 5 days of rhinorrhea and congestion, which resolved prior to presentation. On the day of presentation, she felt lightheaded and lost consciousness for a few seconds at work. She was taken to the emergency department for further evaluation. The young woman was otherwise healthy and did not take any medications. Family history was unremarkable. In the emergency department, her temperature was 102°F, and laboratory evaluation revealed a hemoglobin of 5 g/dL, platelet count of 7×10^9/L, and an elevated lactate dehydrogenase (LDH); electrolytes, BUN, and creatinine were normal and urine pregnancy test was negative. Peripheral blood smear showed a significant number of schistocytes (3–5/hpf). Further evaluation revealed ADAMTS13 activity of 9% (reference range >65%) and ADAMTS-13 inhibitor of 81% (reference range <30%) consistent with TTP. The patient was transferred to the ICU and started on plasma exchange and high-dose corticosteroids.

Introduction

The classic pentad observed in TTP is thrombocytopenia, hemo-lytic anemia, fever, neurologic involvement, and renal impairment; however, these features are variably present with some found more commonly than others (27). TTP is caused by ADAMTS13 (a disintegrin and metalloprotease with thrombospondin type 1 repeats, member 13) deficiency (26,27). ADAMTS13 is respon-sible for cleaving ultra large von Willebrand factor (ULVWF), the multimeric form of VWF (26). ULVWF is typically cleaved by ADAMTS13 before being released into plasma (26,27). When ADAMTS13 activity is low or absent (as seen in TTP), ULVWF remains uncleaved, allowing platelets to bind tightly, resulting in platelet thrombi throughout the microvasculature (27). TTP can be congenital or acquired. In both cases, ADAMTS13 activity level is <10%; acquired TTP is caused by an autoantibody inhibitor to ADAMTS13 (26,27).

Clinical Presentation

Patients with congenital TTP present from birth to adulthood with recurrent episodes of microangiopathic hemolytic anemia and thrombocytopenia (26). Patients sometimes exhibit neurologic abnormalities or other signs of organ injury (26). In acquired TTP, patients present with GI symptoms, weakness, purpura, and/or transient focal neurologic abnormalities usually in the late teen years or after (26). Approximately one third of patients have no neurologic abnormalities (26). TTP rarely cause severe acute kidney injury (26).

Diagnosis

Providers should have a high suspicion for TTP in patients with ane-mia and thrombocytopenia with or without neurologic symptoms as TTP has a high mortality. Peripheral blood smear demonstrates schistocytes and red cell fragmentation (27). ADAMTS13 activity level is usually <10% for both congenital and acquired TTP (26,27). For patients with acquired TTP, an ADAMTS13 inhibitor is detected (Figure 10.5) (26,27). Congenital TTP diagnosis is confirmed with ADAMTS13 mutations (27).

Management

Treatment and management for congenital TTP and acquired TTP are different. Because TTP results in platelet-rich thrombi in micro-circulation, platelet transfusion is generally avoided (27). However, platelet transfusion can be considered in patients with overt bleed-ing and also during invasive procedures in patients with severe thrombocytopenia (27).

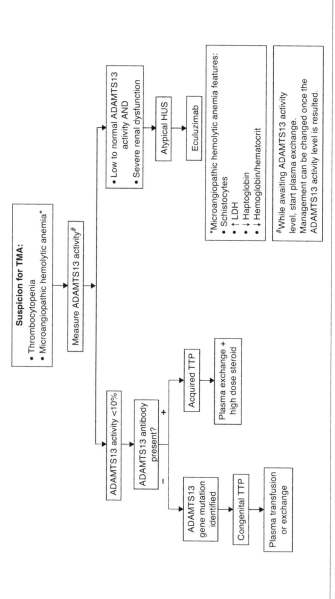

Figure 10.5 Management of TTP and atypical HUS.

+, Present; –, not present; HUS, hemolytic uremic syndrome; TMA, thrombotic microangiopathy; TTP, thrombotic thrombocytopenic purpura.

Congenital TTP

Patients with congenital TTP have mutations in *ADAMTS13* gene, resulting in the inability to make functional ADAMTS13 protein (27). Thus, treatment with plasma infusion is just as effective as plasma exchange to treat acute TTP (27). These patients should receive prophylactic plasma infusion every 2 weeks to prevent acute episodes (27). Other novel therapies are being investigated to treat congenital TTP; one therapy that shows promise is recombinant ADAMTS13 (rADAMTS13) (28). Clinical trials using rADAMTS13 in the treatment of congenital TTP are currently underway (28).

Acquired TTP

In acquired TTP, treatment is focused on removal of the antibodies directed against ADAMTS13, which is achieved by using a combination of therapeutic plasma exchange (TPE) and high-dose steroids (27,28). Other immunosuppressive therapies, such as vincristine, cyclophosphamide, cyclosporine, rituximab, or bortezomib, may be prescribed as an adjuvant therapy to eliminate antibody formation and sustain a long-term remission (27). Rituximab is gaining attention as a potential adjuvant therapy for acquired TTP (28). A phase 2 multicenter, non-randomized trial in the UK comparing standard therapy (plasma exchange and steroids) versus standard therapy with rituximab showed that patients treated with standard therapy with rituximab had reduction in the number of plasma exchanges required to achieve remission, reduction in overall inpatient stay, and reduction in relapse rates (28). The French TMA Reference Center Network and the Oklahoma TTP registry showed fewer and later relapses when rituximab was used as an adjuvant therapy (28). However, up to 50% of acquired TTP cases recover with standard therapy alone and adding rituximab may expose patients to overtreatment (28). Therefore, use of rituximab as part of upfront therapy is still debated and requires further study to determine if it improves outcome. At this time, rituximab is recommended for refractory TTP treatment (28).

Once patients are treated and have recovered from acquired TTP, they need close monitoring because approximately 40% of patients experience two or more relapses (28).

Hemolytic Uremic Syndrome

The classical presenting triad of HUS is hemolytic anemia, thrombocytopenia, and acute kidney injury (AKI) (23,26). HUS can be caused by infection (90% of the HUS cases) or by complement dysregulation (atypical HUS) (23,26). Because initial presenting symptoms are similar to TTP, it is important to measure ADAMTS13 activity and inhibitor to exclude TTP from the differential diagnosis (27).

Infection-Induced HUS

Approximately 85% of infection-induced HUS cases are caused by Shiga toxin-producing *Escherichia coli* (STEC) and several other bacteria, including *Streptococcus pneumonia* (23). For STEC-HUS, severe abdominal pain and diarrhea (often bloody) begin after consuming contaminated food (26). Thrombocytopenia and renal failure begin as the GI symptoms improve (26). Currently, TPE is not recommended and therapy remains supportive with aggressive hydration (23,26).

Atypical HUS

Atypical HUS cases (approximately 10% of HUS cases) are due to a complement pathway genetic mutation (23,26). Individuals present with an elevated serum creatinine level, microangiopathic hemolytic anemia, thrombocytopenia, ADAMTS13 activity >10%, and negative stool tests for Shiga toxin producing infection (26,27). Complement levels should be obtained, but normal plasma levels of complement C3, C4, factor H, factor B, and factor I do not exclude the diagnosis of atypical HUS (26). Recommended therapy is eculizumab—a monoclonal complement C5 inhibitor—and data suggest that rapid initiation of eculizumab is associated with greater improvements in renal function (27). Another therapy option is TPE (23,27). Usually, TPE is initiated due to difficulty differentiating atypical HUS from TTP at the time of presentation. However, as soon as atypical HUS is diagnosed, eculizumab should be initiated (27).

There are other complement pathway inhibitors in development. These inhibitors are being studied to improve management of paroxysmal nocturnal hemoglobinuria (PNH) and should potentially be utilized in the management of HUS. These new complement pathway inhibitors are organized in Table 10.15 (29).

Key Points

- TTP and HUS are part of the thrombotic microangiopathy syndromes (TMA).
- TTP is caused by ADAMTS13 deficiency, while HUS can be caused by infection or by complement dysregulation.
- Because initial presenting symptoms are similar between TTP and HUS, it is important to test for ADAMTS13 activity and inhibitors on initial evaluation.

ACQUIRED PLATELET DISORDERS

Medication

Medication can cause acquired platelet disorders by affecting the platelet function or by thrombocytopenia. NSAIDs and aspirin are

Table 10.15 Novel Complement Inhibitors in Development

Agent Name	Target	Agent Information
ALXN1210	C5	• Anti-C5 monoclonal antibody • IV injection • Phase 1 study in healthy volunteers: Showed immediate, complete, and sustained C5 inhibition • Longer half-life than eculizumab • Phase 1/2 trials on untreated PNH patients: No serious adverse events leading to withdrawal documented. Demonstrated sustained reduction in hemolysis • Phase 3 trials are ongoing
Coversin	C5	• Prevents C5 cleavage by its convertases • Subcutaneous injection • Phase 1 study in healthy volunteers: Showed good pharmacokinetics and pharmacodynamics • Phase 2 study in untreated PNH patients: Only adverse event reported was mild injection site reactions; noted residual hemolysis, but no red cell transfusion needed during the study period
Compstatin (AMY-101)	C3 and C3b	• Disulfide peptide which binds to C3 and C3b, preventing C3 cleavage and C3b incorporation in C3/C5 convertase • Phase 1 study in healthy volunteer completed and waiting for data presentation

Source: From Risitano A, Marotta S. Toward complement inhibition 2.0: next generation anticomplement agents for paroxysmal nocturnal hemoglobinuria. *Am J Hematol.* 2018;93(4):564–577. doi:10.1002/ajh.25016

well known to inhibit platelet function and are used to treat or prevent thrombosis (1). However, NSAIDs or aspirin is not recommended if an individual has a high risk for bleeding. Medications can induce thrombocytopenia by either bone marrow toxicity or immune-mediated platelet destruction (19). Quinine was the first reported case of drug-induced thrombocytopenia, and currently there are several hundred medications that cause thrombocytopenia (19). Providers should suspect medication-induced thrombocytopenia when other causes of thrombocytopenia have been excluded, thrombocytopenia develops after initiation of the new drug, thrombocytopenia improves after discontinuing the drug, and re-exposure to the drug results in recurrent thrombocytopenia (19).

Renal Failure

Platelet abnormalities are reported in renal failure, presenting as thrombocytopenia and/or platelet dysfunction (30). Thrombocytopenia is a common finding in uremic patients, with overconsumption or inadequate production as proposed etiologies (30). Platelet counts are rarely <80 × 10^9/L (30). Platelet dysfunction can result in bleeding or thrombotic tendencies (30). Patients with chronic renal failure have prolonged bleeding due to abnormalities of platelet alpha-granules (reduction in ADP and serotonin), likely contributing to a platelet activation defect (30). Patients with chronic renal failure have normal binding of VWF to GPIb surface receptors on platelets, but have a decrease in the total content of platelet GPIb (30). GPIIb/IIIa surface receptors on platelets, responsible for binding fibrinogen and VWF, are also defective (30). Platelet dysfunction is due to several dialyzable uremic toxins such as urea, creatinine, phenol, or phenolic acids (30). Therefore, dialysis improves platelet abnormalities and reduces the risk of bleeding. Chronic renal failure can cause thrombotic complications, most commonly thrombosis of vascular access (30). The etiology of thrombosis includes increased levels of fibrinogen, factor VIII, and VWF, decreased protein C and protein S, impaired fibrinolysis, increased plasma lipoprotein(a), and the presence of lupus anticoagulant (30).

Cardiopulmonary Bypass, Extracorporeal Membrane Oxygenation

Cardiopulmonary bypass (CPB) and extracorporeal membrane oxygenation (ECMO) result in thrombocytopenia and platelet dysfunction (1). Platelet dysfunction is thought to be due to lack of availability of platelet agonists and to the use of anticoagulants during CPB and ECMO (1).

Key Point

Platelet dysfunction can be acquired secondary to medication or organ dysfunction such as renal failure. Therefore, obtaining a thorough history is important.

REFERENCES

1. Krishnegowda M, Rajashekaraiah V. Platelet disorders: an overview. *Blood Coagulation Fibrinolysis*. 2015;26(5):479. doi:10.1097/01.mbc.0000469521.23628.2d
2. Lambert M. What to do when you suspect an inherited platelet disorder. *Ash Educ Program Book*. 2011;2011(1):377–383. doi:10.1182/asheducation-2011.1.377

3. Candotti F. Clinical manifestations and pathophysiological mechanisms of the Wiskott-Aldrich syndrome. *J Clin Immunol.* 2018;38(1):13–27. doi:10.1007/s10875-017-0453-z

4. Balduini C, Pecci A, Savoia A. Recent advances in the understanding and management of MYH9-related inherited thrombocytopenias. *Brit J Haematol.* 2011;154(2):161–174. doi:10.1111/j.1365-2141.2011.08716.x

5. Chou ST, Kacena MA, Weiss MJ, et al. GATA1-related X-linked cytopenia. In: Adam MP, Ardinger HH, Pagon RA, et al., eds. *GeneReviews® [Internet].* Seattle, WA: University of Washington, Seattle; 1993–2018. https://www.ncbi.nlm.nih.gov/books/NBK1364

6. Pham A, Wang J. Bernard-Soulier syndrome: an inherited platelet disorder. *Arch Pathol Lab Med.* 2007;131(12):1834–1836.

7. Carubbi C, Masselli E, Nouvenne A, et al. Laboratory diagnostics of inherited platelet disorders. *Clin Chem Lab Med.* 2014;52(8):1091–1106. doi:10.1515/cclm-2014-0131

8. Othman M. Platelet-type Von Willebrand disease: three decades in the life of a rare bleeding disorder. *Blood Rev.* 2011;25(4):147–153. doi:10.1016/j.blre.2011.03.003

9. Geddis AE. Congenital amegakaryocytic thrombocytopenia and thrombocytopenia with absent radii. *Hematol Oncol Clin North Am.* 2009;23(2):321–331. doi:10.1016/j.hoc.2009.01.012

10. Thompson A, Woodruff K, Feig S, et al. Congenital thrombocytopenia and radio-ulnar synostosis: a new familial syndrome. *Brit J Haematol.* 2001;113(4):866–870. doi:10.1046/j.1365-2141.2001.02834.x

11. Kaplan J, Domenico I, Ward D. Chediak-Higashi syndrome. *Curr Opin Hematol.* 2008;15(1):22. doi:10.1097/MOH.0b013e3282f2bcce

12. El-Chemaly S, Young L. Hermansky-Pudlak syndrome. *Clin Chest Med.* 2016;37(3):505–511. doi:10.1016/j.ccm.2016.04.012

13. Poon M-C, Minno G, d' Oiron R, Zotz R. New insights into the treatment of Glanzmann thrombasthenia. *Transfus Med Rev.* 2016;30(2):92–99. doi:10.1016/j.tmrv.2016.01.001

14. Neunert C, Lim W, Crowther M, et al. The American Society of Hematology 2011 evidence-based practice guideline for immune thrombocytopenia. *Blood.* 2011;117(16):4190–4207. doi:10.1182/blood-2010-08-302984

15. Journeycake JM. Childhood immune thrombocytopenia: role of rituximab, recombinant thrombopoietin, and other new therapeutics. *Hematology Am Soc Hematol Educ Program.* 2012;2012:444–449.

16. Lambert M, Gernsheimer T. Clinical updates in adult immune thrombocytopenia. *Blood.* 2017;129(21):2829–2835. doi:10.1182/blood-2017-03-754119

17. Cuker N. How I treat refractory immune thrombocytopenia. *Blood*. 2016;128(12):1547–1554. doi:10.1182/blood-2016-03-603 365

18. Peterson J, McFarland J, Curtis B, Aster R. Neonatal alloimmune thrombocytopenia: pathogenesis, diagnosis and management. *Brit J Haematol*. 2013;161(1):3–14. doi:10.1111/bjh.12235

19. Cines D, Liebman H, Stasi R. Pathobiology of secondary immune thrombocytopenia. *Semin Hematol*. 2009;46(1 Suppl 2):S2–S14. doi:10.1053/j.seminhematol.2008.12.005

20. Lee G, Arepally G. Heparin-induced thrombocytopenia. *Ash Educ Program Book*. 2013;2013(1):668–674. doi:10.1182/asheducation-2013.1.668

21. Cuker A, Arepally GM, Chong BH, et al. American Society of Hematology 2018 guidelines for management of venous thromboembolism: heparin-induced thrombocytopenia. *Blood Adv*. 2018;2(22):3360–3392. doi:10.1182/bloodadvances.2018024489

22. Nagler M, Bachmann LM, ten Cate H, ten Cate-Hoek A. Diagnostic value of immunoassays for heparin-induced thrombocytopenia: a systematic review and meta-analysis. *Blood*. 2016;127(5):546–557. doi:10.1182/blood-2015-07-661215

23. Nguyen T, Cruz M, Carcillo J. Thrombocytopenia-associated multiple organ failure and acute kidney injury. *Crit Care Clin*. 2015;31(4):661–674. doi:10.1016/j.ccc.2015.06.004

24. Levi M, Scully M. How I treat disseminated intravascular coagulation. *Blood*. 2018;131(8):845–854. doi:10.1182/blood-2017-10-804096

25. Levi M, Meijers J. DIC: Which laboratory tests are most useful. *Blood Rev*. 2011;25(1):33–37. doi:10.1016/j.blre.2010.09.002

26. George J, Nester C. Syndromes of thrombotic microangiopathy. *New Engl J Medicine*. 2014;371(7):654–666. doi:10.1056/NEJMra1312353

27. Saha M, McDaniel J, Zheng X. Thrombotic thrombocytopenic purpura: pathogenesis, diagnosis and potential novel therapeutics. *J Thromb Haemost*. 2017;15(10):1889–1900. doi:10.1111/jth.13764

28. Joly BSS, Coppo P, Veyradier A. Thrombotic thrombocytopenic purpura. *Blood*. 2017;129(21):2836–2846. doi:10.1182/blood-2016-10-709857

29. Risitano A, Marotta S. Toward complement inhibition 2.0: next generation anticomplement agents for paroxysmal nocturnal hemoglobinuria. *Am J Hematol*. 2018;93(4):564–577. doi:10.1002/ajh.25016

30. Boccardo P, Remuzzi G, Galbusera M. Platelet dysfunction in renal failure. *Semin Thromb Hemost*. 2004;30(5):579–589. doi:10.1055/s-2004-835678

11 Disorders of Coagulation

Stephanie Holdener, Samer Al-Hadidi, Young-na Lee-Kim, Iberia Romina Sosa, and Meredith Reyes

HEMOPHILIA DISORDERS

Clinical Case 11.1

A 17-year-old male presents to an urgent care clinic complaining of swelling and pain in his left knee after a fall from a bicycle. He has a history of recurrent swelling and pain in multiple joints as well as prolonged bleeding after mild trauma throughout his lifetime. Laboratory studies demonstrate platelet of 240 k/μL (reference range: 150–440 K/μL), a prothrombin time (PT) of 13.5 seconds (reference range: 11.8–15 seconds), and a partial thromboplastin time (PTT) of 48 seconds (reference range: 23.6–36.4 seconds). Fibrinogen and thrombin time are found to be normal.

Introduction

Hemophilias A and B are inherited in an X-linked recessive pattern, thereby occurring almost exclusively in males. Female carriers may experience bleeding symptoms of varying degrees, with rare cases of women with symptomatic hemophilia, as an offspring of an affected male and a female carrier or due to loss or inactivation of the normal X chromosome (1). Though hemophilias A and B are primarily inherited disorders, approximately one third of cases occur as spontaneous mutations. Hemophilia A occurs in approximately 1:5,000 live male births and hemophilia B in approximately 1:30,000 live male births.

Comprehensive mutational analysis of the factor VIII (*FVIII*) and factor IX (*FIX*) genes have identified DNA variants in 98% and 99% of cases, respectively. The most common mutation in hemophilia A is an inversion of part of the long arm of the X chromosome within intron 22 of the *FVIII* gene, which is seen in nearly half of the cases and is associated with severe deficiency. Large deletions and stop mutations are more often associated with severe disease and a predilection for inhibitor development than small deletions or missense mutations. A rare, autosomal recessive, combined deficiency of FVIII and factor V is caused by a mutation in the *LMAN1* gene, which is associated with a moderate bleeding tendency and plasma levels of 5% to 30% for both factors, respectively.

Hemophilia B can result from deletions, point mutations and, rarely, gene insertions in the *FIX* gene, thereby resulting in decreased synthesis or activation of FIX protein. The incidence of inhibitor development in hemophilia B is approximately 3%. A rare form of hemophilia B, known as hemophilia B Leyden, is caused by point mutations in the FIX promoter rather than in the coding region. In these patients, *FIX* expression increases after puberty, leading to a milder clinical phenotype by adulthood (2).

Distinguishing hemophilia from other bleeding disorders (such as von Willebrand disease [VWD] or acquired factor deficiencies), as well as the distinction between hemophilia A and B is crucial to the successful treatment of patients. Age at presentation can vary depending on disease severity and can range from easy bruising, hemarthroses, or prolonged bleeding after injury/surgery (3). Spontaneous bleeding can occur in severe cases (3).

Diagnosis

Screening for hemophilia should include routine coagulation tests (PT and PTT) as well as platelet counts. Patients with hemophilia will usually present with a prolonged PTT. In cases of very mild hemophilia, PTT may be normal. In mixing studies, where a patient's plasma is equally mixed with normal plasma, prolonged PTT corrects as the normal plasma serves as a sufficient source of FVIII or IX to produce a normal result. If a mixing study corrects and suggests factor deficiency, factor levels should be measured. In patients who have been treated with factor replacement, antibodies (inhibitors) specific for FVIII or IX may form and no correction of prolonged PTT will occur in mixing studies. If the patient has never been treated with factor replacement and the PTT fails to correct in mixing studies, an alternative diagnosis must be sought (lupus anticoagulant, heparin, or other acquired inhibitors).

Diagnosis depends on a measured factor level (VIII or IX) of <40% of normal (4). When a factor level of ≥40% is found, a diagnosis is still possible when a pathologic mutation of the *FVIII* or *FIX* gene is identified. Classification of hemophilia is based on residual or baseline factor levels (4,5):

- Severe hemophilia—factor activity <1% (<0.01 IU/mL)
- Moderate hemophilia—factor activity 1% to 5% (0.01–0.05 IU/mL)
- Mild hemophilia—factor activity >5%, but <40% (0.05–0.40 IU/mL)

Factor inhibitors are autoantibodies that form in response to treatment of patients with infused factor and are often found in patients with very low factor levels. These autoantibodies to FVIII or FIX neutralize the function of infused factor concentrates and occur in approximately 30% of patients with severe hemophilia A and 3% to 5% of patients with severe hemophilia B. It is important to distinguish the presence of autoantibody inhibitors, as their presence will change management. Bethesda assay is used to quantitate factor inhibitors and is based on the ability of the patient's plasma to inactivate the factor present in normal plasma. By definition, 1 Bethesda Unit (BU) is equivalent to the amount of inhibitor that can neutralize 50% of the factor activity. If an inhibitor is suspected, a Bethesda assay using the Nijmegen modification should be performed. To be considered relevant, inhibitors must be documented on at least two separate occasions within a 1- to-4-week period and must have a level >0.6 BU (4).

Measurement of von Willebrand activity and antigen level is important to distinguish hemophilia from VWD. Patients with VWD may present with low FVIII levels as von Willebrand factor (VWF) is the carrier protein for FVIII in plasma. Likewise, measurement of factor XI and/or XII levels may be done to distinguish from other causes of prolonged PTT. Genetic testing may also be performed to identify specific gene mutations.

Key Diagnostic Dilemma

Hemophilia A and VWD may present with similar laboratory findings as VWF is the carrier protein for FVIII in vivo. Comparison of laboratory testing in type 3 VWD and hemophilia A is presented in Table 11.1. VWF normally functions as a binding and stabilizing protein for FVIII. When VWF levels are decreased, FVIII stability is affected and FVIII levels may be decreased.

Table 11.1 Comparison of Laboratory Testing in von Willebrand Disease and Hemophilia A

	VWD, Type 3	Hemophilia A
Platelet count	Normal	Normal
PFA 100	**Abnormal**	Normal
RIPA	**Abnormal**	Normal
PT	Normal	Normal
PTT	Normal or ↑	**Increased**
Factor VIII	Decreased	Decreased
VWF:Ag	**Decreased**	Normal

PFA, platelet function assay; PT, prothrombin time; PTT, partial thromboplastin time; RIPA, ristocetin-induced platelet aggregation; VWD, von Willebrand disease; VWF:ag, von Willebrand factor:antigen.

Other intrinsic pathway factor deficiencies may present with a similar bleeding history and may be distinguished by measuring the factor levels. Factor XI deficiency, also known as hemophilia C, tends to present with heterogeneous bleeding patterns, which are often less severe than hemophilia A or B. Factor XII deficiency usually presents with a prolonged PTT with no history of bleeding.

As FVIII is an acute-phase reactant, testing of patients with mild hemophilia A may reveal a normal FVIII level if tested while the patient has concurrent illness or stress. Testing should be repeated when the patient is back to baseline health if suspicion for hemophilia is high.

FIX is reduced in newborns due to delayed synthesis of vitamin K–dependent coagulation factors. Age-specific reference ranges must be used when testing patients during the newborn period.

Inhibitors to FVIII or IX may be present as a result of treatment with factor replacement therapy in patients with very low factor levels, or they may be present as an acquired inhibitor in patients with normal FVIII levels. Age of presentation, bleeding history, and factor level that increases with dilution testing can help to distinguish these entities. Factor inhibitors will be covered in greater detail in the section, "Acquired Inhibitors."

Lupus anticoagulants will often prolong the PTT and have the appearance of a factor inhibitor when factor studies are performed. Instead of a bleeding history, these patients will have no history of bleeding or a history of thrombotic events. The Dilute Russel Viper Venom time can be helpful to distinguish the presence of a lupus anticoagulant.

Prognosis

As FVIII and FIX products have replaced blood products as the standard of care in resource-rich settings, the life expectancy of patients with hemophilia is now approaching that of the general population. Care through a Hemophilia Treatment Center has also been associated with a longer life expectancy. Patients with severe hemophilia have reported decreased quality of life related to occupational disability, repeated bleeding events, chronic hemarthroses, and treatment-related sequelae such as inhibitor development (3).

Hemophilia treatment with fresh frozen plasma in the 1960s resulted in transfusion-related infections including hepatitis C and HIV. As a result, many older patients with hemophilia suffer from chronic liver disease and HIV infection. Unfortunately, >50% of hemophilia patients in the United States had HIV infection during the period 1981 to 1984 (6,7). These patients would continue to have clinical symptoms of HIV and many would die secondary to it (7).

Management

The mainstay of treatment for hemophilia is factor replacement therapy (4,5,8,26). In general, one unit of FVIII concentrate increases FVIII activity by 2% and one unit of FIX concentrate increases FIX activity by 1%. Though product half-lives vary among age groups (i.e., longer in adults) and individuals, extended half-life factor products, in general, may allow less-frequent dosing regimens for treatment and prophylaxis (Tables 11.2, 11.3). Antifibrinolytic drugs such as aminocaproic acid (EACA) and tranexamic acid are useful adjunctive therapies, especially for mucosal bleeding. In some patients with mild or moderate hemophilia A, desmopressin (DDAVP), administered intravenously or intranasally, may increase FVIII activity.

Routine prophylaxis with factor replacement frequency depends on the patient and the factor used (Table 11.4) (8). Treatment of bleeding and perioperative management of hemophilia patients are summarized in Table 11.5 (9).

Treatment of Inhibitors in Congenital Hemophilia

Prevention and treatment of bleeding in patients with FVIII inhibitors can be achieved with higher doses of FVIII concentrates if the inhibitor titer is low (e.g., <5 BU) or may require bypass agents such as activated recombinant factor VII or activated prothrombin

Table 11.2 Different Factor VIII Products With Their Half-Lives

Factor VIII Products	Approximate Half-Life (hours)
Standard half-life products	
Advate (recombinant)	9 to 12
Hemophil M (plasma derived, monoclonal antibody purified)	15
Koate (plasma derived, chromatography purified)	16
Kogenate FS (recombinant)	11 to 15
Kovaltry (recombinant)	12 to 14
Novoeight (recombinant)	8 to 12
Nuwiq (recombinant)	12 to 17
Recombinate (recombinant)	15
Xyntha (recombinant)	8 to 11
Extended half-life products	
Adynovate (recombinant, PEGylated)	13 to 16
Afstyla (recombinant, single chain)	10 to 14
Eloctate (recombinant, Fc fusion)	13 to 20

Table 11.3 Different Factor IX Products With Their Half-Lives

Factor IX Products	Approximate Half-Life (hours)
Standard half-life products	
Alphanine SD (plasma derived, solvent/detergent treated)	18
BeneFIX (recombinant)	16 to 19
Ixinity (recombinant)	24
Mononine (plasma-derived, monoclonal antibody purified)	23
Rixubis (recombinant)	23 to 26
Extended half-life products	
Alprolix (recombinant, Fc fusion)	54 to 90
Idelvion (recombinant, albumin fusion)	104

complex concentrates (aPCCs; e.g., factor VIII inhibitor bypassing activity [FEIBA]) if the inhibitor titer is high. The long-term goal should be to eradicate the FVIII inhibitor, since it is associated with increased morbidity and mortality. This is primarily achieved by immune tolerance induction (ITI), which is based on repetitive high dosing of the factor to overwhelm the patient's immune system and reduce antibody production. There are a variety of published ITI protocols using various dosing regimens and factor products (e.g., recombinant, plasma-derived, VWF-containing products) (10).

Table 11.4 Routine Prophylaxis to Prevent or Reduce the Frequency of Bleeding Episodes

Type of factor replacement	Infusion guidelines
Factor VIII concentrate (standard half-life)	20 to 40 units/kg IV push two to four times per week
Extended half-life factor VIII concentrates	30 to 50 units/kg IV push twice weekly to every 5 days; check specific product information for dosing recommendations
Factor IX concentrate (standard half-life)	15 to 30 units/kg IV push twice weekly or 25 to 40 units/kg twice weekly or 40 to 100 units/kg administered two to three times weekly
Extended half-life factor IX concentrates	50 units/kg once weekly or 100 units/kg once every 10 days; check specific product information for dosing recommendations

IV, intravenous.

Table 11.5 Treatment of Bleeding and Perioperative Management of Hemophilia

Type of Bleeding/ Surgery	Factor VIII Concentrate (~50% Longer for EHL Products)	Factor IX Concentrate (Up to 4x Longer for EHL Products)	Bypass Agent for Inhibitors: Recombinant Activated Factor VII (Novoseven®)	Bypass Agent for Inhibitors: Activated Prothrombin Complex Concentrate (FEIBA®)
Severe bleeding (e.g., joint, muscle, CNS) or major surgery	50 units/kg q 8 to 12h	100 to 140 units/kg q 12 to 24h	90 mcg/kg q 2 to 4 h OR 270 mcg/kg as the initial dose	100 units/ kg q 6 to 12h (max 200 units/kg/d)
Minor bleeding or minor surgery	35 units/kg q 8 to 12h	40 to 70 units/kg q12 to 24h	90 mcg/kg q 2 to 4 h	50 to 100 units/kg q 6 to 12h (max 200 units/ kg/d)

EHL, extended half-life; FEIBA, factor VIII inhibitor bypassing activity.

In general, ITI has a higher likelihood of success if the inhibitor titer at the start of ITI is <10 BU; therefore, the initial goal should be to remove all exposure to exogenous FVIII until the inhibitor level declines to <10 BU. Once this is achieved, an ITI regimen should be started. One example of an ITI protocol is a high-dose regimen of 100 units/kg/d using the product that the patient had been receiving when the inhibitor developed.

Immunosuppression (e.g., rituximab) is included in some ITI protocols or can be given if the patient fails to respond to ITI. The overall success rate for ITI in hemophilia A with inhibitors is approximately 70%. For hemophilia B patients with inhibitors, ITI is successful in only 30% of cases and may be associated with anaphylaxis to FIX infusions and the development of nephrotic syndrome.

Future Directions/Clinical Trials

In addition to improvements in factor replacement products (e.g., extended half-life, decreased immunogenicity, subcutaneous administration), there are new treatment strategies in various stages of development for hemophilia, including gene therapy, cellular therapy, monoclonal antibody against tissue factor pathway inhibitor (TFPI), and gene silencing of anticoagulant proteins. These novel agents, by mimicking instead of replacing the deficient factor, do not lead to inhibitor development against the factor. Emicizumab, a recently approved humanized recombinant bispecific (anti- FIXa/FX) IgG4 antibody that restores the missing cofactor activity of activated FVIII, is an appealing option for hemophilia patients with or without inhibitors (11). Fitusiran RNA reduces antithrombin (AT) expression by interference (RNAi) therapy. Concizumab is a monoclonal antibody targeted at anticoagulant TFPI. Gene therapy using adeno-associated virus 8 and lentiviral vectors has shown initial success in increasing coagulation factor levels to varying degrees for both hemophilia A and B patients.

Key Points

- Hemophilia A and B are X-linked recessive diseases that present at various ages, and the extent of clinical presentation is dependent on disease severity, which is defined by factor activity levels.
- Hemophilia A is a deficiency of FVIII, while hemophilia B is a deficiency of FIX.
- Disease severity is classified by factor activity level, with severe disease defined as <1% of normal, moderate as 1% to 5%, and mild as >5% of normal.
- Hemophilia may present as spontaneous bleeding if severe disease is present. Common sites of bleeding include intracranial hemorrhage, joints and soft tissues, and oral mucosa.
- Hemophilia A must be distinguished from VWD by testing of VWF antigen levels.
- Patients with severe hemophilia A or B may develop inhibitors to factors VIII or IX after factor replacement therapy.

VON WILLEBRAND DISEASE

Clinical Case 11.2

A 69-year-old male with a recent upper respiratory tract infection (URTI) presents with recurrent nosebleeds.

Labs:

PT	PTT	TT	Fibrinogen	VWF antigen	FVIII activity
13.7 sec	27 sec	19 sec	524 mg/dL	203%	251%

PT: normal 11 to 15.5 sec, PTT: normal 22 to 35 sec, TT: 14 to 25 sec, fibrinogen: normal 150 to 450 mg/dL, VWF antigen: normal 50% to 150%, FVIII activity: normal 50% to 150%.

Interpretation: PT, PTT, and TT are within normal limits. The fibrinogen is elevated. The next appropriate tests would be VWF antigen and FVIII activity. The VWF antigen and FVIII activity are both elevated, which may be seen in an acute-phase response (e.g., infectious illnesses, autoimmune diseases, exercise, stress, pregnancy). This patient had a recent URTI explaining why the VWF antigen and FVIII are elevated. Retesting when the patient is no longer in acute phase is recommended if clinical concern persists.

Clinical Case 11.3

A 63-year-old male with spinal stenosis presents for elective decompressive laminectomy.

Labs:

PT	PTT	TT	Fibrinogen	VWF antigen	FVIII activity	VWF function (RCoF)
15.3 sec	38.8 sec	13.8 sec	205 mg/dL	42%	46%	48%

VWF Multimers:

High-molecular-weight multimers	Present
Intermediate-molecular-weight multimers	Present
Low-molecular-weight multimers	Present

Interpretation: The PTT is prolonged, while the PT, TT, and fibrinogen are normal. Initial workup should include a mixing study to determine if there is a factor deficiency or factor inhibitor. The mixing study in this case would correct indicating a possible factor deficiency. The more common factor deficiencies contributing to a prolonged PTT should be tested, including factors VIII, IX, and XI activities. A VWD panel should be included in the prolonged PTT workup after the mixing study proves an inhibitor is not present. In this case, the VWF antigen, RCoF, and FVIII activity are decreased and VWF multimers are all present. Since the VWF antigen falls between 30% and 50%, VWD cannot be diagnosed in this case. However, this patient may have a slightly increased bleeding risk given the decreased levels.

Clinical Case 11.4

An 8-year-old female presents with gum bleeding after brushing teeth.

Labs:

PT	PTT	TT	Fibrinogen	VWF antigen	FVIII activity	VWF function (RCoF)
12.5 sec	47 sec	19 sec	277 mg/dL	9%	10%	4%

RCoF: normal 50% to 150%.

VWF Multimers:

High-molecular-weight multimers	Decreased
Intermediate-molecular-weight multimers	Decreased
Low-molecular-weight multimers	Decreased

Interpretation: The PTT is prolonged with normal PT, TT, and fibrinogen. As in the previous case, a mixing study would correct indicating a factor deficiency. Given the presentation, PTT-derived factor activity levels (i.e., VIII, IX, XI) and a VWD panel will be the most helpful. The VWF antigen activity is well below 30% at 9% with a corresponding borderline low FVIII activity of 10%. Follow-up multimer analysis shows decreased multimers of all sizes. These results fit most with a type 1 VWD.

Clinical Case 11.5

A 17-year-old male presents for a preoperative visit for tonsillectomy.

Labs:

PT	PTT	TT	Fibrinogen	VWF antigen	FVIII activity	VWF function (RCoF)
13 sec	38 sec	17 sec	271 mg/dL	29%	27%	8%

VWF Multimers:

High-molecular-weight multimers	Absent
Intermediate-molecular-weight multimers	Absent
Low-molecular-weight multimers	Abnormal bands

Interpretation: The PTT is slightly prolonged with a normal PT, TT, and fibrinogen. The VWD panel shows decreased VWF antigen, FVIII activity, and low VWF function. The RCoF to VWF antigen ratio (RCoF:VWF antigen) is approximately 0.3 suggestive of a type 2 VWD, primarily type 2A. Multimer analysis should be performed in this case and would show absent intermediate- and

high-molecular-weight multimers with abnormal low-molecular
-weight multimers. This pattern correlates well with type 2A VWD.

Clinical Case 11.6

A 23-year-old presents to hematology clinic with a history of menorrhagia and a family history of nosebleeds.

Labs:

PT	PTT	TT	Fibrinogen	VWF antigen	FVIII activity	VWF function (RCoF)
12.6 sec	32 sec	20 sec	398 mg/dL	90%	56%	39%

VWF Multimers:

High-molecular-weight multimers	Absent
Intermediate-molecular-weight multimers	Present
Low-molecular-weight multimers	Present

Interpretation: This patient has a normal PT, PTT, TT, and fibrinogen. Since the patient has a significant personal and family bleeding history, VWD should be considered. The VWF antigen is within normal limits; however, the FVIII activity and VWF function are both decreased. A multimer analysis demonstrates absent high-molecular-weight multimers, which is highly suggestive of type 2B VWD. A RIPA assay is recommended in this case to confirm. RIPA will be increased in type 2B VWD. Of note, the complete blood count may also show thrombocytopenia.

Introduction

VWD is the most common bleeding disorder and is caused by a quantitative or qualitative deficiency of VWF. VWF has two major roles in hemostasis. First, it mediates platelet adhesion to injured endothelium via glycoprotein Ib (GPIb), the first step in the formation of the platelet plug. Second, it binds and protects FVIII, a labile coagulation factor used to form the fibrin clot. VWF is produced and secreted into the plasma by endothelial cells and is also present in platelets. The protein subunits are cross-linked to form multimers, which range in size from dimers to 100 subunits. Shear stress or exposure to extracellular matrix components (i.e., collagen, prostacyclin) induces a conformational change, similar to a ball of yarn unraveling, in the multimers, exposing the GPIb binding site, and the platelets bind to this receptor, eventually leading to a clot. The VWF is cleaved by **a d**isintegrin **a**nd **m**etalloprotease with **t**hrombo**s**pondin-1-like domains (ADAMTS13). Deficiencies in

ADAMTS13 impair the breakdown of VWF and may lead to thrombotic thrombocytopenic purpura (TTP), which is discussed in further detail in Chapter 10, Platelet Disorders (12,13).

The most common presentations of VWD are bleeding after dental extractions, easy bruising, and epistaxis; however, patients may also present with menorrhagia, bleeding after trauma or surgery, gingival bleeding, and postpartum bleeding. VWD can present at any age, and incidence varies immensely ranging from 1.3 per 100 persons to one per 33,000 persons (12,13).

There are three types of VWD. Type 1 is the most common causing a mild-to-moderate bleeding disorder. It is characterized by a partial quantitative deficiency with normal functioning multimers.

Type 2 VWD is often mild to moderate, but can be severe. It is characterized by functional or qualitative deficiencies and often has reduced quantity as well. There are four subdivisions of Type 2. Types 2A and 2B are characterized by a loss of high-molecular-weight multimers, reducing overall function. Type 2A is caused by a mutation leading to defective production and secretion of VWF. Type 2B is a consequence of mutations in the *VWF* gene that lead to increased binding of VWF to the GPIb platelet receptor, yielding increased clearance of high-molecular-weight multimers and platelets. Type 2B similarly presents like platelet-type (pseudo-VWD); however, the mutation is in the *GPIb* gene of the platelet. Type 2M has an essentially normal multimer analysis with a qualitative impairment of the binding ability to the GPIb platelet receptor due to a mutation in the *VWF* gene. Type 2N mutations lead to impairment of the FVIII binding ability of VWF; hence, the VWF antigen levels and multimer analysis are normal. Type 2N is a frequent mimicker of hemophilia A (12,13).

Type 3 VWD is rare and characterized by a quantitative deficiency in VWF, which is often undetectable, leading to a severe bleeding disorder.

Acquired VWD (aVWD) usually presents later in life without a personal or family history of bleeding. It can be associated with a variety of causes including hematopoietic malignancies (i.e., lymphomas, myeloproliferative disorders [MPD], leukemias, plasma cell dyscrasias), Wilms' tumor, autoimmune disorders, hypothyroidism, vascular malformations (i.e., gastrointestinal [GI] telangiectasias or angiodysplasia), physical heart conditions (i.e., valvular disease, hypertrophic obstructive cardiomyopathy, ventricular septal defect, and left ventricular assist device), and drugs (i.e., valproic acid, fluoroquinolones or hetastarch). The mechanism for aVWD is diverse. In MPD, the proposed mechanism is proteolysis of VWF or adsorption of VWF onto platelets. In autoimmune disease, it is likely autoantibody production. Cardiovascular disease associated with high sheer stress leads to loss of high-molecular-weight VWF multimers. Drugs may lead to reduced synthesis of VWF (valproic acid) or accelerated proteolysis (ciprofloxacin). The mechanism of VWD in Wilms' is not well understood, but levels of VWF are known to improve after the initiation of chemotherapy (12,13). Another important consideration is thrombocytosis secondary to acute-phase reactions (12,13).

Diagnosis

An appropriate initial evaluation for VWD should include VWF antigen levels, VWF function, and FVIII levels. PT and PTT should also be included to help rule out other coagulation disorders. The ristocetin cofactor (RCoF) assay is often used to measure VWF function by testing the ability of the patient's VWF to bind and agglutinate *normal* platelets. FVIII is often decreased when VWF is decreased, since VWF acts as a carrier protein. VWF antigen levels <30 IU/dL define diagnosis of VWD. Levels of 30 to 50 IU/dL are associated with an increased bleeding risk (12–14).

Type 1 VWD has decreased VWF antigen levels and RCoF, producing a RCoF:VWF antigen ratio of 1. Type 2A VWD lacks higher functioning intermediate- and high-molecular weight multimers; therefore, the RCoF assay is disproportionately lower than the VWF antigen levels, resulting in a low RCoF:VWF antigen ratio (approximately 0.3). Type 2B VWD has a slightly higher RCoF given the presence of intermediate-weight molecular multimers, resulting in an RCoF:VWF antigen ratio of approximately 0.6. Type 2N VWD solely shows low FVIII levels (12–14).

When the aforementioned tests are suggestive of a type 2 or type 3 VWD, VWF multimer analysis is used as a confirmatory test. Multimer analysis purely demonstrates the quantity of each multimer, but does not provide any qualitative information. As previously mentioned, type 2A has only low-molecular-weight multimers, while type 2B has low- and intermediate-molecular-weight multimers. Multimer analysis is normal in types 2M and 2N as the defect is a qualitative one. Type 3 VWD shows complete absence of multimers of all sizes (12–14).

If the multimer analysis is suggestive of type 2B, ristocetin-induced platelet aggregation (RIPA) should be performed to confirm type 2B VWD or platelet-type VWD. Similar to RCoF assay, RIPA tests the ability of the patient's VWF to bind and agglutinate the *patient's* platelets at differing concentrations of ristocetin. Type 2B VWD and platelet-type VWD both show increased RIPA at lower ristocetin concentrations (12–14). Table 11.6 summarizes the differences between different types of VWD (27). Figure 11.1 represents the approach to a patient with history of bleeding.

Table 11.6 Different Types of von Willebrand Disease and Interpretation

	Inheritance	Factor VIII	VWF Antigen	Ristocetin Cofactor	RIPA	Average Ristocetin Cofactor:VWF Antigen Ratio	Multimer Analysis	Pathogenesis
Type 1	Autosomal dominant	Low	Low	Low	Low or normal	1	Normal or all sizes decreased	Decreased production
Type 2A	Autosomal dominant or autosomal recessive	Low	Low	Very low	Low	0.3	Absent large and intermediate size multimers	Defective production and secretion
Type 2B	Autosomal dominant	Low or normal	Low or normal	Very low	Increased	0.6	Absent large multimers	Increased turnover
Type 2M	Autosomal dominant or autosomal recessive	Low or normal	Low	Very low	Low or normal	<1	Normal	Impaired binding to platelets
Type 2N	Autosomal dominant	Very low	Normal	Normal	Normal	1	Normal	Defective FVIII binding
Type 3	Autosomal dominant	<10%	Undetectable	Undetectable	Very low	Both undetectable	All sizes absent	Defective production

(*continued*)

Table 11.6 Different Types of von Willebrand Disease and Interpretation (continued)

	Inheritance	Factor VIII	VWF Antigen	Ristocetin Cofactor	RIPA	Average Ristocetin Cofactor:VWF Antigen Ratio	Multimer Analysis	Pathogenesis
Platelet type	Autosomal dominant	Low or normal	Low or normal	Very low	Increased	<1	Absent large multimers	Abnormal platelet GpIb-IX with increased affinity for large VWF multimers Phenotype similar to type 2B
Acquired	No family history of VWD	Low or very low	Low or very low	Low or very low	Low or very low	≤1	Type 1 or 2 pattern	Examples of clinical conditions associated with acquired VWD—Wilms' tumor, myeloproliferative neoplasms, lymphoproliferative disorders, valve disease, drugs (valproic acid, ciprofloxacin)

FVIII, factor VIII; GPIb, glycoprotein Ib; RIPA, ristocetin-induced platelet aggregation; VWF, von Willebrand factor; VWD, von Willebrand disease.
Source: From Nichols WL, Hultin MB, James AH, et al. von Willebrand disease (VWD): evidence-based diagnosis and management guidelines, the National Heart, Lung, and Blood Institute (NHLBI) Expert Panel report (USA). *Haemophilia.* 2008;14(2):171–232. doi:10.1111/j.1365-2516.2007.01643.x

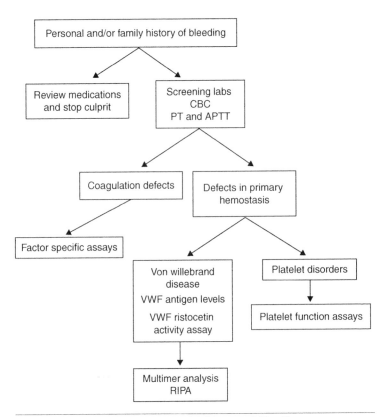

Figure 11.1 Approach to a patient with history of bleeding.

APTT, activated partial thromboplastin time; CBC, complete blood count; PT, prothrombin time; RIPA, ristocetin-induced platelet aggregation; VWF, von Willebrand factor.

Key Diagnostic Dilemma

VWD can be difficult to diagnose as the expression and penetrance are variable, especially in type 1. Workup may require a series of assays including VWF quantity, VWF function, and FVIII activity. FVIII and VWF are often elevated in an acute-phase reaction; therefore, it is important to measure another acute-phase marker such as fibrinogen. Additionally, estrogen use and pregnancy, particularly in the third trimester, can mask mild VWD due to elevations in VWF. Newborns have elevated VWF at birth, which gradually decreases to baseline in the first 6 months. Interestingly, persons with blood type O are known to have lower mean VWF levels, though the mechanism is unclear. Moreover, VWF is more susceptible to proteolysis by the ADAMTS13 metalloprotease in blood type O individuals (12–14).

Management

There are five treatment categories for VWD, which include DDAVP, replacement VWF-concentrates, antifibrinolytic drugs, topical therapy (thrombin or fibrin sealant), and estrogen therapy in women (15,16). Physicians may consider using FVIII activity, ristocetin activity, and/or PFA-100 to monitor response to therapy.

Desmopressin (DDAVP)

Type I VWD, most of type 2 VWD, and some aVWD patients respond to DDAVP, which causes indirect release of VWF from the endothelial cells. A DDAVP trial should be done at the time of diagnosis when the patient is not having an acute bleeding episode to determine effectiveness prior to needing therapy. It is performed by obtaining baseline FVIII activity and RCoF blood levels and then administering 0.3 mcg/kg of IV DDAVP in 50 mL of saline over 20 to 30 minutes. FVIII activity and RCoF are reassessed at 1, 2, and 4 hours. An effective response is an RCoF level of at least 30 IU/dL at 1 hour, with 50 IU/dL being an optimal response. DDAVP is most useful prior to minor surgeries or in minor bleeding episodes (i.e., nosebleeds, menorrhagia, tooth extractions) and can be administered intravenously, subcutaneously, or intranasally (14) (Table 11.7). Side effects include facial flushing, headache, nausea, and occasional tingling. Response is significantly reduced after repeat administrations. DDAVP should be used with extreme caution in patients with type 2B disease

Table 11.7 Desmopressin (DDAVP)

	DDAVP Administration		
Route	Intravenous	Subcutaneous*	Intranasal
Dose	Prophylaxis or acute bleeding episodes: 0.3 mcg/kg diluted in 50 mL of normal saline over 20 to 30 minutes infusion Maximum dose: 20 mcg		Prophylaxis for minor invasive procedure, minor acute bleed, or onset of menses in women: weight <50 kg: 150 mcg or one metered puff; weight >50 kg: 300 mcg or two metered puffs in separate nostrils
	May be used at 12-hour intervals for two to four doses		

*Available in Europe, but not in the United States.

Table 11.8 Replacement von Willebrand Factor Concentrate Administration

Replacement VWF-concentrate administration		
	Initial Dose	**Follow-Up Dosing**
Minor bleeding or surgery	30 to 60 ristocetin cofactor units/kg	20 to 40 ristocetin cofactor units/kg every 12 to 48 hours Goal: VWF level >30 IU/dL for 3 to 5 days
Major bleeding or surgery	40 to 60 ristocetin cofactor units/kg	20 to 40 ristocetin cofactor units/kg every 12 to 24 hours Goal: VWF level 50 to 100 IU/dL for 7 to 14 days

VWF, von Willebrand factor.

as there may be worsening of thrombocytopenia. Additionally, excessive water intake during administration may lead to hyponatremia given the diuretic properties of DDAVP (13,17).

VWF Replacement Therapies

There are several VWF/FVIII replacement therapies often utilized in more severe forms of the disease and when prolonged therapy is required to treat major bleeding or in anticipation of major surgery (Table 11.8). Though cryoprecipitate contains VWF, it is not recommended given the risk of viral transmission. The intermediate purity FVIII concentrates (i.e., Humate P, Alphanate, and Wilate) contain both VWF and FVIII and are labeled with their respective RCoF activity units. These concentrates are pasteurized or treated with solvent detergent and/or heat to reduce the risk of viral transmission (15).

Koate DVI is a hemophilia A product also containing VWF; however, it is not labeled with RCoF activity units as it contains different ratios of VWF and FVIII (13,18). LFB-VWF is a highly pure VWF-concentrate with a much higher VWF activity than FVIII (approximately 10:1) and is available in Europe. This treatment initially requires recombinant FVIII; however, subsequent doses sufficiently prolong endogenous FVIII, once these are above 20% (13,18).

Recombinant human VWF products (i.e., rVWF, Vonicog Alfa, and Vonvendi) are highly effective and they contain a range multimers including the ultra-high-molecular-weight multimers (Table 11.9). Experience is limited and more studies are needed to evaluate patients with differing severity and optimize therapy (13,18).

Table 11.9 Recombinant Human von Willebrand Factor Administration

Recombinant Human VWF Administration		
	Initial Dose	**Follow-Up Dosing**
Minor bleeding or surgery	40 to 50 IU/kg	40 to 50 IU/kg every 8 to 24 hours as needed
Major bleeding or surgery	50 to 80 IU/kg	40 to 60 IU/kg every 8 to 24 hours to keep the VWF level at 50 to 100 IU/kg for 2 to 3 days as needed
VWF, von Willebrand factor.		

Others

The two major antifibrinolytic therapies are EACA and tranexamic acid, which work to prevent the breakdown of the fibrin plug. They are most effective in mucous membrane areas in cases of mild bleeding and work well in conjunction with other medications. EACA is administered at a dose of 25 to 50 mg/kg up to four times daily, with the maximum dose being 5 g. Tranexamic acid is given intravenously up to three times daily at a dose of 10 mg/kg (18,19).

Topical agents such as Gelfoam or Surgicel are soaked in topical thrombin and provide relief for localized bleeding (i.e., nosebleeds or oral bleeding). Human thrombin is typically used; however, bovine thrombin may be substituted despite the risk of antibody formation against the bovine factor V which may cross-react with the patient's factor V leading to an increased bleeding risk (18).

Estrogen therapy partially increases the synthesis of VWF and has been shown to improve bleeding in women with type 1 VWD (17,20).

Recombinant factor VIIa is useful in patients with type 3 VWD who have developed alloantibodies to VWF after replacement therapy. Factor VIIa bypasses the intrinsic pathway and binds to activated platelets initiating the extrinsic pathway. Caution should be used in patients with coronary artery disease as these patients are at increased risk of thrombosis (13,18).

Special Circumstances

Delivery and Postpartum

Women presenting for delivery should have VWF and FVIII levels monitored. If available, the type of VWD, history of bleeding episodes, VWF and FVIII activity, and prior therapy response should be elicited. VWF levels should be maintained at 50 IU/dL or higher during delivery and for 3 to 5 days after. Women who are known to have responded to DDAVP in the past may be given a dose after labor has begun and another as close to delivery as possible (18).

Postpartum women may require intermittent DDAVP or VWF replacement therapy over the next 2 to 4 weeks after delivery as the average onset of postpartum hemorrhage in women with VWD is 11 to 23 days after delivery (18).

Minor Bleeding and Minor Surgery

As mentioned in management section, the current recommendation is intravenous or intranasal DDAVP.

Major Bleeding and Major Surgery

The current recommendation is VWF-concentrate replacement therapy.

Future Directions/Clinical Trials

Improvement in diagnosis of VWD is an area of active research. A cutoff of 100 IU/dL for VWF antigen or activity on the first test resulted in >95% negative predictive value for ruling out the diagnosis in pediatric patients (21). Given that VWF and FVIII levels increase with age, a recent study indicated that 20% of studied patients with type 1 VWD had normalization of VWF:Ag with time. A consideration of repeating testing for patients with type 1 VWD 5 to 10 years after the initial lab diagnosis should be entertained (22).

Key Points

- Initial workup should include PT, PTT, VWF antigen, RCoF assay, FVIII, and fibrinogen.
- Secondary testing may include RIPA and multimer analysis.
- VWD may be masked by an acute-phase reaction, pregnancy, estrogen use, or during the newborn period.
- Persons with blood type O may have low mean VWF levels.
- Mainstay treatments include DDAVP, VWF-concentrate replacement therapies, antifibrinolytic therapy, topical therapy, estrogen in women, and recombinant factor VIIa in type 3 VWD with alloantibodies to VWF.

ACQUIRED INHIBITORS

Clinical Case 11.7

A 65-year-old male with no prior history of bleeding presents with severe lower extremity bruising and swelling after he jumped from a small curb into the street while playing baseball with his grandchildren. He reports no other trauma and has no external bleeding. Over the last day, his bilateral legs have become increasingly bruised, swollen, and "feel tight." Laboratory evaluation reveals a normal PT and an elevated PTT. Fibrinogen and thrombin time are found to be normal. A PTT mixing study is performed, which shows modest correction, but fails to correct the PTT into the normal range. Incubation of the mixing study for 2 hours shows a further prolongation of the PTT. Lupus anticoagulant testing is negative.

Introduction

Acquired coagulation inhibitors are antibodies that develop spontaneously and either inhibit clotting factor activity or increase the clearance of clotting factor. Patients clinically present with bleeding due to minor trauma or spontaneous bleeding, bruising, or soft tissue bleeding (23). Importantly, these patients lack a previous history of bleeding diathesis.

Acquired autoantibodies to FVIII are the most common, a condition called acquired hemophilia A. These autoantibodies may increase the clearance of FVIII or interfere with its function. The development of acquired FVIII autoantibodies is spontaneous and the reasons for their appearance are unclear, but the presence of certain gene polymorphisms has been associated with their inception.

The incidence of acquired FVIII inhibitors has been estimated to be approximately 1.3 to 1.5 cases per million population per year (13). Patients are usually over the age of 50 (median age of presentation is 78) and there is an equal distribution between males and females (13). One exception is the development of acquired FVIII inhibitors in younger pregnant or postpartum women. The development of inhibitors has been associated with pregnancy, malignancy, autoimmune diseases such as rheumatoid arthritis and systemic lupus erythematosus, and drug reactions. In as many as 50% of patients, no underlying disorder or cause is ever discovered (23).

Patients may present with extensive ecchymoses, large hematomas, or mucosal bleeding, which is severe and requires immediate attention. There are disorders with other rare acquired inhibitors for which the treatment approach is different (Table 11.10).

Diagnosis

Laboratory evaluation should include routine clotting assays including PT, PTT, fibrinogen, and platelet count. Patients classically have a prolonged PTT with all other values being normal. Mixing studies should be performed with 2 hours of incubation if an acquired inhibitor is suspected. Mixing studies may show correction

Table 11.10 Other Types of Acquired Inhibitors

Type	PT	PTT	Comments
Factor IX	Normal	Prolonged, does not correct with mixing	Need to exclude lupus anticoagulant
Factor XI	Normal	Prolonged, does not correct with mixing	Need to exclude lupus anticoagulant
Factor XII	Normal	Prolonged, does not correct with mixing	Need to exclude lupus anticoagulant
Factor V	Prolonged, does not correct with mixing	Prolonged, does not correct with mixing	-----
Factor II	Prolonged, does not correct with mixing	Prolonged, does not correct with mixing	Prolonged thrombin time, not corrected with mixing
Factor X	Prolonged, does not correct with mixing	Prolonged, does not correct with mixing	------
Fibrinogen	Prolonged, does not correct with mixing	Prolonged, does not correct with mixing	Prolonged thrombin time, not corrected with mixing
Factor VII	Prolonged, does not correct with mixing	Normal	Need to exclude vitamin K antagonist intake
Factor XIII	Normal	Normal	Specific assay with measurements on the patient sample and with mixing is needed to identify inhibitors

PT, prothrombin time; PTT, partial thromboplastin time.

immediately, but because the inhibitor is time dependent, the PTT will show prolongation after 2 hours of incubation (23). Heparin should be excluded by performing thrombin time. While lupus anticoagulants typically do not present with bleeding but thrombosis, a complete workup should include evaluation immunoassays for immunoglobulin G and immunoglobulin M antibodies to cardiolipin and beta-2 glycoprotein I and a functional assay for the lupus anticoagulant for exclusion of antiphospholipid antibodies. Factor assays should be performed for the intrinsic pathway factors including VIII, IX, and XI as well as von Willebrand antigen and activity tests. Factor assays for FVIII demonstrate a low level of FVIII and an "inhibitor pattern": With increasing dilution of factor testing, increased factor activity is demonstrated. This can be explained by dilution of the inhibiting factor with dilution of the sample, allowing more factor activity. Levels of factors IX, XI, and XII may also show a low-level decrease due to artifact caused by the FVIII inhibitor (13).

Once a low level of factor is demonstrated, the level of inhibitor should be evaluated. This is accomplished with the Bethesda assay where serial dilutions of patient plasma are incubated with normal pooled plasma of known factor level. Residual FVIII activity is measured and compared to known curves. One BU is defined as the amount of inhibitor that neutralizes 50% of factor activity.

Key Diagnostic Dilemmas

Acquired inhibitors in patients with normal FVIII levels must be distinguished from inhibitors that develop in congenital hemophilia patients after factor replacement therapy, although clinical history is quite different in these patient populations. Prolonged bleeding history and hemarthroses are suggestive of congenital factor deficiencies. Hemarthroses are rarely seen in cases with acquired factor inhibitors. Most patients with acquired inhibitors have no previous bleeding history and most commonly present with massive ecchymoses, muscle bleeds, GI bleeds, and retroperitoneal bleeds.

Lupus anticoagulants may also present with prolongation of PTT. These patients are easily distinguished from those with acquired factor inhibitors as patients usually have a history of thrombosis and no history of bleeding, and laboratory testing with 1:1 mixing of patient and normal plasma shows persistent prolongation of the clotting time with both immediate and 2-hour incubation. Laboratory testing with slow-acting inhibitors, such as anti-FVIII, shows correction of immediate incubation, but not 2-hour plasma incubation.

Prognosis

Spontaneous regression of the acquired inhibitor is experienced by 25% to 30% of patients (13). The relapse rate after a first complete remission has been estimated at about 20%; 70% of such relapsing patients achieve a second complete remission. Immediate survival is related to severity of bleeding and rate of control. Mortality rate from hemorrhage is reported at 9.1% and is mostly due to GI and retroperitoneal bleeds (13). Patients also suffer from a high rate of secondary infection due to immunosuppressive treatment. Neither FVIII level nor inhibitor titer is predictive of the severity of bleeding (13).

Management

Treatment strategies vary depending on the nature of the inhibitor. For those acquired inhibitors in the absence of congenital hemophilia, the goal of treatment is to control active bleeding and prevent bleeding complications. Depending on the bleeding risk, the physician may use desmopressin, FVIII concentrates, aPCCs (e.g., FEIBA), recombinant human factor VIIa, and recombinant FVIII concentrates.

While some inhibitors regress spontaneously, many require the use of immunosuppressive agents such as prednisone, cyclophosphamide, IV immunoglobulin and/or anti-CD20 (rituximab) to eradicate their presence.

Key Points

- Patients with acquired coagulation inhibitors are usually older and have no previous bleeding history.
- Fifty percent of inhibitors are idiopathic with no underlying cause.
- Patients present with ecchymoses, GI bleeding, or retroperitoneal bleeds.
- Diagnosis is dependent on the findings of prolonged PTT and prolongation of the PTT in a 1:1 mix with normal plasma after a 2-hour incubation. For anti-FVIII inhibitors, the FVIII levels are found to be low and the mixing study demonstrates an inhibitor pattern.
- Treatment for acquired inhibitors involves treatment of associated bleeding, factor replacement, bypassing agents, and immunosuppression.
- Spontaneous regression of the acquired factor inhibitor is experienced by 25% to 30% of patients.

OTHER CONGENITAL FACTOR DEFICIENCIES

Rare inherited bleeding disorders are transmitted most likely as autosomal recessive. The incidence is one to two cases per million. Though such conditions are rare, improvement in knowledge of their presentation and treatment will help in optimal patient management (24,25). Table 11.11 summarizes diagnosis and treatment of these disorders.

Table 11.11 Rare Inherited Bleeding Disorders

Type of Factor Deficiency	Most Common Clinical Features	Laboratory Findings	Comments on Treatment
I (Fibrinogen)	Umbilical cord bleeding Epistaxis First trimester abortion	Prolonged TT, PT, and PTT	May use cryoprecipitate or fibrinogen concentrate for treatment or prophylaxis
II (Prothrombin)	Subcutaneous hematoma Muscle hematoma Mucosal bleeding Hemarthrosis Menorrhagia Prolonged post-injury bleeding	Prolonged PT and PTT. Normal TT	May use PCC for treatment or prophylaxis
V	Epistaxis Mucosal bleeding Menorrhagia	Prolonged PT and PTT. Normal TT	May use plasma for treatment or prophylaxis
VII	Epistaxis Easy bruising Menorrhagia	Prolonged PT. Normal PTT and TT	Can use factor VII or PCC. Recombinant activated factor VII can be used
X	Umbilical cord bleeding Epistaxis Hemarthrosis Menorrhagia Subcutaneous hematoma Muscle hematoma	Prolonged PT and PTT. Normal TT	Can use plasma or PCC for treatment
XI	Postoperative bleeding Menorrhagia	Prolonged PTT. Normal PT and TT	Can use plasma or factor XI concentrates
XIII	Umbilical cord bleeding Subcutaneous hematoma Menorrhagia Miscarriages Intraperitoneal bleeding	Normal PT, PTT, and TT Requires specific assays	May use cryoprecipitate or PCC. Factor XIII concentrates can be used

(*continued*)

Table 11.11 Rare Inherited Bleeding Disorders (*continued*)

Type of Factor Deficiency	Most Common Clinical Features	Laboratory Findings	Comments on Treatment
Combined V and VIII	Epistaxis Post-dental extraction bleeding Menorrhagia Postpartum bleeding	Prolonged PT and PTT Normal TT	Limited data Treatment as of factor V deficiency
Vitamin K–dependent coagulation factors	Intracranial bleeding Umbilical cord bleeding Retroperitoneal bleeding May have skeletal abnormalities	Prolonged PT and PTT Normal TT	Vitamin K and PCC can be used for treatment where vitamin K is used for prophylaxis

PCC, prothrombin complex concentrate; PT, prothrombin time; PTT, partial thromboplastin time; TT, thrombin time.

REFERENCES

1. Espinós C, Lorenzo JI, Casaña P, et al. Haemophilia B in a female caused by skewed inactivation of the normal X-chromosome. *Haematologica*. 2000;85(10):1092–1095.

2. Reijnen MJ, Maasdam D, Bertina RM, Reitsma PH. Haemophilia B Leyden: the effect of mutations at position +13 on the liver-specific transcription of the factor IX gene. *Blood Coagul Fibrinolysis*. 1994;5(3):341–348.

3. Mauser Bunschoten EP, Van Houwelingen JC, Sjamsoedin Visser EJ, et al. Bleeding symptoms in carriers of hemophilia A and B. *Thromb Haemost*. 1988;59(3):349–352. doi:10.1055/s-0038-1647493

4. Blanchette VS, Key NS, Ljung LR, et al. Definitions in hemophilia: communication from the SSC of the ISTH. *J Thromb Haemost*. 2014;12(11):1935–1939. doi:10.1111/jth.12672

5. White GC, Rosendaal F, Aledort LM, et al. Definitions in hemophilia. Recommendation of the scientific subcommittee on factor VIII and factor IX of the scientific and standardization committee of the International Society on Thrombosis and Haemostasis. *Thromb Haemost*. 2001;85(3):560. doi:10.1055/s-0037-1615621

6. Evatt BL. The tragic history of AIDS in the hemophilia population, 1982-1984. *J Thromb Haemost*. 2006;4(11):2295–2301. doi:10.1111/j.1538-7836.2006.02213.x

7. Chorba TL, Holman RC, Clarke MJ, Evatt BL. Effects of HIV infection on age and cause of death for persons with hemophilia A in the United States. *Am J Hematol.* 2001;66(4):229–240. doi:10.1002/ajh.1050

8. Hay CR, Dimichele DM. The principal results of the International Immune Tolerance Study: a randomized dose comparison. *Blood.* 2012;119(6):1335–1344. doi:10.1182/blood-2011 -08-369132

9. Neufeld EJ, Solimeno L, Quon D, et al. Perioperative management of haemophilia B: A critical appraisal of the evidence and current practices. *Haemophilia.* 2017;23(6):821–831. doi:10.1111/ hae.13279

10. Dimichele D. Immune tolerance therapy for factor VIII inhibitors: moving from empiricism to an evidence-based approach. *J Thromb Haemost.* 2007;5 Suppl 1:143–150. doi:10.1111/j.1538-7836.2007.02474.x

11. Mahlangu J, Oldenburg J, Paz-priel I, et al. Emicizumab prophylaxis in patients who have Hemophilia A without inhibitors. *N Engl J Med.* 2018;379(9):811–822. doi:10.1056/NEJMoa1803550

12. Kottke-Marchant K. Algorithmic approaches to hemostasis testing. *Semin Thromb Hemost.* 2014;40(2):195–204. doi:10.1055/s-0033-1364187

13. Marder VJ. *Hemostasis and Thrombosis, Basic Principles and Clinical Practice*. Philadelphia, PA: Lippincott Williams & Wilkins; 2012.

14. Roberts JC, Flood VH. Laboratory diagnosis of von Willebrand disease. *Int J Lab Hematol.* 2015;37 Suppl 1:11–17. doi:10.1111/ ijlh.12345

15. Goudemand J, Negrier C, Ounnoughene N, Sultan Y. Clinical management of patients with von Willebrand's disease with a VHP vWF concentrate: the French experience. *Haemophilia.* 1998;4 Suppl 3:48–52. doi:10.1046/j.1365-2516.1998.0040s3048.x

16. Kouides PA, Byams VR, Philipp CS, et al. Multisite management study of menorrhagia with abnormal laboratory haemostasis: a prospective crossover study of intranasal desmopressin and oral tranexamic acid. *Br J Haematol.* 2009;145(2):212–220. doi:10.1111/j.1365-2141.2009.07610.x

17. Harrison RL, Mckee PA. Estrogen stimulates von Willebrand factor production by cultured endothelial cells. *Blood.* 1984;63(3):657–664.

18. National Heart, Lung, and Blood Institute. *The diagnosis, evaluation, and management of von Willebrand disease*. NIH Publication No. 08-5832. Bethesda, MD: Author; 2007.

19. Witmer CM, Elden L, Butler RB, et al. Incidence of bleeding complications in pediatric patients with type 1 von Willebrand disease undergoing adenotonsillar procedures. *J Pediatr*. 2009;155(1):68–72. doi:10.1016/j.jpeds.2009.01.051

20. Alperin JB. Estrogens and surgery in women with von Willebrand's disease. *Am J Med*. 1982;73(3):367–371. doi:10.1016/0002-9343(82)90729-X

21. Doshi BS, Rogers RS, Whitworth HB, et al. Utility of repeat testing in the evaluation for von Willebrand disease in pediatric patients. *Blood*. 2018;132(Suppl 1):981. doi:10.1111/jth.14591

22. Abou-ismail MY, Ogunbayo GO, Secic M, Kouides PA. Outgrowing the laboratory diagnosis of type 1 von Willebrand disease: a two decade study. *Am J Hematol*. 2018;93(2):232–237. doi:10.1002/ajh.24962

23. Franchini M, Lippi G. Acquired factor VIII inhibitors. *Blood*. 2008;112(2):250–255. doi:10.1182/blood-2008-03-143586

24. Peyvandi F, Palla R, Menegatti M, Mannucci PM. Introduction. Rare bleeding disorders: general aspects of clinical features, diagnosis, and management. *Semin Thromb Hemost*. 2009;35(4):349–355. doi:10.1055/s-0029-1225757

25. Palla R, Peyvandi F, Shapiro AD. Rare bleeding disorders: diagnosis and treatment. *Blood*. 2015;125(13):2052–2061. doi:10.1182/blood-2014-08-532820

26. Srivastava A, Brewer AK, Mauser-Bunschoten EP, et al. Guidelines for the management of hemophilia. *Haemophilia*. 2013;19(1):e1–e47. doi:10.1111/j.1365-2516.2012.02909.x

27. Nichols WL, Hultin MB, James AH, et al. von Willebrand disease (VWD): evidence-based diagnosis and management guidelines, the National Heart, Lung, and Blood Institute (NHLBI) Expert Panel report (USA). *Haemophilia*. 2008;14(2):171–232. doi:10.1111/j.1365-2516.2007.01643.x

12 Venous Thromboembolism

Robert Streck, Safiya Joseph, and
Iberia Romina Sosa

VENOUS THROMBOEMBOLISM

Clinical Case 12.1

A 26-year-old female presents to her primary care physician with complaints of tightness in her left lower extremity, accompanied by new erythema and swelling. She recently returned from a family trip to Israel where she was in the middle seat for most of the journey. Two months ago, she started a low-dose oral contraceptive pill (OCP) containing estrogen for irregular menstruation. She denies any trauma to the affected leg. She takes no other medications and has no past medical history. She does not smoke and only has an occasional alcoholic beverage. Her mother suffered a pulmonary embolus 4 weeks after the birth of her first child and was required to take prophylactic anticoagulation with subsequent pregnancies. No other family members have had clots.

Introduction

Venous thromboembolism (VTE) is diagnosed in 1.43 per 1,000 persons each year (1). It includes pulmonary embolism (PE) and deep vein thrombosis (DVT), most often of the lower extremities, although it may also occur in upper extremities and atypical sites (mesenteric, ovarian, and cerebral veins). Depending on the anatomic location, there are important differences in epidemiology, diagnosis, and treatment of VTE; hence, for the purposes of this review, we explore DVT of lower extremities, upper extremities, and PE as distinct entities.

VTE is attributed to disturbances in Virchow's triad, where alterations in blood flow, endothelial injury, and variations in blood components contribute to thrombotic events. Disturbances in Virchow's triad may be inherited or acquired. Risk factors contributing to thromboses can be identified in a majority of patients presenting with VTE, with an amalgamation of risk factors contributing to a thrombotic event. A summary of inherited and acquired risk factors is provided in Table 12.1.

Table 12.1 Risk Factors for Venous Thromboembolism

Acquired	Inherited
Major general or orthopedic surgery	Factor V Leiden mutation
Trauma	Prothrombin gene mutation
Central venous catheter	Protein S deficiency
Chemotherapy	Protein C deficiency
Congestive heart failure	Antithrombin deficiency.
Hormone replacement therapy	Plasminogen deficiency
Malignancy	Dysfibrinogenemia
Oral contraceptive therapy	Factor XII deficiency
Paralytic stroke	
Pregnancy: Antepartum and postpartum	
Previous VTE	
Acquired thrombophilia	
Extended immobility: Long distance travel or bed rest	
Obesity	
Increasing age ≥40	
Antiphospholipid antibody syndrome	
Chronic renal disease	
Nephrotic syndrome	
Inflammatory bowel disease	
Liver disease with portal hypertension	
Paroxysmal nocturnal hemoglobinuria	
Myeloproliferative neoplasms	
Heparin-induced thrombocytopenia	
Hyperhomocysteinemia	
Polycystic ovarian	
Ovarian hyperstimulation syndrome	
Elevated FVIII	
Anatomic:	
Varicose veins	
Paget Schroetter	
May Thurner	

VTE, venous thromboembolism.

Both acquired and hereditary risk factors are important contributors to the development of VTE. The most frequent inherited hypercoagulable states are factor V Leiden (FVL) and the prothrombin gene mutation (PT20210), which together account for 60% of cases associated with inherited risk factors (1). Acquired risk factors or predisposing conditions include prior thrombotic event(s), recent major surgery, placement of central venous catheters (CVC), malignancy, pregnancy, use of OCPs, myeloproliferative neoplasms, and antiphospholipid antibody syndrome (APAS). Most patients have multiple risk factors, as outlined in our case scenario. The MEGA case–control study comparing patients with first-time VTE with asymptomatic subjects revealed that major medical illness increases VTE risk with odds ratio 1.5 to 4.9 (2). The combination of major medical illness and immobilization increased the odds further with a ratio of 10.9, while the combination of major medical illness and thrombophilia increased the odds ratio the most, up to 88 for those specifically with FVL mutation.

Clinical Presentation

The signs and symptoms of lower extremity DVT (LEDVT) are nonspecific and patients may be asymptomatic. Nevertheless, if a patient presents with leg swelling, pain, warmth, or erythema, DVT should be suspected. The symptoms are often unilateral, but bilateral DVT may also occur.

An important clinical presentation to identify is phlegmasia cerulea dolens (PCD). PCD is part of a clinical spectrum that ranges from phlegmasia alba dolens to venous gangrene (3). It is the result of an acute massive thrombus that blocks venous drainage of the extremity resulting in sudden, severe pain, swelling, cyanosis, edema, venous gangrene, and compartment syndrome. Delay in treatment can lead to loss of the limb. PCD occurs more frequently in fifth and sixth decades, with a higher reported incidence in females. The most common triggering factor is malignancy, which has been reported in 20% to 40% of patients. Other associated risk factors for PCD include inherited thrombophilias, surgery, trauma, vena cava filter insertion, and pregnancy.

Diagnosis

A preferred diagnostic approach for patients with suspected first DVT is to estimate the clinical pre-test probability (PTP) and then perform laboratory and imaging studies based on the calculated PTP of DVT. There are several PTP scoring systems available for DVT, but the best studied algorithm is the Wells score (Table 12.2) (4).

The total score for an individual denotes the risk of DVT: 0 points is low probability, 1 to 2 points is moderate probability, and 3 to 8 points suggests a high probability of thrombotic event. Validation of this score with ultrasonography in the outpatient setting showed that patients with low probability had 3% incidence of sonographic-confirmed DVT and those with moderate probability had 17% incidence, and high probability scores had 50%–75% incidence (4). A revision of the original score, the modified Wells score, allots an additional point for a prior history of DVT and scores patients based on whether DVT is likely ($\geq$2 points) or unlikely ($\geq$1 point).

Table 12.2 Wells Criteria

Clinical Findings and History	Points
Paralysis, paresis, orthopedic cast	+1
Immobile for >3 days or major surgery within the past 4 weeks	+1
Localized tenderness in deep vein system	+1
Swelling of leg	+1
Calf swelling 3 cm greater than the other leg (measure 10 cm above tibial tuberosity)	+1
Pitting edema of symptomatic leg	+1
Collateral non-varicose superficial veins	+1
Active cancer or cancer treated within 6 months	+1
Alternative diagnosis other than DVT (Baker's cyst, cellulitis, muscle damage, postphlebitic syndrome, inguinal lymphadenopathy)	−2

DVT, deep vein thrombosis.

In patients with low or moderate PTP for first LEDVT, a D-dimer is obtained. A D-dimer has a moderate to high sensitivity for acute DVT. It should not be done if it is expected to be elevated due to another condition (Table 12.3). Patients with a normal D-dimer (<500 ng/mL) and a low PTP do not need further testing. Those with positive D-dimer and moderate PTP should undergo compression ultrasonography (CUS) of whole or proximal leg. For patients with moderate PTP, a negative D-dimer assay is considered insufficient to rule out DVT, unless the assay is a "high-sensitivity" assay. Since

Table 12.3 Clinical Disorders Associated With Elevated Plasma D-Dimers

Pregnancy

Arterial thromboembolic disease

Venous thromboembolic disease

Disseminated intravascular coagulation

Preeclampsia/eclampsia

Infection/sepsis/inflammation

Liver disease

Renal disease

Cardiovascular disease

these are not always readily available, the recommendation is that the patient proceed to CUS. Patients with high PTP for first LEDVT should always go directly to ultrasonography.

The imaging modality of choice for patients with suspected DVT is CUS with Doppler, which offers a sensitivity and specificity of >95% for the diagnosis of proximal DVT. Proximal CUS assesses the proximal veins down to the calf vein trifurcation (Figure 12.1). A whole leg ultrasound is necessary to identify distal DVTs (Figure 12.1). Lack of compressibility of the vein with the ultrasound probe is a sensitive and specific (>95%) sonographic sign for proximal vein thrombosis; however, the sensitivity decreases with examination of calf and iliac veins as the compression maneuver is difficult to elicit given the anatomic accessibility of these vessels. Experts disagree on the benefit of diagnosing a distal DVT as these have lower risk of embolization and may not require treatment; hence, many institutions only offer the more reliable, proximal CUS. Alternative imaging such as CT or MRI may be more useful at identifying iliac vein or inferior vena cava thromboses.

At the time of diagnosis, it is important to determine whether the cause of VTE is provoked or unprovoked. The term unprovoked implies that no discernable environmental event or individual risk factor is evident. In contrast, a provoked DVT has an underlying inciting factor such as surgeries, hospitalization, or travel. For those patients with clear risk factors, an analysis of these will determine the patient's length of anticoagulation treatment, risk of recurrence, and risk of other complication.

Key Diagnostic Dilemma

Nondiagnostic studies present a challenge to physicians, especially when there is a moderate to high PTP of DVT. Nondiagnostic studies occur when the presence or absence of DVT cannot be adequately assessed due to:

1. Patient's body habitus (obesity, edema, trauma)
2. Presence of chronic thrombi or
3. Difficulty interpreting small extension of existing DVT (5)

It is important to understand the limitations of our routine imaging modalities. The specificity of a CUS to diagnose ipsilateral recurrence decreases when compared to its specificity for "first" DVT. After acute DVT, thrombus will slowly resorb, with a decrease in residual venous diameter of about 50% to 60% over the first 3 months in the common femoral and popliteal veins (5). However, it is not uncommon for ultrasound findings to remain abnormal after 3 months (5). For this reason, an ultrasound abnormality detected

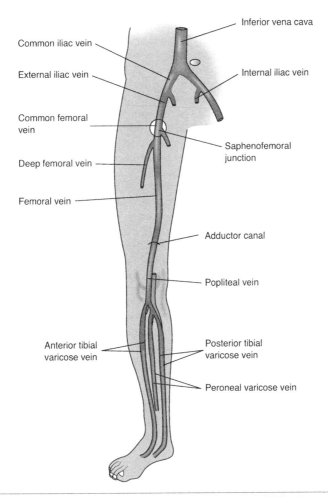

Figure 12.1 Deep veins of the lower extremity. The paired tibial veins (anterior tibial, peroneal, and posterior tibial) are shown with their adjacent arteries. The bridging veins between the paired veins are also demonstrated. The popliteal and femoral veins are also sometimes duplicated (omitted from the diagram) with one of the duplicated segments frequently larger in caliber than the other.

in a suspected recurrence may be difficult to interpret as a new or old DVT. If a patient has a suspected recurrence of ipsilateral DVT, the clinician should proceed directly to ultrasonography rather than performing initial D-dimer. Radiographic evidence of the following is considered to be sonographic evidence of recurrent DVT (5):

1. New noncompressibility in a previously uninvolved segment
2. An increase in compressed venous diameter of >4 mm or
3. Evidence or an extension in thrombus length >10 cm in a previously involved segment

A patient with an increase of 2 to 4 mm in residual vein diameter is unlikely to have experienced recurrent DVT. A conservative approach may be adopted, whereby the patient is reimaged in a week (5). If the findings are stable, no treatment changes are necessary. If the CUS reveals extension, new treatment or modifications to existing treatment should be pursued.

Prognosis

The estimated rate of recurrence following cessation of anticoagulation in patients with a first unprovoked episode of VTE is 10% for the first year and approximately 5% per year after the first year (3). The highest rates of recurrence have been reported with those with unprovoked proximal DVT and PE. The rate of recurrence for those who suffer a provoked event is harder to estimate. A meta-analysis suggested that all patients with transient risk factor have an estimated 3.3% per patient-year, with those having a nonsurgical risk factor, having a higher risk than those with a surgical risk factor (4.2% per patient-year and 0.7% per patient-year, respectively) (3). Overall, a good rule of thumb is to estimate the risk of recurrence from a provoked DVT at 1% to 5% after 1 year and 3% to 15% at 5 years.

Complications

A common complication following acute DVT is post-thrombotic syndrome (PTS). Patients develop chronic venous insufficiency as a result of valvular incompetence and venous hypertension due to thrombotic obstruction. Patient characteristics, as well as DVT-specific characteristics play an important role in the development of PTS. Individuals with primary venous insufficiency, older age, obesity, and preexisting varicose veins are at higher risk (6). A proximal DVT, inadequate anticoagulation during initial treatment of DVT, residual thrombus in the vein, and recurrent DVT, all increase the likelihood of PTS. The diagnosis is often a clinical one and is made when the patient experiences extremity pain, vein dilation, edema, skin pigmentation, and venous ulcers following a DVT. It is a burdensome and costly complication for which therapeutic options are limited to symptomatic relief.

Management

The mainstay of therapy for patients with DVT is anticoagulation. All patients should be assessed at the time of anticoagulant initiation and throughout the course of treatment for potential bleeding risk. For those patients who already have preexisting factors for bleeding, administration of blood thinners will increase the bleeding risk, so these factors must be carefully considered in a patient with new diagnosis of DVT. If the patient's 3-month bleeding risk is <2%, anticoagulation is pursued (3). For those patients with a 3-month bleeding risk >13%, anticoagulation should not be initiated (3). For patients with an estimated bleeding risk between these values, the decision needs to be based on a careful consideration of that patient's risk–benefit ratio (3). Clinicians often use their own experience to develop a "best estimate" of the bleeding risk in their patients. Despite the existence of several tools to estimate the bleeding risk (i.e., HAS-BLED, ATRIA), none has been validated in patients receiving anticoagulation for DVT, and are therefore not routinely used for this purpose.

Traditionally, patients with new diagnosis of DVT were admitted for 5 to 10 days of systemic anticoagulation with a heparin-based therapy (Table 12.4) and then transitioned to oral anticoagulation with vitamin K antagonists (VKAs). The introduction of the new direct oral anticoagulants (DOACs) has changed this paradigm as a subset of newly diagnosed DVT patients can be treated as outpatients. DOAC medications are given at a fixed dose, do not require titration or lab monitoring, and some can be initiated without the typical "bridging" that is required with the VKA medications, making them an attractive option for the initial treatment of PE (Table 12.5) (3). Outpatient therapy is considered for patients who are hemodynamically stable, have a low risk of bleeding, have no renal insufficiency, and have a good support system for the administration and surveillance of anticoagulation at home. Those patients with massive DVT, concurrent PE, comorbid conditions, and a high bleeding risk should still be admitted to the hospital for initial systemic anticoagulation.

An inferior vena cava (IVC) filter should be considered for patients with acute proximal DVT with an absolute contraindication to anticoagulation, such as intracranial hemorrhage, gastrointestinal bleeding, or aortic dissection. There is no clear benefit for IVC filter placement in patients with isolated distal DVT regardless of symptomatology. Ideally, IVC filters are utilized as bridges until the patient can tolerate anticoagulation. They are not meant to be standalone or adjunct therapy to anticoagulation. Retrievable filters are preferred to prevent long-term complications of filter placement, such as recurrent DVT and PTS (7).

Table 12.4 Nomogram for Unfractionated Heparin Administration

Initial Dose	80 units/kg bolus, then 18 units/kg/hr*	
aPTT result	Action	Next aPTT check
aPTT <35 sec (<1.2 × control)	80 units/kg bolus, then increase the infusion rate by 4 units/kg/hr	6 hours
aPTT 35 to 45 sec (1.2–1.5 × control)	40 units/kg bolus, then increase the infusion rate by 2 units/kg/hr	6 hours
aPTT 46 to 70 sec (1.5–2.3 × control)	No change (therapeutic range)	6 hours (when two consecutive values are within therapeutic range, then next aPTT in the morning)
aPTT 71 to 90 sec (2.3–3.0 × control)	Decrease the infusion rate by 2 units/kg/hr	6 hours
aPTT >90 sec (>3.0 × control)	Hold infusion for 1 hour, then decrease the infusion rate by 3 units/kg/hr	6 hours

aPTT, activated partial thromboplastin time.

Table 12.5 Direct Oral Anticoagulant Dose Recommendations

Anticoagulant	Dosage
Rivaroxaban	Initial: 15 mg/BID for the first 3 weeks Maintenance: 20 mg qdaily with food
Apixaban	Initial: 10 mg/BID for the first 7 days Maintenance: 5 mg BID
Edoxaban	Initial: 5–10 days of parenteral anticoagulation Maintenance: 60 mg/QD or 30 mg/QD in patients with a body weight >60 kg
Dabigatran	Initial: 5–10 days of parenteral anticoagulation Maintenance: 150 mg BID

BID, twice a day; QD, one per day.

The optimal length of anticoagulation is not clearly defined, but most experts agree that the presence or absence of provoking factors, bleeding risk, recurrence risk, and the patient's lifestyle and preferences (occupation, life expectancy, burden of therapy, etc.) should be taken into account. For most patients with a first episode of DVT, a minimum of 3 months of therapy is recommended as this time period represents the highest risk of recurrence.

Most patients with a first episode of VTE will be anticoagulated for a finite period of 3 to 12 months. However, there is a minority of patients for whom the risk of recurrence is significant and would benefit from indefinite anticoagulation. Experts agree that patients with a first unprovoked DVT and/or PE or those with recurrent, unprovoked VTE would benefit from indefinite anticoagulation. In patients with a first, unprovoked episode of DVT or PE, it has been shown that gender and D-dimer levels may be useful in better selecting those patients who would benefit from extended anticoagulation. Patients with a positive D-dimer have double the risk of recurrence than those with negative D-dimers posttreatment (3). The risk of recurrence for a woman who experienced an unprovoked VTE and has a negative posttreatment D-dimer is equivalent to that of a patient with a proximal VTE provoked by a transient risk factor (15% recurrence at 5 years); hence, the D-dimer is useful in preventing the general recommendation of extended anticoagulation for female patients. Men have a 1.75-fold higher risk of recurrence than women. The risk of recurrence for a male with a negative D-dimer (25% at 5 years) is not less than the estimated risk for recurrence of patients with unprovoked VTE (30% at 5 years); so, posttreatment D-dimers are less useful in males (3). Patients with a provoked VTE due to transient risk factors or those with high risk of bleeding complications should not pursue indefinite anticoagulation. Less clear is what to do with those patients who suffer recurrent provoked VTE, provoked VTE with persistent risk factors, or those with multiple major risk factors.

Special Populations

May–Thurner syndrome (MTS) is an anatomic condition characterized by extrinsic venous compression by the arterial system of the iliocaval venous system, usually the right common iliac artery compressing on the left common iliac vein. MTS may be asymptomatic, but it accounts for 2% to 5% of LEDVT. The classic presentation of thrombotic MTS is a young female in the second or third decade of life presenting with left lower extremity swelling. Risk factors for progression from asymptomatic anatomic anomaly to chronic venous hypertension or thrombosis include: (a) female gender, particularly postpartum, multiparous, or using oral contraceptives;

(b) scoliosis; (c) dehydration; and (d) hypercoagulable disorders. Patients with DVT suspected to be tied to underlying MTS should receive full-dose anticoagulation if not contraindicated. Catheter-directed thrombolysis or pharmacomechanical thrombolysis may be indicated to reduce thrombotic burden (8). If intrinsic venous stenosis is present, angioplasty and stenting of the diseased ilioca-val segment should be considered (8).

Patients with malignancy constitute a therapeutic challenge. Cancer patients have increased rates of VTE recurrence due to a hypercoagulable state associated with malignancy and cancer treatments (catheters and chemotherapy), while also having high-er-than-normal bleeding risk (cytopenias associated with malig-nancy or chemotherapy). A cancer patient with a newly diagnosed VTE, a reasonable life expectancy, acceptable bleeding risk, and adequate renal function should be treated with low-molecu-lar-weight heparin (LMWH) (3). Recent studies suggest that DOACs may be an adequate alternative which provides better quality of life (9). In patients with renal insufficiency who have active malignancy, VKA is the recommended alternative. The use of low-dose DOACs to prevent VTE is under investigation in high-risk cancer patients (Khorana risk score >2), but no consensus exists on the benefit of prophylactic anticoagulation or the type of anticoagulant (9).

The anticoagulant of choice for pregnant women is LMWH because it has a predictable response, does not require monitor-ing, and is safe for the fetus as it does not cross the placenta (10). During the final weeks of pregnancy, around 36 to 37 weeks, obste-tricians prefer to switch the patient to unfractionated heparin (UFH) in case rapid reversal of therapy is required, although this practice is variable. DOACs have not been tested in pregnant women and the safety for the fetus is unclear. DOACs are excreted in breast milk and are not considered safe for breastfeeding women (10). VKAs have demonstrated teratogenic effects on animal studies and are consequently not used antepartum. However, VKAs are accept-able in the postpartum period as they are not excreted in breast milk and can be safely used by a breastfeeding mother.

Patients with heparin-induced thrombocytopenia (HIT) should not be further exposed to heparin-based products. Immediate anticoagulation with parenteral non–heparin-based therapy (direct thrombin inhibitors or anti-Xa) should be implemented. This is fur-ther discussed in Chapter 10, Platelet Disorders. The use of DOACs has been recently endorsed in the American Society of Hematology (ASH) guidelines, but their use should be reserved for long-term management and not acute treatment of HIT episode (10).

Patients with APAS should be treated with heparin overlapped with VKA. At this time, VKAs are still preferred over DOACs. A recent study demonstrated superiority of VKAs over DOACs for high-risk APAS patients with triple-positive laboratory values (11). It is unclear if DOACs afford equivalent efficacy for lower-risk APAS patients. Anticoagulation therapy is not recommended for patients with laboratory values consistent with lupus inhibitor who do not meet the clinical criteria for APAS because they have not had a thrombotic event. The clinical and laboratory criteria for APAS are discussed further in the section "Hypercoagulable Disorders" in this chapter.

Patients with inherited thrombophilia receive similar treatment to those without. Chest guidelines do not recommend primary prevention of VTE for patients with inherited thrombophilia due to a lack of clinical trials to support its use (12). Patients with recurrent VTE are candidates for indefinite anticoagulation regardless of their inherited thrombophilia.

Weight-based therapy is the standard of care for obese patients. This can be achieved with UFH and VKAs. DOACs have not been studied in patients with a body mass index (BMI) of >40 kg/m^2 or a weight of >120 kg; so, it is unclear if therapeutic anticoagulation is reliably achieved in obese patients.

Recommendations for anticoagulation in other special scenarios are outlined in Table 12.6.

Emerging Therapies

The finding that humans with hereditary factor XI deficiency have mild bleeding tendencies but exemplify a significant protection against certain thrombotic diseases has sparked interest in factor XI as a target for novel antithrombotic treatments. Currently, MAA868, a novel antibody against FXI, is investigated for its potential to prevent and treat thrombosis with a minimal risk of bleeding. Following successful preclinical studies, the drug has moved to investigation in humans in phase 1, demonstrating that in healthy subjects, single SC doses of MAA868 are safe and well tolerated.

Key Points

- For patients with provoked DVT, there is often more than one risk factor contributing to thrombosis; often, these can be a combination of acquired and hereditary factors.
- The imaging of choice for diagnosis of proximal DVT is CUS, with a high specificity and sensitivity for first-time DVT.
- Recurrence risk is higher for patients with an unprovoked DVT (Table 12.7), and indefinite anticoagulation must be considered in this high-risk population.
- The anticoagulant of choice is dependent on the clinical scenario.

Table 12.6 Anticoagulation of Choice in Special Populations

Factor	Preferred Anticoagulation	Qualifying Remarks
Malignancy	LMWH	Recent trials suggest that DOACs may be useful in prophylactic and therapeutic settings for high-risk patients
Oral therapy preferred or need to avoid parenteral therapy	Rivaroxaban, apixaban	VKA, edoxaban, and dabigatran require initial parenteral therapy
Liver disease and coagulopathy	LMWH	DOACs contraindicated if baseline INR elevated due to liver disease. VKA therapeutic effect is also difficult to monitor with baseline elevated INR levels.
Renal disease (creatinine clearance <30 mL/min)	VKA	DOACs and LMWH contraindicated due to significant renal excretion of these agents
CAD	VKA, rivaroxaban, apixaban, edoxaban	CAD events appear to occur more often with dabigatran than with VKA
Dyspepsia or history of GI bleeding	VKA, apixaban	Dabigatran associated with increased dyspepsia Rivaroxaban associated with increased GI bleeding risk
Thrombolytic therapy use	UFH infusion	
Reversal agent needed	VKA, heparin, DOACs	Reversal agents available for all DOACs but they are costly.
Pregnancy	LMWH	Other anticoagulants may potentially cross the placenta
Antiphospholipid antibody syndrome	VKA	DOACs continue to be studied. Recent studies on high-risk patients (triple-positive laboratory disease) do not support DOAC use over VKA
Heparin-induced thrombocytopenia	VKA	New society guidelines have endorsed the use of DOACs in long-term therapy, but not in acute setting

CAD, coronary artery disease; DOAC, direct oral anticoagulant; LMWH, low-molecular-weight heparin; UFH, unfractionated heparin; VKA, vitamin K antagonist.

Table 12.7 Rate of Venous Thromboembolism Recurrence

VTE Risk Factor	First Year Recurrence (%)	Annual Rate After First Year (%)
First episode: Unprovoked	10	5
Second episode: Unprovoked	15	7.5
First episode: Provoked due to surgical risk factor	1 to 2	0.5
First episode: Provoked due to nonsurgical risk factor	5	2 to 3

VTE, venous thromboembolism.

PULMONARY EMBOLISM

Clinical Case 12.2

A 54-year-old man with a past medical history of treatment for naïve renal cell carcinoma presents to the emergency department with complaints of acute-on-set shortness of breath and right-sided pleuritic chest pain starting earlier that day. Vital signs are remarkable for a heart rate of 112 beats per minute, blood pressure of 92/58 mmHg, respiratory rate of 28 breaths per minute, and pulse oximetry showing an oxygen saturation of 87%, which improves to 92% with 4 L/min of supplemental oxygen delivered via nasal cannula. His exam is notable for regular tachycardia, the absence of heart murmurs, the presence of jugular venous distension, and a clear lung exam without wheezes or rales. Labs are remarkable for a mild elevation in serum troponin and brain natriuretic peptide (BNP). Plain radiography of the chest is unremarkable and shows bilaterally clear lung fields. An EKG obtained at presentation shows sinus tachycardia. Subsequently, a CT scan with pulmonary angiography (CTPA) is ordered and shows an increased right-to-left ventricular diameter ratio, suggesting right ventricular (RV) overload as well as a filling defect in the right main pulmonary artery consistent with PE.

Introduction

PE is a manifestation of VTE and is frequently encountered by clinicians with an estimated incidence of 60 to 112 per 100,000 people in the United States (13). It is the third most common acute cardiovascular syndrome following stroke and myocardial infarction and carries with it a significant burden of morbidity and mortality (14). In recent decades, the rate of diagnosis of PE has been increasing with a higher proportion being segmental or subsegmental (15). Advanced imaging modalities have improved diagnostic capabilities. In fact, approximately 3% of PEs are found incidentally on CT imaging ordered for other reasons (15). Meanwhile, mortality and length of hospital stays have been on the decline, which is not only likely due to the diagnosis of smaller emboli of undetermined clinical significance, but also improvements in antithrombotic management (15). Despite these improvements, PE remains a diagnostic challenge owing to its nonspecific presentation. As many as 94% of patients die from PE prior to being diagnosed (13).

Diagnosis

The presentation of PE is nonspecific. Patients may present with some degree of chest pain and/or dyspnea, though these symptoms are associated with other common conditions such as acute coronary syndromes, acute exacerbation of chronic obstructive pulmonary disease, or pneumonia (14). The most specific symptoms of PE are hemoptysis and calf pain, but these are present only 10% and 42% of the time, respectively (13). The clinician must maintain a high index of suspicion to make the correct diagnosis.

If PE is suspected, the next step is to risk-stratify the patient into either "high-risk" or "non–high-risk" categories, thereby delineating the extent of further testing (Figures 12.2 and 12.3) (13). This early risk stratification is simple and rapidly performed by assessing the hemodynamic status of the patient with suspected PE. Patients presenting with hypotension or shock fall under the suspected high-risk category, whereas normotensive patients are considered to be non–high-risk patients (13).

Patients in the "high-risk" category should be assessed with CTPA to confirm the diagnosis of PE (Figure 12.2) (13). If CT imaging is not available or is contraindicated, the preferred imaging modality is echocardiography, which may reveal acute-onset pulmonary hypertension (PH) or RV overload (13). These findings may merit the need for thrombolysis or embolectomy, which is discussed later. Catheter pulmonary angiography was at one time considered the gold standard in diagnosis of acute PE. It has been replaced by CTPA owing mostly to the morbidity and mortality associated with invasive angiography (16). Currently, invasive angiography is reserved for catheter-based interventions, such as mechanical thrombectomy and possibly, the diagnosis of chronic thromboembolic pulmonary hypertension (CTEPH). Along with right heart catheterization (RHC), concurrent pulmonary angiography allows for diagnosis and assessment of disease severity of CTEPH at the same time (16).

Hemodynamically stable patients are considered non-high risk, which allows for more in-depth assessment of PE probability prior to confirmatory testing with the aid of a standardized clinical

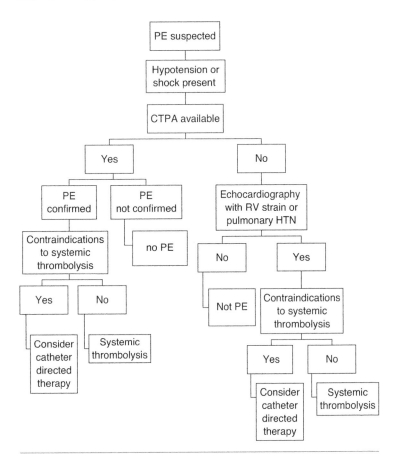

Figure 12.2 Approach to suspected high-risk PE.

CTPA, CT pulmonary angiography; HTN, hypertension; PE, pulmonary embolism; RV, right ventricular.

Source: Adapted from Meyer G. Effective diagnosis and treatment of pulmonary embolism: improving patient outcomes. *Arch Cardiovasc Dis.* 2014;107(6–7):406–414. doi:10.1016/j.acvd.2014.05.006

prediction tool (Figure 12.3). The modified Wells score (Table 12.8) is one such validated tool and assigns patients to one of two groups: "pulmonary embolism likely" and "pulmonary embolism unlikely" (17). Patients in whom PE is likely should have confirmatory testing preferably with CTPA. Patients in whom PE is unlikely should proceed to D-dimer level testing, similar to what was described for DVT. Patients with a D-dimer <500 ng/mL are considered to have a low probability of PE, whereas patients with a D-dimer concentration

Table 12.8 Modified Wells Score—Clinical Prediction Tool

Variable	Points
Clinical signs/symptoms of DVT	3
Alternative diagnoses less likely than PE	3
Heart rate >100/min	1.5
Immobilization >3 days or surgery in past 4 weeks	1.5
History of prior PE or DVT	1.5
Hemoptysis	1
Malignancy (active or treated within 6 months)	1
Score ≤4 – PE unlikely	
Score >4 – PE likely	
DVT, deep vein thrombosis; PE, pulmonary embolism.	

>500 ng/mL are considered indeterminate, requiring additional workup (Figure 12.3) (17).

Currently, the standard diagnostic modality for confirmation of PE is CTPA, but acceptable alternatives include lung ventilation/perfusion (V/Q) scan and CUS of the lower extremities (13). A V/Q scan is a nuclear medicine scan that uses injected Tc-99m macroaggregated albumin to measure perfusion defects in the lung. (16). V/Q scan is a tool that has been available for decades and a negative result is effective at eliminating the diagnosis of PE with 97% specificity (13). In patients with a high PTP, a positive result is likely to be diagnostic of PE. However, roughly 50% of V/Q scans are nondiagnostic, so their use should be limited to carefully selected patient populations. V/Q scans involve a lower exposure to radiation when compared to CTPA and avoid the use of iodinated contrast, making it appropriate for pregnant patients, patients with severe renal disease, and those who are allergic to contrast media (16). For patients in whom chronic PE or CTEPH is of consideration, V/Q scan remains the diagnostic study of choice (18).

Risk Stratification

Once a diagnosis of PE has been made, additional assessment and testing are recommended to further risk-stratify patients into either low- or intermediate-risk categories (14), which allow for selection of patients who may be safely managed at home and those who require hospitalization for observation and additional workup (13,15). The most validated tools for this purpose are

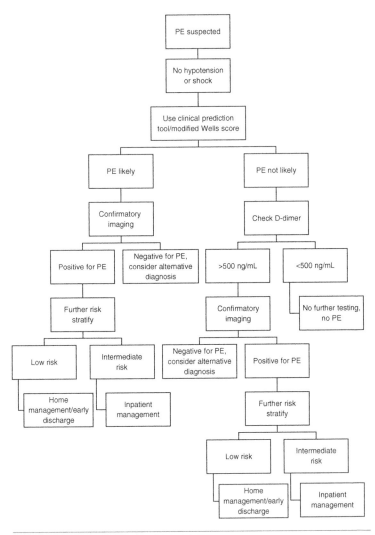

Figure 12.3 Approach to non–high-risk PE.

Source: Adapted from Meyer G. Effective diagnosis and treatment of pulmonary embolism: improving patient outcomes. *Arch Cardiovasc Dis.* 2014;107(6–7):406–414. doi:10.1016/j.acvd.2014.05.006

PE, pulmonary embolism.

the Pulmonary Embolism Severity Index (PESI; Table 12.9) and the simplified Pulmonary Embolism Severity Index (sPESI; Table 12.10) (15). The PESI stratifies patients into one of five categories: very low, low, intermediate, high risk, or very high risk. The sPESI

Table 12.9 Pulmonary Embolism Severity Index

	Variable	Points
Demographics	Age	1 per year
	Male	10
Comorbidities	History of cancer	30
	History of heart failure	10
	History of chronic lung disease	10
	Heart rate ≥110/minute	20
	Systolic blood pressure <100 mmHg	30h
	Respiratory rate ≥30/min	20
Clinical findings	Temperature <36°C	20
	Altered mental status	60
	Arterial oxygen saturation <90%	20
Very low risk	Class I – <65 points	
Low risk	Class II – 66 to 85 points	
Intermediate risk	Class III – 86 to 105 points	
High risk	Class IV – 105 to 125 points	
Very high risk	Class V – >125 points	

stratifies patients into low- or high-risk category. Patients who are assigned to the low-risk category may be safely discharged home with appropriate therapy and without the need for additional testing (14). Patients assigned to the intermediate or high-risk category should have additional testing with imaging and biochemical markers with the aim of identifying those with RV dysfunction who are at high risk of decompensation (14). Imaging modalities to be considered are CTPA and echocardiography with attention to quantitative measures of RV dysfunction (15). Biochemical markers that suggest RV dysfunction or injury include BNP, pro-BNP, and troponin (15). The presence of either imaging or biochemical markers suggestive of RV dysfunction would classify a patient as intermediate-low risk and the presence of both would classify a patient as intermediate-high risk. Of importance, the intermediate-risk classification may be used to guide clinical decision-making, but there is currently no data showing that it alters patient outcomes (15).

Table 12.10 Simplified Pulmonary Embolism Severity Index

Variable	Points
Age >80 years	1
History of cancer	1
History of chronic cardiopulmonary disease	1
Heart rate ≥110/minute	1
Systolic blood pressure <100 mmHg	1
Arterial oxygen saturation <90%	1
Low risk	0
High risk	≥1

Complications

A rare complication of acute PE is the development of CTEPH which occurs in 0.5% to 4% of patients with an acute PE (18). CTEPH is thought to be secondary to ineffective resolution of a thrombus leading to chronic occlusion of pulmonary arteries and in some cases, progression to distal vessel arteriopathy (18). Risk factors for the development of CTEPH include a history of splenectomy, the presence of ventriculoatrial shunts, presence of a pacemaker, and chronic inflammation (18). Interestingly, an inherited hypercoagulable state does not predict a higher likelihood of developing CTEPH compared to normal controls (18). The signs and symptoms of CTEPH are not specific and mirror those of PH and, in more severe cases, right heart failure. They may include dyspnea, chest pains, general fatigue, and leg edema. A degree of hypoxemia can exist in these patients due to increased dead space ventilation. Spirometry, if performed, often demonstrates a mild to moderate reduction in diffusing capacity of the lungs for carbon monoxide (DLCO); severe reductions in DLCO are not expected for CTEPH alone. Often, echocardiography is the first test performed that raises suspicion for the presence of CTEPH (18). Additional workup includes an RHC to confirm elevated pulmonary artery pressures. Diagnosis can be made with a number of different imaging modalities, but a V/Q scan is the recommended study as discussed. A normal V/Q scan effectively rules out most cases of CTEPH. Despite the increasing ubiquity of CTPA for the diagnosis of acute PE, it is not recommended as first-line testing as the sensitivity is higher with a V/Q scan. CTPA is still useful in the workup of CTEPH as it provides more definition of the heart and lung parenchyma, helping to also evaluate alternative diagnoses that mimic CTEPH.

Gold standard diagnostic testing remains pulmonary angiography, although some centers are replacing this imaging procedure with MRI and magnetic resonance angiography (MRA) (18).

Key Diagnostic Dilemma

Controversy exists over the clinical significance of smaller PEs which are now detected with increasing frequency due to the improved sensitivity of CTPA, specifically subsegmental PEs (15). Healthy patients will pass small PEs as the pulmonary capillary bed has fibrinolytic activity that can break down these clots (19). It has been suggested that an isolated subsegmental PE (i.e., single PE and no concurrent DVT) is likely a "false-positive" finding. Consequently, the need to treat these "small" PEs is often debated and considered unnecessary (20).

Occasionally, clinicians will be faced with the challenge of managing a PE that was diagnosed on an imaging study ordered for reasons other than for confirmation of suspected PE (19,20). This is typically seen with patients who have a CT scan ordered for pulmonary diseases or cancer staging (20). Roughly half of the incidental PEs are found in the main or lobar arteries, and between 11% and 27% are found in the subsegmental, smaller arteries (19). Importantly, incidental PE does not equate with "asymptomatic" PE. With close scrutiny, patients discovered to have an "incidental" PE have reported symptoms typically associated with acute PE, most notably, fatigue, shortness of breath, and cough (19). Retrospective studies have found conflicting results on the prognosis of incidental PE, specifically in comparison to "symptomatic" PE diagnoses. Since the prognoses of incidental PEs and symptomatic PEs appear to be similar, current recommendations by the American College of Chest Physicians (ACCP) (grade 2B) and the American Society of Clinical Oncology (ASCO) (informal consensus, moderate strength recommendation) advocate for a similar treatment strategy (3,19).

Prognosis

Prognosis of PE varies considerably and is dependent on individual patient factors, existing comorbidities, and clinical presentation (14). As mentioned earlier, the overall mortality of PE has been decreasing in recent years, likely due to an increasing proportion of PE diagnoses being segmental and subsegmental as well as advances in anticoagulant therapy (15). Still, PE remains the third leading cause of death among patients with cardiovascular diseases (13).

The most influential factors on a patient's risk of short-term mortality are a patient's hemodynamics, RV function, and the

Table 12.11 Pulmonary Embolism Severity Index Class and 30-Day Mortality

PESI Class and Approximate 30-day Mortality	
Class I	1%
Class II	3%
Class III	6.5%
Class IV	10.5%
Class V	24.5%

presence or absence of myocardial injury (15). This risk for mortality can be estimated in patients using a validated tool, one of which, the PESI, has already been discussed in the section "Risk Stratification." Using the PESI, patients can be assigned to classes that range from the least severe, Class I, and the most severe, Class V, with 30-day mortality rates of about 1% and 24.5%, respectively (Table 12.11) (15).

Management

Anticoagulation is the mainstay treatment for PE, and the conventional approach, as in DVT, consisted of UFH infusion with overlapping treatment of a VKA, such as warfarin, for a minimum of 5 days until a goal INR of 2 to 3 is achieved (14). The introduction of LMWH and fondaparinux, subcutaneous, fixed-dose agents that do not require titration, shifted the treatment of low-risk PE from the hospitals to home (15). These conventional approaches are still acceptable and are recommended in some cases, but with the advent of DOACs, treatment options have once again shifted (13). Several studies have demonstrated similar efficacy of DOACs when compared to conventional therapy with a more favorable safety profile, given lower rates of major or clinically significant bleeding (13).

Patients diagnosed with high-risk PE (i.e., patients presenting with hemodynamic instability) have a more complicated treatment than the sole decision of which type of anticoagulant to use. Unstable patients without a contraindication carry a recommendation for systemic thrombolytic therapy (3). Instability in these patients is a result of right heart failure or cardiogenic shock secondary to poor left ventricular filling leading to systemic hypotension which, if left untreated, may precipitate death (14). The rationale for thrombolytic therapy is to rapidly dissolve the thrombus, reducing RV afterload and restoring forward blood flow and left ventricular filling (14). In addition to thrombolytics, immediate anticoagulation should be started while awaiting confirmation of the diagnosis to reduce recurrence of thromboembolic events and held briefly during the time of thrombolysis (15). Patients receiving thrombolytics carry a significant risk of hemorrhage, especially intracranial bleeding, making UFH the initial anticoagulant of choice in this instance, given its short half-life and the ability to monitor its level of anticoagulation (14). A reasonable approach is to continue these patients on UFH for at least 12 hours after completion of thrombolysis or until there is reasonable confidence that a risk of major bleeding is minimized (15). Once these patients are stabilized, they may be transitioned to a DOAC, with caution, as these agents have long half-lives relative to UFH. Antidotes, while now available, are not easily accessible in small or remote facilities and are costly (15).

Additional considerations in patients with high-risk PE are for interventional approaches such as mechanical thrombectomy and catheter-directed thrombolytic therapy (15). Current recommendations are to reserve these procedures for patients who are evaluated at medical facilities with the expertise to execute these procedures and meet at least one of the following criteria (3):

• High risk of bleeding
• Failure to respond to systemic attempts at thrombolysis
• Imminent life-threatening shock likely to decompensate before systemic thrombolysis can take effect

Not all patients require hospitalization for treatment of PE after initial diagnosis. Patients with low-risk PE who have no contraindications to use of a DOAC or LMWH may be managed entirely at home or with short hospital stays (3). Patients with intermediate-risk PE should be admitted to the hospital for anticoagulation, but more importantly for close observation. These patients have already exhibited some risk or evidence of RV dysfunction and/or injury and may require additional treatments and supportive care specific to this finding (Table 12.12) (14).

Choice of anticoagulant may depend on many patient- and clinical-specific factors as described in Table 12.6.

On occasion, patients will have PE and absolute contraindications to anticoagulation. It is reasonable to consider the placement of an IVC filter to prevent further VTE in these patients (14) However, long-term placement of an IVC filter is not recommended, and they should be removed when anticoagulation can be safely instituted. It is not recommended to place an IVC filter in a patient who is otherwise capable of receiving anticoagulants (3).

The duration of therapy varies from patient to patient, but generally patients should be on anticoagulation for at least 3 months

Table 12.12 Summary of Diagnostic Algorithms With Prognostication and Treatment Recommendations

PE Risk	PESI Class	Biochemical Markers of RV Strain	Radiographic Markers of RV Strain	Hypotension	Treatment	Treatment Location
Low risk	I to II	Testing not recommended		No	Anticoagulation	Home
Intermediate-low risk	III to V	Positive biochemical OR radiographic markers		No	Anticoagulation	Hospital
Intermediate-high risk	III to V	Positive	Positive	No	Anticoagulation	Hospital or intensive care unit
High risk	Any	Positive	Positive	Yes	Thrombolysis then anticoagulation	Intensive care unit

PE, pulmonary embolism; PESI, Pulmonary Embolism Severity Index; RV, right ventricular.

(3). There are recommendations for many specific situations, but most can be summarized as follows:

- Patients with a PE provoked by surgery or another transient risk factor should be treated for at least 3 months.
- Patients with a first unprovoked PE should be treated for at least 3 months; then an assessment of bleeding risk should be done and those at a low risk should continue indefinitely, while those at a high risk should discontinue therapy at that 3-month mark.
- It is reasonable to test D-dimer levels 1 month after discontinuing therapy to help guide a possible decision to extend therapy or continue observation off therapy. Please note that gender plays a role in this decision as outlined in earlier sections.
- Patients on extended/indefinite therapy should be reassessed at least annually for considerations of continuing versus discontinuing therapy.
- Patients with a second unprovoked PE and at low or intermediate bleeding risk should be continued on indefinite anticoagulation and patients at a high risk of bleeding should be treated for 3 months.
- Once patients with an unprovoked PE are off anticoagulation, they should be started on aspirin for continued prevention of recurrence if they are unable to receive anticoagulation due to bleeding risk.
- Patients with a PE and an active cancer should be continued on indefinite anticoagulation regardless of bleeding risk.

With increasing frequency, patients are being diagnosed with subsegmental PE (15). In this situation, patients should be assessed for a proximal DVT with CUS and if there is no proximal DVT, and the risk of recurrent VTE is low, no anticoagulation therapy is recommended (3). The likelihood of a subsegmental PE being a false-positive result is high in the absence of a DVT or VTE risk factors (20). For this reason, current recommendations are that isolated subsegmental PE should go untreated unless there is a high risk of recurrent VTE or there is a concurrent DVT (3). However, patients with a high risk of recurrent VTE or with a concurrent DVT require anticoagulation (3).

Treatment for CTEPH begins with referral to a surgical center with experience in pulmonary thromboendarterectomy (PTE) (3,18). Indefinite anticoagulation is recommended in all patients who have been diagnosed with CTEPH, even in those post-PTE (18). Choice of anticoagulant in patients with CTEPH is controversial, but warfarin remains the most commonly used agent despite a lack of randomized clinical trials supporting its use. The only medication that is U.S. Food and Drug Administration (FDA) approved for treatment specifically for CTEPH is riociguat, a guanylate cyclase stimulator, which is used to treat distal, inoperable CTEPH or patients with residual PH after PTE (18). However, many other medications are used off-label, such as prostacyclin analogs and phosphodiesterase-5 inhibitors, which are used routinely for idiopathic PH even though no clinical trials have been completed to support this practice in CTEPH (18). Treatment of right heart failure with diuretics and supplemental oxygen for patients with hypoxemia is recommended.

Additional recommendations regarding more specific clinical scenarios are available in the guidelines published by the ACCP, American Heart Association (AHA)/American College of Cardiologists (ACC), and so forth.

Key Points

- Rapid stratification of patients into high- and non–high-risk categories is vital in treating potentially life-threatening PE in a timely fashion.
- Diagnostic testing varies based on PTP.
- Imaging modalities to diagnose PE have improved in recent years and the capability of diagnosing nonsymptomatic PEs has increased.
- The advent of DOACs has allowed for low-risk PE patients to be safely managed at home.
- Patients who develop CTEPH should be referred to a center with experience in PTE.
- Recent advances in treatment have emerged as have multidisciplinary teams to assess and tailor treatment to individual patient's needs.

UPPER EXTREMITY DVT

Introduction

Upper extremity DVT (UEDVT) constitutes 1% to 4% of all cases of DVT, with thromboses occurring in the deep veins that drain the upper extremity: subclavian, axillary, and brachial veins (Figure 12.4). The clinical presentation may be asymptomatic; however, if symptoms occur, they are consistent with the local effects of obstruction and embolization, such as arm swelling, pain, and a heaviness that may or may not improve with elevation of extremity to the heart level (Table 12.13).

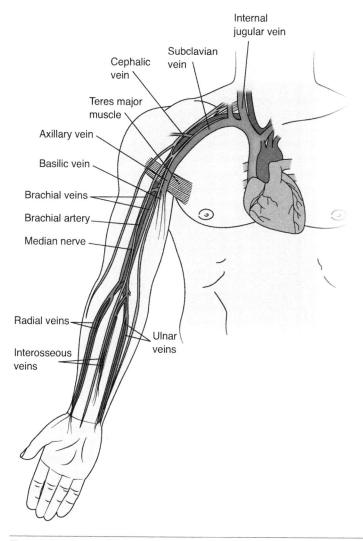

Figure 12.4 Deep veins of the upper extremity. The deep veins of the upper extremity include the paired ulnar, radial, and interosseous veins in the forearm; paired brachial veins of the upper arm; and axillary vein. The axillary vein originates at the lower border of the teres major muscle in continuity with the brachial veins. The basilic and cephalic veins, which are superficial veins, contribute to the axillary vein, though many anatomic variations occur. After passing the outer margin of the first rib, the axillary vein continues as the subclavian vein.

Table 12.13 Symptoms and Signs Associated With Upper Extremity Deep Vein Thrombosis

Arm swelling and pain
Neck swelling
Paresthesias or pain in ulnar nerve distribution (brachial plexus compression)
Wasting of intrinsic hand muscles
PCD
PCD, phlegmasia cerulea dolens.

Most cases of UEDVT are secondary to central catheter placement or prothrombotic states such as malignancy and thrombophilia. Catheter-related thrombosis (CRT) accounts for 70% to 80% of the cases of UEDVT. Primary or spontaneous UEDVT is rare and may be due to an underlying anatomic anomaly, such as venous thoracic syndrome or Paget–Schroetter syndrome, a type of effort thrombosis that occurs due to strenuous and/or repetitive use of the arm and shoulder (21).

Both congenital and acquired anatomic abnormalities of the thoracic outlet may result in compression of the vein. Congenital abnormalities include cervical ribs, supernumerary muscles, or abnormal tendinous insertions. Acquired abnormalities include bony overgrowth secondary to fracture or hypertrophy of the scalene muscle, which usually occurs secondary to repetitive movements. Approximately 60% to 80% of patients with primary UEDVT report a history of exercise or strenuous activity such as weight lifting, rowing, or other activities which result in hyperabduction of upper extremity muscles, typically in the dominant arm, thereby leading to perivenous fibrosis and narrowing of the affected vein (22).

Risk factors for primary UEDVT include young age, male gender, anatomic abnormality, strenuous upper extremity activity, and repetitive arm movements (22). Intravenous (IV) catheters, including percutaneously inserted central line catheters (PICC), tunneled and non-tunneled central venous lines, port devices, and pacemakers, all have the potential to cause secondary UEDVT (22) (Table 12.14).

Diagnosis

Regardless of the underlying etiology for UEDVT, confirmation of the thrombosis is necessary. The preferred imaging modality is a noninvasive CUS. As in the case of LEDVT/PE, a D-dimer may

Table 12.14 Risk Factors for Upper Extremity Deep Vein Thrombosis

Primary	Catheter Associated
Young age (children, adolescents)	Diameter of catheter
Male gender	PICC insertion
Anatomic abnormalities of thoracic outlet	Malposition of tip
Repetitive arm hyperabduction, i.e.,	Catheter Infection
pitching	Prior DVT
Thrombophilia	Chemical irritation

DVT, deep vein thrombosis; PICC, percutaneously inserted central line catheter.

be useful in excluding thrombosis as an etiology, but it will not exclude vein stenosis/compression as a source of symptoms (23).

Catheter-based venography provides the best definition of abnormal venous anatomy (24). However, it is an invasive modality, requiring cannulation of either a peripheral or a central vein, as well as instillation of IV contrast into the lumen of the catheter. This modality is usually reserved for those cases in which noninvasive studies are equivocal, but the clinical suspicion for venous obstruction remains high (24). Other less-invasive methods of venography include CT and MR-based venography. Both modalities are useful to evaluate central veins and surrounding structures, but limited studies exist to demonstrate their usefulness in primary diagnosis (24).

Due to the high prevalence of underlying thrombophilia in cases of primary UEDVT, some experts recommend including a hypercoagulable workup in the clinical evaluation. Specifics of a hypercoagulable workup are covered in the section "Hypercoagulable Disorders."

Key Diagnostic Dilemma

Acute presentations of UEDVT typically manifest with pain and swelling in the affected arm or neck. However, not all cases of venous obstruction are related to thrombosis, especially in primary cases where anatomic defects contribute to the clinical presentation. In these cases, establishing a diagnosis may not be possible with standard D-dimer and CUS. Catheter venography, as detailed in the section "Diagnosis," provides the best definition of abnormal venous anatomy.

Prognosis

Possible complications that may arise from UEDVT are recurrent thromboembolism, PE, fatal PE, and PTS. Chances of developing

PE are higher in patients with catheters, cancer, and underlying thrombophilia.

Management

There is a lack of randomized controlled trials to guide the treatment of UEDVT. Current management is extrapolated from treatment of LEDVT. Following the ACCP guidelines, anticoagulation is primary recommendation, with a goal to maintain patency of collateral veins, reduce thrombus propagation, and reduce the risk of pulmonary embolization. The length of anticoagulation is typically a minimum of 3 months or for those with a catheter, for the tenure of the catheter (3).

The choice of anticoagulant should be similar to that used for LEDVT. A parenteral anticoagulant, such as LMWH, fondaparinux, and UFH, is initiated. Thereafter, a transition can be made to VKA or continuation with LMWH. The use of DOACs has not been studied in UEDVT, but once again, extrapolation from LEDVT means these are now frequently utilized for acute management of UEDVT with adequate results (3).

Primary Thrombosis

An aggressive approach that includes thrombolysis, thoracic outlet decompression, and venoplasty appears to improve the long-term outcomes in patients with primary UEDVT. If thrombolysis is performed within 2 weeks of the onset of symptoms, restoration of subclavian vein patency is nearly always successful (3). The ACCP current recommendation is that catheter-directed thrombolysis be performed over systemic thrombolysis. Patients most likely to benefit from this intervention include those with the following: severe symptoms at presentation, thrombus involving most of the subclavian vein and the axillary vein, symptoms for <14 days, good functional status, life expectancy of ≥1 year, and low risk for bleeding (3).

Due to the risk of reocclusion even after successful thrombolysis, some experts favor thoracic outlet decompression to provide more space for neurovascular structures of the upper extremity (22). The choice of procedure depends on the specific abnormality. For patients identified with a cervical rib, a cervical rib resection is pursued. If cervical rib is not present, first rib resection is pursued along with dissection of other structures deemed to be contributing to compression of the thoracic outlet (Table 12.15).

The role of venoplasty in the management of primary UEDVT is less clear. There is uniform agreement that thoracic outlet decompression should be done early on, but once this is achieved, there are insufficient data to support the need for venoplasty or vein

Table 12.15 Thoracic Outlet Decompression Procedures
Cervical rib resection
First rib resection
Division of anomalous bands
Division of anomalous musculotendinous insertions
Scalenectomy

repair (21). Overall, if residual or recurrent stenosis occurs, percutaneous transluminal angioplasty may be beneficial.

The ACCP recommends continuation of anticoagulation for a minimum of 3 months regardless of interventions. Longer duration therapy is recommended for those who have had recurrence.

Catheter-Related Thrombosis

When treating CRT, it is essential to consider the status of the catheter, the ongoing need for central access, the presence of prothrombotic states, and contraindications to anticoagulants. CRT is managed more conservatively than primary UEDVT, as the latter has a higher rate of PTS and risk of residual thrombosis. Despite the lack of direct studies to support its safety and efficacy, anticoagulation remains the cornerstone of therapy. For axillary and more proximal vein DVT, the recommendation is to anticoagulate, with or without catheter removal, provided there are no contraindications (3). For isolated brachial vein thrombosis, where the risk of embolization is lower, the intensity and duration of therapy is individualized to the patient and clinical scenario (3).

In patients who have ongoing need for a catheter, its removal is not routinely recommended if the line is functional, not infected, and remains well positioned. Occluded catheters should be replaced, but for patients with limited access sites, salvage may be attempted with fibrinolytic agents. The local instillation of alteplase can restore catheter function in up to 90% of patients (following two doses of 2 mg (25,26). The use of catheter-directed fibrinolytic therapy is more controversial and a risk–benefit assessment should be performed, as this modality is expensive and may increase morbidity. The potential benefit to the patient's clinical status and quality of life should be determined.

Treatment of asymptomatic CRT is controversial. The risk of embolization from asymptomatic subclavian vein thrombosis is unknown, so a risk–benefit analysis is difficult to establish. An argument for pursuing treatment is that an untreated UEDVT may result in permanent obstruction of the affected vein and compromise future central venous access.

Superficial Vein Phlebitis

The risk of pulmonary embolus is quite low from upper extremity superficial vein thrombi. Management is directed toward pain control and comfort. Superficial IV should be removed and all infusions through the vein discontinued. Nonsteroidal anti-inflammatory drugs (NSAIDs), extremity elevation, and warm or cool compresses are used to offer symptomatic relief.

Prophylactic Anticoagulation

The benefit of prophylactic anticoagulation to prevent CRT has not been demonstrated. Current society recommendations do not advocate the use of prophylactic anticoagulation for the sole purposes of preventing CRT, even in high-risk populations such as those with cancer.

Key Points

- CVCs cause endothelial trauma and vein wall inflammation, which can result in thrombosis.
- Risk factors for CRT include catheter-related factors (e.g., catheter malposition, catheter size), the presence of prothrombotic states (congenital or acquired), hormonal therapy, and infusion of irritating substances.
- Primary spontaneous UEDVT is rare and may be associated with underlying thrombophilia or anatomic abnormality.
- Primary UEDVT is best managed by a multidisciplinary approach which includes thrombolysis, thoracic outlet decompression, venoplasty, and anticoagulation—a combination that appears to improve long-term outcomes.

HYPERCOAGULABLE DISORDERS

Clinical Case 12.3

A 32-year-old woman presents to clinic to discuss her recent diagnosis of DVT in her right leg. She has a medical history significant for a prior DVT, which occurred 5 years ago after she returned from a transcontinental flight, for which she was treated with 3 months of warfarin. She expresses a concern because both her mother and sister have a history of DVT. Her mother had a DVT at the age of 43 when she was recovering from an appendectomy, and her sister had a DVT at the age of 28 when she was pregnant with her first child. She wonders if she has an inherited condition that predisposes her to recurrent DVTs and asks if she should be tested.

Introduction

Hypercoagulability, or thrombophilia, refers to a group of conditions that increase the risk of developing venous or arterial thrombi (27). Hypercoagulability is classified as either acquired or inherited, and a careful history and physical exam are paramount to identifying the presence of any risk factors which help to guide the clinician's differential diagnosis and subsequent testing or treatment. Hypercoagulability is a complex condition and its etiologies are not limited to the conventional tests typically ordered in a "hypercoagulable workup," (28) although this is what will be primarily covered in this section. A thorough physical exam should be performed to focus on findings which can elucidate an undiagnosed underlying medical condition. Information to elicit in the interview includes, but is not limited to, the following (27):

- Site of thrombosis
- Previous history of thrombosis
- History of easy bruising or bleeding
- Comorbid medical conditions
- Pregnancy
- Detailed medication list
- Surgical history
- Smoking status
- Family history of thrombotic events
- Results of any previous age-appropriate cancer screening

Laboratory testing is only a portion of the evaluation of a hypercoagulable disorder and comes at a considerable potential cost, both economical and psychological (12). As such, it is reserved for specific situations, and the focus should be on attaining results that have the potential to alter management (28).

Whom to Select for Additional Testing?

Estimates for the monetary cost of hypercoagulability testing can be staggering. One study estimated that to prevent one fatal PE associated with FVL heterozygotes taking OCPs, 92,000 carriers of the gene would need to be identified in the general population and have OCPs withheld with a cost upward of $300 million (28). This example highlights the need to carefully assess the population that will benefit from testing to prevent undue economic and psychological burden.

A history of VTE increases the risk of a second VTE by approximately 30% in 5 to 8 years and is one of the best predictors for future VTE risk (12). However, in the setting of a well-described transient major risk factor, the risk of recurrence is very low (Table 12.7) (12). A history of provoked VTE is not an indication for testing.

Generally speaking, testing may be indicated for the following populations:

- Patients with idiopathic thromboembolism
- Patients with recurrent thromboembolism without discernable transient risk factors
- Age <40 at the time of first thrombosis
- Venous thrombosis in the setting of strong family history of VTE in first-degree relatives
- VTE in an unusual site: cerebral, hepatic, mesenteric, renal
- Warfarin-induced skin necrosis
- Recurrent pregnancy loss
- Neonatal purpura fulminans

Typical Workup

Testing should be done in steps, beginning with the highest yield screening studies performed first, and more focused confirmatory testing done second (Table 12.16) (27). When possible, the workup should be as focused as possible, especially in the setting of workup for guiding decision-making on primary prevention measures (28). The following are the most frequently evaluated etiologies for the typical hypercoagulability workup.

Protein C

Inherited protein C deficiency is an autosomal dominant disorder occurring approximately in 0.14% to 0.5% of the general population (27). Heterozygosity increases the risk of thrombosis by about sevenfold (27). Homozygosity is rare and has severe manifestations, often with neonatal purpura fulminans or disseminated intravascular coagulation (DIC) (27). Typically, patients with this disorder will experience their first VTE at a young age, between 10 and 50 years (27). These patients are at an elevated risk of warfarin-induced skin necrosis, and protein C deficiency should be considered in patients presenting with this condition (27).

There are two types of protein C deficiency: type I is a quantitative deficiency and type II is a qualitative deficiency (27). There are also two types of assays to test for protein C deficiency: functional and antigenic (27). When testing, it is important to first start with the functional assay and follow-up with the quantitative antigenic assay (27). If one were to begin with the quantitative assay, type II deficiencies, which comprise approximately 20% to 25% of all protein C deficiencies, would be missed as the dysfunctional protein would still be detected in normal concentrations.

Table 12.16 Screening and Confirmatory Testing for Hypercoagulable States

Disorder	Protein C Deficiency	Protein S Deficiency	Antithrombin Deficiency	Factor V Leiden	Prothrombin G20210A	Antiphospholipid Syndrome		Hyperhomo-Cysteinemia
Screening test	Protein C functional assay	Protein S functional assay	Antithrombin functional assay	Activated protein C resistance assay	None	PT/aPTT, hexagonal phase phospholipid neutralization	Anticardiolipin antibody assay	Homocysteine level
Confirmatory test	Protein C antigenic assay	Protein S antigenic assay	Antithrombin antigenic assay	Factor V Leiden SNP analysis	Prothrombin G20210A SNP analysis	Lupus anticoagulant testing (DRVVT PNP, incubated aPTT mixing study)	B2GP1 antibody assay	MTHFR SNP analysis*

*Not recommended to test for this as it does not alter management.

aPTT, activated partial thromboplastin time; B2GP1, beta-2 glycoprotein I; DRVVT, dilute Russell's viper venom test; MTHFR, methylenetetrahydrofolate reductase; PNP, platelet neutralization procedure; SNP, single-nucleotide polymorphism.

Acquired protein C deficiencies are more common than inherited ones and should be excluded prior to diagnosing a patient with inherited protein C deficiency (27). Protein C is dependent on vitamin K for synthesis in the liver; also, as such, liver dysfunction and VKA (i.e., warfarin) may alter the results of testing (27). Testing for protein C should be deferred until at least 10 days after discontinuing warfarin therapy to get a reliable result (27). Additional conditions that may transiently depress protein C levels include current or recent thrombosis, intra/postoperative periods, nephrotic syndrome, DIC, and L-asparaginase therapy (27). If initial testing for protein C is abnormal with any of these conditions present, testing should be repeated at a future date when these confounders are no longer present to confirm the initial result. Additionally, pregnancy and OCP use have been associated with elevated levels of protein C, so when testing is normal or inconclusive in the setting of a very high suspicion of disease, repeat testing is also reasonable.

Protein S

Inherited protein S deficiency is an autosomal dominant mutation that affects roughly 0.2% to 0.5% of the general population (27). Homozygosity is rare and presents with DIC or newborn purpura fulminans, similar to those with protein C homozygosity. There are three types of protein S deficiency with types I and III being quantitative and type II being qualitative (Table 12.17). Types I and III both have a low free (unbound) protein S and low protein S activity; however, type I has a low total protein S level and type III has a normal total protein S level (27). Free or unbound protein S is the active form, and it is thought that type III deficiency is likely a problem with excess binding of protein S to C4bBP, reducing the overall active form while keeping a normal total level (27). Type II deficiency is qualitative, and thus, it has a normal total and free protein S level but shows reduced activity (27).

Testing can be done with either functional or antigenic assays. The best test to commence workup is unclear. Functional assays identify all three types of deficiency, but are not specific for protein

Table 12.17 Protein S Deficiency Subtypes

	Type of Defect	Functional Activity	Total Protein	Free/ Unbound
Type I	Quantitative	Decreased	Decreased	Decreased
Type II	Qualitative	Decreased	Normal	Normal
Type III	Quantitative	Decreased	Normal	Decreased

S deficiency, and the presence of FVL mutations or lupus anticoagulant can give a false-positive result (27). This being the case, some opt to use an antigenic assay that identifies type I and III deficiencies, which comprise 95% of all protein S deficiencies (27). While antigenic assays are more specific, they will not identify 5% of protein S deficiencies, namely the Type II subtype (27).

The same conditions that cause acquired protein C deficiency can cause acquired protein S deficiency and should be excluded (27). Protein S can be bound to C4bBP, which is an acute-phase reactant (27). Acute inflammatory or infectious states increase the levels of C4bBP, thus increasing the proportion of bound, or the inactive, protein S, resulting in abnormal functional assay results (27). Interpretation of protein S results can be particularly challenging (28). Women may have lower levels of protein S in the setting of OCP use, hormone replacement therapy, or during the last two trimesters of pregnancy (27). Testing that is positive during any of these situations must be repeated when these conditions have resolved to confirm a true protein S deficiency (27). One should also give attention to age- and sex-specific reference ranges for the particular assay being used for more accurate interpretation (28).

Antithrombin

Inherited antithrombin deficiency is autosomal dominant, present in 0.05% to 0.1% of the general population, and carries the highest risk of thrombosis of any of the heritable hypercoagulable disorders (27). Like proteins C and S, antithrombin is made in the liver, but differs in that it is not vitamin K dependent (27). As expected, antithrombin deficiency is associated with DVTs and PEs, but may also present with thromboses in unusual veins (27). Cerebral, mesenteric, portal, or renal vein thrombosis should raise suspicion for the presence of an antithrombin deficiency (27). Patients often experience their first thrombosis at a young age, but it is atypical for the first episode to occur in those <20 years old unless another heritable risk factor, like FVL, is present (27). A little over half of patients experience a spontaneous thrombosis as their first manifestation, while the others have at least one transient, preventable risk factor.

Like proteins C and S, both functional and antigenic assays are there for antithrombin. Typically, functional assays are run first for screening purposes and if the functional level is low, another sample is run for confirmation with both a functional assay and an antigenic assay (27). This allows for differentiation of the two types of deficiency: type I, a quantitative deficiency, or type II, a qualitative deficiency. Both types of deficiency have low levels on a functional assay, but type II has higher antigen levels relative to functional levels when compared to type I.

Acquired deficiencies of antithrombin must be ruled out when testing is positive. The list of causes is extensive and includes use of drugs (like heparin, OCPs, or L-asparaginase), liver disease, nephrotic syndrome, protein-losing enteropathies, DIC, sepsis, burns, trauma, pregnancy, metastatic tumors, hematomas, surgery requiring cardiopulmonary bypass, hepatic veno-occlusive disease, or thrombotic microangiopathies; deficiencies even occur in premenopausal women (27). As with other hypercoagulable disorders, repeat testing should be done to confirm positive results upon resolution of any of the previously listed conditions (27).

Factor V Leiden

The FVL mutation is a heritable hypercoagulability and is the most common cause of activated protein C (APC) resistance (27). Heterozygosity for the mutation is the most common hereditary risk factor for VTE with a high overall prevalence (27). It is estimated that 3% to 5% of Caucasians carry at least one copy of the gene. The mutation is rare in other ethnicities, namely, African, Australian, and South Asian populations (27). Heterozygosity for this gene increases VTE risk from fourfold to eightfold, while homozygosity raises the risk of thrombosis 80-fold (27). Additional risk factors for thrombosis dramatically increase the risk of thrombosis in this population. For example, females who are heterozygous for the FVL mutation have increased thrombotic risk from 30- to 60-fold while using OCPs (27).

Screening for FVL is done by running an APC resistance assay and, if abnormal, performing confirmatory testing with DNA analysis (27). False-positive results with an APC assay can occur in the setting of other causes of prolonged aPTT, such as anticoagulant medication use, liver disease, and in patients with low protein S or elevated factor VIII levels (27). Of note, DNA analysis for FVL will not detect other hereditary mutations that contribute to APC resistance, such as FV Cambridge, FV Liverpool, FV Nara and FV Bonn.

Prothrombin G20210A

Another heritable hypercoagulability is a gain-of-function mutation in prothrombin gene G20210A (PT20210) which results in increased prothrombin levels, also called factor II (27). While the mechanism is unclear, studies have found an estimated threefold increase in the risk of thrombosis in those who are heterozygous for the mutation (27). The prevalence is lower than FVL in the general population and can be found in 1% to 3% of individuals. Like FVL, prevalence varies based on ethnicity: 2% to 4% of Europeans carry the mutation and it is rarely found in Asians, Native Americans, and Africans (27). There is no initial screening test for PT20210, and the initial testing uses DNA/polymerase chain reaction (PCR)-based methods for diagnosis.

Antiphospholipid Antibody Syndrome

Antiphospholipid syndrome is a common acquired hypercoagulable disorder and is present in 3% to 5% of the population (27). This condition has an association with venous or arterial thrombosis as well as recurrent pregnancy loss. Diagnosis requires clinical and laboratory criteria as outlined in the following (27):

Clinical criteria (either/or):

- Vascular thrombosis: One or more clinical episodes of arterial, venous, or small vessel thrombosis in any tissue or organ. Thrombotic changes need to be confirmed by imaging studies or pathology
- Pregnancy morbidity as determined by:
  1. One or more unexplained deaths in a morphologically normal fetus at or beyond 10 weeks of gestation
  2. One or more premature births of a morphologically normal neonate before 34th week of gestation due to preeclampsia or placental insufficiency
  3. Three or more unexplained consecutive spontaneous abortions before 10 weeks of gestation, with maternal anatomic and/or hormonal abnormalities and paternal and maternal chromosomal causes excluded

Laboratory criteria require one of the following on at least two separate occasions at least 12 weeks apart:

- Positive lupus anticoagulant
- Cardiolipin antibody, IgM, or IgG, in medium or high titer
- Beta-2 glycoprotein I (B2GP1) antibodies, IgM, or IgG, in medium or high titer

The following four criteria must all be met in the interpretation of laboratory findings to confirm the presence of lupus anticoagulant as well.

- Prolongation of at least one phospholipid-dependent clotting test (aPTT, dilute Russell's viper venom test [DRVVT], hexagonal phospholipid neutralization screen)
- Inhibitory activity demonstrated by a mixing study

- Demonstrated phospholipid inhibitor dependence with reduction of clotting time after addition of more phospholipid
- Presence of specific factor inhibitors, including anticoagulants, should be excluded

False-negative lupus anticoagulant results may be found if tested in the acute phase of a thrombosis or in responses with elevated factor VIII levels. Additionally, patients on warfarin should not be tested until they have been off the medication for 1 to 2 weeks and when the INR is <1.5. False positives are also common and careful selection of patients for lupus anticoagulant testing reduces the likelihood of obtaining a false-positive result. There are three grades of recommendation for patients who should be tested (27):

- Low grade: Elderly patients with venous or arterial thrombosis
- Moderate grade: Young patients with a provoked VTE, asymptomatic patients with a prolonged aPTT, or those with recurrent early pregnancy loss
- High grade: Unprovoked VTE and arterial thromboses in patients under 50 years old, thrombosis at unusual sites, late pregnancy loss, thrombosis or pregnancy morbidities in the setting of an autoimmune disease

Transient positivity for anticardiolipin and B2GP1 antibodies secondary to infection or drugs is common; thus, it is recommended to retest in 12 weeks to confirm persistent positivity (27). It should be noted that these transient positive results have not been shown to be associated with elevated thrombotic risk.

Homocysteine

Homocysteine is an intermediate amino acid in the folate cycle and is the product of methionine demethylation by methylenetetrahydrofolate reductase (MTHFR). Very high levels of homocysteine, which occur in homocystinuria, an inborn error of metabolism, have been associated with not only VTE, but also coronary heart disease, acute myocardial infarction, peripheral artery disease, strokes, aneurysm, migraines, hypertension, male infertility, neural tube defects of offspring, and recurrent pregnancy loss (27).

Mild hyperhomocysteinemia can be acquired or hereditary. The etiologies of mild acquired hyperhomocysteinemia include deficiency of vitamin B6, vitamin B12, or folate; renal failure; hypothyroidism; rheumatoid arthritis; or the use of certain drugs (methotrexate, niacin, anticonvulsants, theophylline, L-dopa, thiazides, cyclosporine A, or phenytoin) (27). Mild hereditary hyperhomocysteinemia is caused due to mutations in the *MTHFR* gene.

Polymorphisms of *MTHFR* are common, and alterations are found in up to 40% of the general population with 10% to 13% of the population being homozygous for these mutations (29). Two polymorphisms, known as c.665C->T and c.1286A->C, have been associated with a mildly increased risk of venous thrombosis and recurrent pregnancy loss. Most recent studies have revealed that the thrombotic risk associated with mild hyperhomocysteinemia is lower than previously thought, with some epidemiologic studies reporting no increased risk when confounding variables were included in the analysis (29). Moreover, reducing the levels of homocysteine with vitamin B supplementation, as is a traditional practice, does not reduce VTE incidence. Hence, newest recommendations are against the routine testing for *MTHFR* mutations in patients with VTE.

Additional Testing

When appropriate, additional testing may be warranted based on a patient's clinical presentation, such as atypical thrombi sites (Table 12.18). Myeloproliferative neoplasms (MPNs), paroxysmal nocturnal hemoglobinuria (PNH), or malignancies can all increase the risk of thrombosis (28). Testing directed to specific conditions which will further guide management should be done in the appropriate clinical context. Furthermore, a hypercoagulable workup should always include age-appropriate cancer screening as part

Table 12.18 Atypical Venous Thromboembolism Sites

Specified Site of VTE	Associated Hypercoagulable States
Budd–Chiari	MPN, IBD, OCPs, abdominal infection, abdominal malignancy, hereditary hypercoagulable state, Behcet's
Splanchnic vein thrombosis	MPN, PNH, APA, hormonal therapy, abdominal malignancy, IBD
Ovarian vein thrombosis	Pregnancy, postpartum state, surgical manipulation
Cerebral venous sinus thrombosis	OCPs, autoimmune disease (SLE, sarcoidosis, Behcet's), MPN, hereditary hypercoagulable state, nephrotic syndrome, malignancy, head injury

APA, antiphospholipid antibody; IBD, inflammatory bowel disease; MPN, myeloproliferative neoplasm; OCPs, oral contraceptive pills; PNH, paroxysmal nocturnal hemoglobinuria; SLE, systemic lupus erythematosus; VTE, venous thromboembolism.

of the standard workup as patients with undiagnosed malignancy have high risk of "unprovoked" VTE (30). More extensive cancer screening with CT imaging may be warranted in patients with unprovoked DVT (30).

Timing of Testing

As discussed with several of the conditions presented herein, multiple factors can affect the reliability of testing. Much of the hypercoagulable workup uses assays and tests affected by acute thrombosis or anticoagulant therapy, with the exception of genetic testing and antibodies for cardiolipin and β2GP1 (28). Due to inconsistencies among labs, it is recommended to defer testing during acute thrombosis and anticoagulant therapy. Alternatively, a two-step approach can be taken. Step one would be molecular testing for FVL and PT20210, as well as serology testing for cardiolipin and β2GP1 antibody titers, since these are unlikely to be affected by acute VTE or anticoagulation. Anticoagulation can be held after 3 months of therapy. Step 2 is when the remainder of the workup is sent, the gamut of functional protein assays, preferably 2 to 4 weeks after anticoagulation has been held. This timeline also allows for optimal testing of D-dimer, if this is pursued for future VTE risk assessment (28). Once the results of testing are available, the decision to resume anticoagulation can be made.

Goal of Testing

Overall, positive test results rarely affect long-term management. Most studies suggest that after a first episode of VTE, testing for a heritable hypercoagulable condition does not reduce the risk of having a second VTE (12). Having a thrombophilia also does not change the likelihood that a person will survive a thrombotic event and it does not predict or change the odds that a patient will develop PTS (28). Testing should be pursued only if it can improve or modify management.

In patients with an identifiable, transient risk factor that caused a "provoked" VTE, the risk of recurrence is no different between a patient with a heritable hypercoagulability and one without an identifiable hypercoagulability (28). Even with a positive test, a 3- to 6-month course of anticoagulation for treatment of a first thrombosis is still the initial treatment recommendation because the benefit of continuing indefinite anticoagulation does not outweigh the overall risk of bleeding complications (12). In other words, the recommendation for a time-limited course of treatment remains the same, regardless of the presence of a hypercoagulability (28). In instances when testing is performed and positive, clinicians tend to overestimate the risk of recurrence, subsequently prescribing extended courses of anticoagulation, potentially exposing patients to excessive risk of bleeding complications (28). For this reason, testing for a hypercoagulable disorder is not recommended after an episode of provoked VTE.

In patients without an identifiable transient risk factor leading to an episode of VTE ("unprovoked"), the 5-year risk of recurrence is close to 30% (28). Again, there is no conclusive evidence that testing for heritable hypercoagulable disorders changes the rates of recurrent VTE. With this in mind, the current recommendation is for indefinite anticoagulation in the absence of contraindications regardless of negative hypercoagulability testing (12). Thus, hypercoagulability testing after unprovoked DVT will not change management. One exception is the patient with an unprovoked VTE and low bleeding risk whose preference it is to stop anticoagulation despite recommendations. Testing may uncover additional, non-modifiable risk factors that suggest higher thrombotic risk (28). That being said, it is important to note that negative thrombophilia testing in an unprovoked DVT does not reduce the aforementioned recurrence risk.

Often, patients with no personal history but a strong family history of VTE will request testing for hypercoagulable disorders. A family history of VTE is a significant risk factor for VTE (28). Yet, the overall risk of bleeding complications from anticoagulation for primary prevention generally outweighs the risk of a first unprovoked VTE; so, anticoagulation for primary prevention is not recommended. However, appropriate prophylaxis in the presence of transient provoking factors for VTE may be indicated for patients with a strong family history of VTE (28). Some studies have shown that testing positive for a hypercoagulable disorder may improve compliance with prophylaxis in high-risk situations; however, the converse is also true. Patients with negative testing are less likely to comply with prophylaxis despite their family history, resulting in false sense of security and potential harm. Overall, testing is still not recommended for patients with strong family history. Instead, counseling is provided to patients on using prophylaxis when exposed to high-risk situations (i.e., immobility, extended travel), given their increased risk of VTE (28).

A well-described risk factor for VTE is the use of estrogen-containing medications. Their use in the setting of heritable hypercoagulable disorders increases the relative risk of VTE; so, some have suggested testing patients with a family history of VTE to guide use of primary prevention in patients using these medications (28). However, the absolute risk of thrombosis remains low, especially in the younger population of patients who are likely to be considering OCP use (28). Moreover, family history of VTE in one or more first-degree relatives predicts an elevated risk of estrogen-associated VTE regardless of thrombophilia findings. Hence, thrombophilia testing is not recommended and instead, the use of estrogen-sparing OCP preparations, such as progestin-based intrauterine devices, should be considered for these patients (28).

Pregnancy increases the relative risk of VTE by fivefold to 10-fold in the general population, and a hypercoagulability increases this risk by another sevenfold (28). Women with a history of unprovoked VTE or a prior VTE provoked by pregnancy or estrogen-containing medications should be placed on VTE prophylaxis during pregnancy. Thrombophilia testing will not alter this recommendation. Pregnant patients with a first-degree relative with VTE do not appear to be at significant risk of VTE in the absence of thrombophilia; hence, routine thrombophilia testing is not recommended in asymptomatic family members who are considering pregnancy. On the other hand, if there is a known thrombophilia diagnosis, and that thrombophilia (i.e., homozygous FVL, homozygous PT20210, combined heterozygote FVL/PT20210, and antithrombin deficiency) would alter VTE prophylaxis recommendations, then testing is a reasonable course of action (Table 12.19).

Hypercoagulable disorders are a complicated and complex group of diseases and can pose a challenge to even well-seasoned clinicians. When the results of testing are indeterminate or the recommendations for treatment or prophylaxis are not clear, referral to a specialist with experience in VTE is preferred (12).

Key Points

- Testing for hereditary hypercoagulable conditions rarely changes clinical management of most patients with VTE; hence, routine testing is not recommended for primary or secondary prevention.

- An exception would be an asymptomatic woman of fertile age, with family history of VTE and *known* thrombophilic defect, as testing may lead to a decision to instill prophylactic anticoagulation in the antepartum or postpartum period as well as the individual decision to not use estrogen-containing OCPs.

- Testing for a hypercoagulable disorder is not recommended after an episode of provoked VTE.

- Clinical history and site of thrombosis are important considerations, as they may indicate the need to test for acquired hypercoagulable conditions, which are important to identify as they would affect long-term management for the patient: malignancy, MPNs, PNH, and APAS.

Table 12.19 Anticoagulation Recommendations for Pregnant Women With Inherited Thrombophilias

Clinical Scenario	Antepartum Management	Postpartum Management
Low-risk thrombophilia No personal or family history of VTE	Surveillance	Surveillance
Low-risk thrombophilia with a family history of VTE	Surveillance	Prophylactic anticoagulation
Low-risk thrombophilia with a previous episode of VTE, not taking long-term anticoagulation therapy	Prophylactic LMWH/ UFH or surveillance	Prophylactic anticoagulation
High risk thrombophilia without a previous VTE and positive family history	Prophylactic anticoagulation	Prophylactic anticoagulation
High-risk thrombophilia, with no prior personal or family history of VTE	Surveillance	Prophylactic anticoagulation
No thrombophilia with previous single episode of VTE associated with transient risk factor that is no longer present, excluding pregnancy- or estrogen-related risk factor	Surveillance	Prophylactic anticoagulation
No thrombophilia with previous single episode of VTE associated with transient risk factor that was pregnancy or estrogen related	Prophylactic anticoagulation with LMWH/UFH	Prophylactic anticoagulation
No thrombophilia with previous single episode of unprovoked VTE not receiving long-term anticoagulation therapy	Prophylactic anticoagulation with LMWH/UFH	Prophylactic anticoagulation
Thrombophilia or no thrombophilia with more than two episodes of VTE, not receiving long-term anticoagulation therapy	Prophylactic or therapeutic dose of LMWH or UFH	Prophylactic or therapeutic dose anticoagulation

(*continued*)

Table 12.19 Anticoagulation Recommendations for Pregnant Women With Inherited Thrombophilias (*continued*)

Clinical Scenario	Antepartum Management	Postpartum Management
Thrombophilia or no thrombophilia with more than two episodes of VTE, receiving long-term anticoagulation therapy	Therapeutic dose LMWH or UFH	Resume long-term anticoagulation therapy

- Low-risk thrombophilia: FVL heterozygosity, PT20210 heterozygosity, protein C and protein S deficiency
- High-risk thrombophilia: FVL homozygosity, PT20210 homozygosity, heterozygosity for combined FVL/PT20210, and AT deficiency
- Suggested period of anticoagulation for postpartum management is 6 weeks
- For postpartum anticoagulation, it is not necessary to utilize LMWH or UFH; however, if DOACs are used, the clinician must confirm that the mother will not be breastfeeding, as these agents are excreted in breast milk

Note: Recommendations listed in this table are a summary of those made by the American College of Obstetricians and Gynecologists and the ACCP. The specific guidelines for both these organizations may sometimes document the use of prophylactic or intermediate-dose anticoagulation. Since there is no consensus on what intermediate-dose anticoagulation constitutes, this aspect has not been summarized in this table.

LMWH, low-molecular-weight heparin; UFH, unfractionated heparin; VTE, venous thromboembolism.

REFERENCES

1. Naess IA, Christiansen SC, Romundstad P, et al. Incidence and mortality of venous thrombosis: A population-based study. *J Thromb Haemost*. 2007;5(4):692–699. doi:10.1111/j.1538-7836.2007.02450.x
2. Ocak G, Vossen CY, Verduijn M, et al. Risk of venous thrombosis in patients with major illnesses: Results from the MEGA study. *J Thromb Haemost*. 2013;11(1):116–123. doi:10.1111/jth.12043
3. Kearon C, Akl EA, Ornelas J, et al. Antithrombotic therapy for VTE disease: CHEST guideline and expert panel report. *Chest*. 2016;149(2):315–352. doi:10.1016/j.chest.2015.11.026
4. Wells PS, Anderson DR, Bormanis J, et al. Value of assessment of pretest probability of deep-vein thrombosis in clinical management. *Lancet*. 1997;350(9094):1795–1798. doi:10.1016/S0140-6736(97)08140-3
5. Le Gal G, Kovacs MJ, Carrier M, et al. Validation of a diagnostic approach to exclude recurrent venous thromboembolism. *J Thromb Haemost*. 2009;7(5):752–759. doi:10.1111/j.1538-7836.2009.03324.x

6. van Dongen CJ, Prandoni P, Frulla M, et al. Relation between quality of anticoagulant treatment and the development of the postthrombotic syndrome. *J Thromb Haemost*. 2005;3(5):939–942. doi:10.1111/j.1538-7836.2005.01333.x

7. Decousus H, Leizorovicz A, Parent F, et al. A clinical trial of vena caval filters in the prevention of pulmonary embolism in patients with proximal deep-vein thrombosis. *N Engl J Med*. 1998;338(7):409–415. doi:10.1056/NEJM199802123380701

8. Hurst DR, Forauer AR, Bloom JR, et al. Diagnosis and endovascular treatment of iliocaval compression syndrome. *J Vasc Surg*. 2001;34(1):106–113.doi:10.1067/mva.2001.114213

9. Khorana AA, Francis CW. Risk prediction of cancer-associated thrombosis: appraising the first decade and developing the future. *Thromb Res*. 2018;164(Suppl 1):S70–S76. doi:10.1016/j.thromres.2018.01.036

10. Bates SM, Rajasekhar A, Middeldorp S, et al. American Society of Hematology 2018 guidelines for management of venous thromboembolism: venous thromboembolism in the context of pregnancy. *Blood Adv*. 2018;2(22):3317–3359. doi:10.1182/bloodadvances.2018024802

11. Pengo V, Denas G, Zoppellaro G, et al. Rivaroxaban vs warfarin in high-risk patients with antiphospholipid syndrome. *Blood*. 2018;132(13):1365–1371. doi:10.1182/blood-2018-04-848333

12. Middeldorp S. Inherited thrombophilia: a double-edged sword. *ASH Education Book*. 2016;1:1–9. doi:10.1182/asheducation-2016.1.1

13. Meyer G. Effective diagnosis and treatment of pulmonary embolism: improving patient outcomes. *Arch Cardiovasc Dis*. 2014;107(6–7):406–414. doi:10.1016/j.acvd.2014.05.006

14. Barco S, Konstantinides SV. Risk-adapted management of pulmonary embolism. *Thromb Res*. 2017;151(Suppl 1):S92–S96. doi:10.1016/S0049-3848(17)30076-2

15. Becattini C, Agnelli G. Risk stratification and management of acute pulmonary embolism. *ASH Education Book*. 2016;1:404–412. doi:10.1182/asheducation-2016.1.404

16. Ruggiero A, Screaton NJ. Imaging of acute and chronic thromboembolic disease: state of the art. *Clin Radiol*. 2017;72(5):375–388. doi:10.1016/j.crad.2017.02.011

17. van Belle A, Büller HR, Huisman MV, et al. Effectiveness of managing suspected pulmonary embolism using an algorithm combining clinical probability, D-dimer testing, and computed tomography. *JAMA*. 2006;295(2):172–179. doi:10.1001/jama.295.2.172

18. Robbins IM, Pugh ME, Hemnes AR. Update on chronic thromboembolic pulmonary hypertension. *Trends Cardiovasc Med*. 2017;27(1):29–37. doi:10.1016/j.tcm.2016.05.010

19. Chiu V, O'Connell C. Management of the incidental pulmonary embolism. *AJR Am J Roentgenol.* 2017;208(3):485–488. doi:10.2214/AJR.16.17201

20. Klok FA, Huisman MV. Management of incidental pulmonary embolism. *Eur Respir J.* 2017;49(6):1700275. doi:10.1183/13993003.00275-2017

21. Illig KA, Doyle AJ. A comprehensive review of Paget-Schroetter syndrome. *J Vasc Surg.* 2010;51(6):1538–1547. doi:10.1016/j.jvs.2009.12.022

22. Mustafa S, Stein PD, Patel KC, et al. Upper extremity deep venous thrombosis. *Chest.* 2003;123(6):1953–1956. doi:10.1378/chest.123.6.1953

23. Kleinjan A, Di Nisio M, Beyer-Westendorf J, et al. Safety and feasibility of a diagnostic algorithm combining clinical probability, d-dimer testing, and ultrasonography for suspected upper extremity deep venous thrombosis: a prospective management study. *Ann Intern Med.* 2014;160(7):451–457. doi:10.7326/M13-2056

24. Di Nisio M, Van Sluis GL, Bossuyt PMM, et al. Accuracy of diagnostic tests for clinically suspected upper extremity deep vein thrombosis: a systematic review. *J Thromb Haemost.* 2010;8(4):684–692. doi:10.1111/j.1538-7836.2010.03771.x

25. Rajasekhar A, Streiff MB. How I treat central venous access device-related upper extremity deep vein thrombosis. *Blood.* 2017;129(20):2727–2736. doi:10.1182/blood-2016-08-693671

26. Semba CP, Deitcher SR, Li X, et al. Treatment of occluded central venous catheters with alteplase: results in 1,064 patients. *J Vasc Interv Radiol.* 2002;13(12):1199–1205. doi:10.1016/S1051-0443(07)61965-4

27. Nakashima MO, Rogers HJ. Hypercoagulable states: an algorithmic approach to laboratory testing and update on monitoring of direct oral anticoagulants. *Blood Res.* 2014;49(2):85–94. doi:10.5045/br.2014.49.2.85

28. Stevens SM, Woller SC, Bauer KA, et al. Guidance for the evaluation and treatment of hereditary and acquired thrombophilia. *J Thromb Thrombolysis.* 2016;41(1):154–164. doi:10.1007/s11239-015-1316-1

29. Ospina-Romero M, Cannegieter SC, den Heijer M, et al. Hyperhomocysteinemia and risk of first venous thrombosis: the influence of (unmeasured) confounding factors. *Am J Epidemiol.* 2018;187(7):1392–1400. doi:10.1093/aje/kwy004

30. Carrier M, Le Gal G, Wells PS, et al. Systematic review: the Trousseau syndrome revisited: should we screen extensively for cancer in patients with venous thromboembolism? *Ann Intern Med.* 2008;149(5):323–333. doi:10.7326/0003-4819-149-5-200809020-00007

13 Lymphoid Disorders

Elaine Chang and Samer A. Srour

LYMPHADENOPATHY

Clinical Case 13.1

A 28-year-old male presented with a 2-week history of bilateral cervical lymphadenopathy (LAD) and 1 week of fever, decreased appetite, epigastric discomfort, and shortness of breath. His past medical and family histories were unremarkable. On examination, he had enlarged bilateral neck and supraclavicular lymph nodes and the largest one measured 1.5 cm and was firm and mobile. The spleen was palpated 3 cm below the costal margin. Initial laboratory examination revealed a white blood cell (WBC) count of 4,700 cells/mm³, hemoglobin 11.8 g/dL, mean corpuscular volume (MCV) 89 fL, platelets 462,000/µL, creatinine 1.0 mg/dL, alanine aminotransferase (ALT) 51 U/L, and aspartate aminotransferase (AST) 56 U/L.

Introduction

The differential diagnosis for a patient presenting with LAD (defined as size >1 cm in adults) is broad. Only 1.1% of patients presenting to a primary care physician with unexplained LAD are diagnosed with a malignancy (1,2). In addition to history and physical exam, age has the highest impact on cancer risk. Even so, only 4% of patients with unexplained LAD above the age of 40 will have a malignant neoplasm (1,2). In healthy children, 45% to 57% may have palpable LAD at any one time (3).

LAD is best approached by location (Table 13.1). Detailed history is important (Table 13.2). The major categories to consider when evaluating LAD are infectious, autoimmune, malignant, and idiopathic (Box 13.1). Medications are a cause of generalized LAD, which is frequently overlooked by clinicians. Phenytoin and carbamazepine are the most notorious offenders, with hypersensitivity reaction being the explanatory mechanism (4,5).

Table 13.1 Common Causes of Lymphadenopathy, by Location

Location	Benign Causes	Malignant Causes
Cervical	EBV, CMV, toxoplasmosis, mycobacteria (typical and atypical), dental abscess, cat scratch disease	Lymphoma, head and neck squamous cell carcinoma, thyroid cancer
Preauricular	Viral or bacterial conjunctivitis, cat scratch disease	
Postauricular, suboccipital	Rubella infection, bacterial or fungal infections of parietotemporal scalp	
Supraclavicular	(High risk of malignancy, especially in patients over the age of 40.) Fungal and mycobacterial infections	Right: Lung, esophagus Left: Abdominal (stomach, gallbladder, pancreas, kidneys, testicles, ovaries, lymphoma, prostate)
Axillary	Cat scratch disease and other infections of the arm, thoracic wall, and breast; silicone breast implants (inflammatory foreign body reaction)	Breast cancer or metastases from other primary cancer sites
Epitrochlear	Forearm or hand infections, tularemia, secondary syphilis	Lymphoma, sarcoidosis
Inguinal	Lower extremity infection, sexually transmitted diseases	Cancer of the skin of lower extremities or trunk, anogenital, rectal, ovarian

CMV, cytomegalovirus; EBV, Epstein–Barr virus.

Highlighted in the following are a few clinical points and a comparison table for rare idiopathic-inflammatory causes:

- **Infection**: LAD is a common presentation of HIV infection in any stage of the disease. Biopsy should be considered in HIV patients, given the increased risk of lymphomas and opportunistic infections (particularly, fungal infections).
- **Immune:** Generalized LAD can be the presenting symptom of systemic lupus erythematosus.
- **Malignant**: Differential diagnosis includes lymphoma (non-Hodgkin and Hodgkin) and metastases from carcinoma, sarcoma, or melanoma.

Table 13.2 Approach to Lymphadenopathy by Epidemiologic Clues

Risk Factor	Suggested Diagnoses
High-risk sexual behavior	Chancroid (*Haemophilus ducreyi*), HIV infection, lymphogranuloma venereum (*Chlamydia trachomatis*), syphilis
Joint stiffness or swelling, rash, muscle weakness	Rheumatoid arthritis, systemic lupus erythematosus, Sjögren syndrome, dermatomyositis
Animal or food contact	
Cats	Bartonellosis (cat scratch disease), toxoplasmosis
Rabbits, sheep, cattle	Anthrax, brucellosis, tularemia
Undercooked meat	Anthrax, brucellosis, toxoplasmosis
Travel	
Southwestern United States	Coccidioidomycosis, bubonic plague (*Yersinia pestis*)
Southeastern United States	Histoplasmosis
Asia	Scrub typhus (*Orientia tsutsugamushi*)
Africa	African trypanosomiasis (sleeping sickness), leishmaniasis (kala-azar)
Any developing country	Typhoid fever (*Salmonella eneterica*), extrapulmonary tuberculosis

- **Posttransplant lymphoproliferative disorder (PTLD)**: The majority of cases are associated with Epstein–Barr virus (EBV) and the intensity of the immunosuppressive regimen impairing T-cell–mediated EBV-directed immunity.

   Approximately 90% of the U.S. population is infected with EBV by age 25. In immunocompromised hosts, EBV can manifest with LAD. In patients with solid organ or hematologic transplant, PTLD can range from an infectious mononucleosis-like syndrome (with fever, pharyngitis, cervical LAD, hepatosplenomegaly, atypical lymphocytosis) to monomorphic PTLD which is considered a lymphoma.

- **Idiopathic-inflammatory**: See Table 13.3.

Diagnosis

The history and physical examination frequently identify the underlying cause of LAD. Location helps to narrow the differential to a specific etiology. Key features include: duration of LAD, associated

Box 13.1 Causes of Lymphadenopathy

I. Infection: The differential varies depending on the immunocompetence of the host, but may include bacterial diseases (atypical mycobacteria, *Bartonella*, chancroid, syphilis, tuberculosis, tularemia, *Rickettsia*), viruses (Epstein–Barr virus, cytomegalovirus, adenovirus, rubella, hepatitis), fungal (histoplasmosis, cryptococcosis), and parasitic (filariasis, toxoplasmosis, trypanosomiasis)

II. Immune Disorders: Immunodeficiency (autoimmune lymphadenopathy/Canale–Smith syndrome), HIV, posttransplant lymphoproliferative disorder, and rheumatologic (dermatomyositis, granulomatosis with polyangiitis, mixed connective tissue disease, rheumatoid arthritis, Sjögren syndrome, Still's disease, systemic lupus erythematosus)

III. Malignant: Hodgkin lymphoma, non-Hodgkin lymphoma, dermatopathic lymphadenitis, metastases from solid tumors

IV. Idiopathic-Inflammatory: Castleman's (unicentric and multicentric), IgG4-related disease, inflammatory myofibroblastic tumor, Kikuchi–Fujimoto disease, Kimura's disease, Rosai–Dorfman disease, sarcoidosis

V. Drugs: Allopurinol, antiepileptics (carbamazepine, phenytoin, primidone), aspirin, atenolol, captopril, erythromycin, gold, hydralazine, penicillins, pyrimethamine, quinidine, sulindac, trimethoprim/sulfamethoxazole, and other sulfa drugs

VI. Metabolic: Lipid storage diseases (Niemann–Pick)

VII. Endocrine Disorders: Hyperthyroidism

VIII. Other: Amyloidosis (usually AL subtype), severe hypertriglyceridemia, dermatopathic lymphadenitis, vascular transformation of lymph node sinuses, silicosis, berylliosis

symptoms (local and/or constitutional symptoms), age, distribution, and history of immunodeficiency or autoimmune disease (Figure 13.1, Tables 13.1, 13.2, and Box 13.1). In a young patient with LAD for <2 weeks or resolving LAD, the concern for malignancy is low and biopsy is not as critical. Workup of the patient in the case scenario revealed infectious mononucleosis. If a patient has multiple risk factors for malignancy (older patient with smoking history, weight loss, supraclavicular location), a lymph node (LN) biopsy is indicated.

For patients with localized LAD, attention to the anatomic drainage and clinical symptoms and signs of skin/soft tissue infection or malignancy should guide evaluation and LN biopsy (Table 13.1). If there is suspicion for an underlying malignancy, then a biopsy should be pursued without delay (Figure 13.1).

In generalized LAD, the history and physical exam provide a framework for diagnostic evaluation. If there are any concerns of

Table 13.3 Benign Idiopathic-Inflammatory Causes of Lymphadenopathy

	Epidemiology	Signs/Symptoms	Diagnostic Pearls	Prognosis
UCD (6)	• Usually younger age (fourth decade) compared to multicentric disease • **Not typically associated with HHV-8**	• Often asymptomatic and discovered incidentally, usually in the mediastinum or hilum • Laboratory abnormalities uncommon	Differential diagnosis (depending on the histological variant) includes: • HIV lymphadenitis • Toxoplasma lymphadenitis (more commonly affects peripheral lymph nodes) • Follicular hyperplasia • Non-Hodgkin lymphoma	• **Excision** is the gold standard treatment and curative in 95% of cases
Castleman's, multicentric (7–9)	• Strong association with HIV infection • Associated with HHV-8 in 50% of immune competent and almost **all HIV patients** • Median age of presentation: 50s in immune competent, 40s in HIV patients	• **B symptoms, chest or peripheral LAD, hepatosplenomegaly, and multiorgan dysfunction** • Elevated inflammatory markers (ESR, CRP, polyclonal hypergammaglobulinemia) • Lung pathology (subpleural nodules, interlobular septal thickening, peribronchovascular thickening, ground glass opacities, pleural effusions, patchy consolidations	• Biopsy required • Rule out infection (EBV, histoplasmosis) and lymphoma • PET-CT should demonstrate multiple slightly enlarged nodes with borderline elevated FDG uptake ($SUV_{max} = 2–5$) • International Working Group criteria were published in 2017 for IMCD	• Can be **rapidly progressive** and lead to death within weeks without chemotherapy • **Indolent**, stable but persisting for years • **Episodic**, remitting and relapsing

(continued)

Table 13.3 Benign Idiopathic-Inflammatory Causes of Lymphadenopathy (*continued*)

	Epidemiology	Signs/Symptoms	Diagnostic Pearls	Prognosis
IgG4-RD (10–12)	• More than 60% males affected • Median age: 60s • Found in 80% of patients with autoimmune pancreatitis	• Range of clinical presentations is wide • Usually **subacute, in an organ** • Asthma or allergy symptoms in approximately 40% of patients • Systemic symptoms typically not present, though multiorgan involvement may be associated with weight loss. Often diagnosed incidentally (abnormal radiology or biopsy for another indication) • Symptomatic disease may present with salivary or lacrimal gland enlargement, thyroiditis, interstitial pneumonitis, or tubulointerstitial nephritis	• Histopathologic diagnosis can be difficult because finding **increased numbers of IgG4+ plasma cells is not specific for IgG4-RD** • Biopsy should be performed in organs other than lymph nodes if possible • Assess for key morphology (whorled, dense lymphoplasmacytic infiltrate and mild/moderate eosinophil infiltrate) • In the late phase, fibrosis may predominate • Closest mimicker is lymphoma	• Variable • **Usually remitting and relapsing course** • Some have complications of organ failure (portal hypertension/cirrhosis due to sclerosing cholangitis, diabetes mellitus from autoimmune pancreatitis, etc.)

(*continued*)

Table 13.3 Benign Idiopathic-Inflammatory Causes of Lymphadenopathy (*continued*)

	Epidemiology	Signs/Symptoms	Diagnostic Pearls	Prognosis
IMT, also known as inflammatory pseudotumor, plasma cell granuloma, histiocytoma, fibroxanthoma (13)	• Fifty percent of the patients are <40 years of age • No gender or ethnic predilection	• Variable presentation • **Two thirds of patients are asymptomatic** • Symptoms are **usually respiratory** • Often incidentally detected as **a solitary well-circumscribed mass**	• Differential diagnosis includes cryptogenic organizing pneumonia, IgG4-RD, inflammatory sarcomatoid carcinomas, and "pleomorphic" soft tissue sarcomas (previously termed malignant fibrous histiocytoma) • IMT distinguished by its bland cytologic features and immunohistochemistry	• **Indolent. If localized, most are cured after surgical resection** • Metastatic disease (rare; <5% of cases) may be associated with significant morbidity and mortality • ALK-rearranged disease (which comprises 50%–70% of cases), responds well to ALK inhibitors
Kikuchi–Fujimoto (also known as Kikuchi's disease or histiocytic necrotizing lymphadenitis) (14)	• Most frequently found in East Asians; rare in the United States and Europe • Female-to-male incidence is 4:1	• Onset over 2 to 4 weeks • **Usually cervical lymphadenopathy (occasionally generalized) and fever** • Sore throat, arthralgias, rashes are seen in approximately 10% of patients	• Can be difficult to distinguish from lymphoma	• **Usually resolves without treatment in <6 months.** Steroids and antibiotics may result in improvement • Recurrences are rare, death due to disease also rare (approx. 2% of patients)

(*continued*)

Table 13.3 Benign Idiopathic-Inflammatory Causes of Lymphadenopathy (*continued*)

	Epidemiology	Signs/Symptoms	Diagnostic Pearls	Prognosis
Kimura's disease (15)	• Mainly affects young Asian men	• **Indolent presentation, with painless lymphadenopathy in head and neck**	• Often confused with angiolymphoid hyperplasia with eosinophilia • Serum immunoglobulin E levels may be elevated	• **Remissions in up to 25% with surgery** • Steroids induce responses, but relapses are frequent • High risk of recurrence if: peripheral eosinophils >50%, serum IgE >10,000 IU/mL, and/or multifocal lesions outside the salivary glands
Progressive transformation of germinal centers (reactive hyperplasia) (16)	• Male:female incidence 3:1 • Occurs in children and adults; affects the elderly in Japan but men <30 years of age in the United States	• **Usually solitary asymptomatic lymphadenopathy of head and neck**, but one third have multiple nodes involved • Lymph nodes 1.3 to 4.0 cm	• Not a premalignant condition, but can be mistaken for NLPHL because the immunophenotypes of both are CD45+, CD20+, CD15−, CD30−	• **No clinical sequelae** in the **majority** of cases • At least 20% of cases recur

(continued)

Table 13.3 Benign Idiopathic-Inflammatory Causes of Lymphadenopathy (*continued*)

	Epidemiology	Signs/Symptoms	Diagnostic Pearls	Prognosis
Rosai–Dorfman disease (histiocytosis of group R, under 2016 classification) (17)	• More common in children and young adults (mean age 21) • African descent • Not confined to any age group	• **Massive lymphadenopathy in the head/neck** • **Fevers, elevated inflammatory markers** • Half of the patients have extranodal (sinuses, orbit, CNS, bone, or skin) involvement	• **Histiocytosis in lymph nodes or other locations** • Immunohistochemistry: S100 and CD68+; CD1a will be negative • **Differential diagnosis includes low-grade B-cell lymphomas with marginal zone distribution**	• **Frequently resolves with excision** • Resolves with steroids in some cases
Sarcoidosis	• Rare in patients <20 years old • Elevated risk in African Americans, African-Caribbean, Scandinavians, and Japanese	• Respiratory symptoms are common • Lymphadenopathy in the chest (95% have mediastinal lymphadenopathy) • Peripheral lymphadenopathy occurs in approximately 30% of patients	• Löfgren syndrome (hilar lymphadenopathy with erythema nodosum, with or without arthritis or fever) does not require invasive tissue biopsy if infection or malignancy is not suspected	• **Variable** • Spontaneous remission may occur in 60% of patients • Ten percent experience a chronic or progressive course

ALK, anaplastic lymphoma kinase; CNS, central nervous system; CRP, C-reactive protein; EBV, Epstein–Barr virus; ESR, erythrocyte sedimentation rate; FDG, fluorodeoxyglucose; HHV-8, human herpesvirus-8; IgG4-RD, IgG4-related disease; IMCD, idiopathic multicentric Castleman's disease; IMT, inflammatory myofibroblastic tumor; LAD, lymphadenopathy; NLPHL, nodular lymphocyte predominant Hodgkin lymphoma; PET-CT, positron emission tomography-CT; SUV, standardized uptake value; UCD, unicentric Castleman's disease.

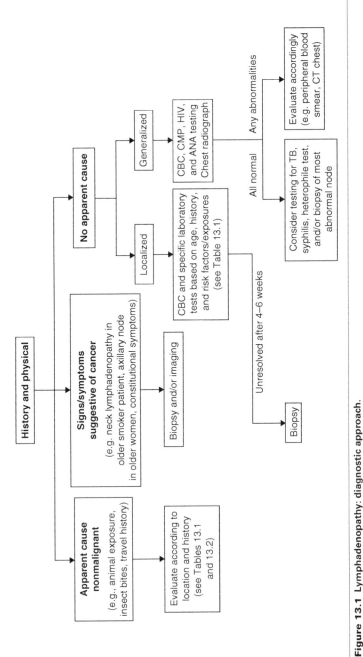

Figure 13.1 Lymphadenopathy: diagnostic approach.

ANA, antinuclear antibody; CBC, complete blood count; CMP, comprehensive metabolic panel; TB, tuberculosis.

malignancy based on symptoms, exam, or location of LAD, clinicians should refer patients for LN biopsy and/or have specific imaging as indicated. Otherwise, a more conservative approach is followed (Figure 13.2). In a patient with history of solid or bone marrow transplant, LN biopsy and peripheral blood EBV viral load by polymerase chain reaction (PCR) should be obtained (about 80% of PTLDs are associated with EBV).

Key Diagnostic Dilemma

LAD without an obvious cause is challenging. Biopsy should be used cautiously and the mode of biopsy should be selected judiciously.

Similar histopathologic patterns and clinical manifestations can be seen across disease categories:

- Large transformed B immunoblasts surrounded by plasma cells with basophilic cytoplasm can be seen in EBV or cytomegalovirus (CMV) infection as well as Hodgkin lymphoma (18).
- Chronic granulomatous inflammation can be seen in infection, malignancy, and immune disorders. *Mycobacterium tuberculosis* and sarcoidosis mimic each other; typically necrotizing in the former and non-necrotizing in the latter, but tuberculosis can be non-necrotizing, and sarcoidosis is thought to be a clinical sequela of tuberculosis in some patients. LAD due to autoimmune diseases

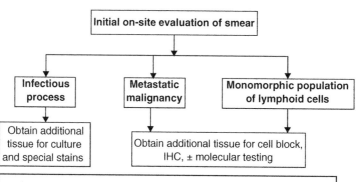

Figure 13.2 Diagnostic process for FNA of abnormally enlarged lymph node.

FISH, fluorescence in situ hybridization; FNA, fine needle aspiration; IHC, immunohistochemistry; PCR, polymerase chain reaction.

such as granulomatosis with polyangiitis (previously known as Wegener's granulomatosis) can be necrotizing or non-necrotizing (although predominantly non-necrotizing). Lymphomas may mimic chronic granulomatous inflammation (19).

- Angioimmunoblastic T-cell lymphoma (AITL) can be difficult to diagnose. Morphologic features of polymorphous infiltrate, prominent vascularity, absence of follicles with extrafollicular proliferation of follicular dendritic cells are seen in many reactive and neoplastic conditions. AITL can resemble Castleman's disease, Hodgkin lymphoma, and T-cell–rich B-cell lymphoma. T-cell receptor (TCR) gene rearrangement studies are often necessary, but not entirely sensitive as only 75% to 80% of cases have TCR gene rearrangements. Immunoglobulin heavy chains may be rearranged in up to 25% due to EBV-expanded B cell clones, which widens the differential diagnosis to B-cell lymphoproliferative disorders (20).

If LAD remains unexplained after initial assessment, there is no standardized diagnostic approach to follow. Figure 13.1 provides one diagnostic algorithm to consider. When there is low suspicion for malignancy, a biopsy should be deferred and an alternative etiology should be sought (Table 13.2). If there are concerns for malignancy and/or the patient has LAD persisting beyond 4 to 6 weeks with no identifiable cause, then an LN biopsy is required for diagnosis and adequate tissue sampling is the key. Steroids can mask or delay the diagnosis of an underlying lymphoma or leukemia and should be avoided.

The mode of biopsy depends on patient, disease, and physician factors. Fine-needle aspiration cytology biopsies are quick and minimally invasive. These can be reliable in diagnosing a recurring disease or as a triaging office-based procedure to rule out a metastatic solid carcinoma or reactive lymph node. The disadvantage of fine needle aspiration (FNA) is the low sensitivity, particularly when hematologic malignancies are in the differential. In such cases, an open incisional or excisional LN biopsy is the preferred diagnostic modality. FNA and multiple core biopsies may substitute for an open LN biopsy, ensuring enough tissue is obtained for immunohistochemistry, flow cytometry, and genetic and molecular testing.

Biopsies of both hematologic and solid malignancies are routinely fixed in formalin, but any suspicion for hematologic malignancy should prompt fresh specimens for flow cytometry which can be important in the diagnosis of lymphoid neoplasms.

Management and Prognosis

Treatment and prognosis of patients with LAD are dependent on the underlying etiology. Management of LAD can be conservative without any specific treatment (e.g., drug-induced or some viral LAD) or may require urgent intervention (chemotherapy for aggressive lymphomas) (Table 13.4). Likewise, prognosis ranges from indolent course with an excellent long-term prognosis (such as drug-induced LAD and early-stage Hodgkin lymphoma) to very aggressive and poor prognosis (e.g., AITL with 5-year overall survival of <35%). Detailed treatment and prognostic discussion for all disease categories that cause LAD is beyond the scope of the current book chapter.

Table 13.4 Treatment of Benign Idiopathic-Inflammatory Causes of Lymphadenopathy

	Surgery is a Mainstay of Treatment	Steroids Have a Role	Other Medications	Self-Resolving
Castleman's, unicentric	✓			
Castleman's, multicentric		✓	Rituximab, cytotoxic chemotherapy, anti–IL-6 therapy	
IgG4-related disease		✓	Rituximab; fewer data for azathioprine, mycophenolate mofetil	
IMT	✓		Crizotinib	
Kikuchi's		✓		
Kimura's	✓	✓	Cetirizine, radiation therapy, topical tacrolimus, thalidomide	
PTGC				✓
Rosai–Dorfman	✓			
Sarcoidosis		✓	Methotrexate, azathioprine, leflunomide, tumor necrosis factor-alpha inhibitors	✓

IL, interleukin; IMT, inflammatory myofibroblastic tumor; PTGC, progressive transformation of germinal centers.

DISORDERS OF THE SPLEEN

Clinical Case 13.2

A 59-year-old female is referred to a hematologist for an incidental finding of splenomegaly. She has a history of diabetes mellitus, hyperlipidemia, and hypertension. She only drinks alcohol socially, approximately one to two drinks every 3 months. Her review of systems is negative for constitutional symptoms. On exam, her vital signs are normal. Her body mass index (BMI) is 37 kg/m². There are no palpable lymph nodes. The liver is palpable 3 cm below the right costal margin and the spleen is palpable 2 cm below the left costal margin. She has trace bilateral leg edema. Her exam is otherwise negative. Prior CT scans of the abdomen and pelvis confirm hepatosplenomegaly along with fatty infiltration of the liver. There is no adenopathy. On labs, basic metabolic panel (BMP) and complete blood count (CBC) are normal. AST is 105 U/L and ALT is 140 U/L. Total bilirubin is 0.8 mg/dL. Alkaline phosphatase is 223 IU/L.

Introduction

The spleen has protective immunologic and hematopoietic functions, which vary during different stages of life. A normal spleen is up to 13 cm in length and is not usually palpable until almost twice its normal size. The main physiologic functions of the spleen include: (a) clearance of antibody-coated bacteria; (b) clearance of senescent or defective erythrocytes; and (c) synthesis of antibodies. In utero, the spleen is a site of hematopoiesis.

The differential diagnosis for splenomegaly is broad. Figure 13.3 and Table 13.5 provide a list of the causes of splenomegaly. A retrospective study including 449 patients demonstrated the causes of splenomegaly as liver disease (33%), hematologic malignancy (27%), infections (23%), congestion or inflammation (8%), primary splenic disease (4%), and other or unknown (5%) (21). Massive splenomegaly, with spleen crossing the midline, is more commonly noted with neoplastic conditions, but can be associated with benign conditions (Figure 13.3). Acute splenomegaly is likely to be caused by infection, with HIV-AIDS–related infections being the commonest. *Mycobacterium avium* complex in these patients has been associated with massive splenomegaly.

The association of liver cirrhosis and splenomegaly is well established, but a less-recognized association is steatohepatitis and splenomegaly, even in the absence of cirrhosis. This correlation was demonstrated in a postmortem analysis of liver and splenic specimens from patients at one institution (22).

On the contrary, hyposplenism and asplenia are less commonly encountered medical conditions. Few conditions have been

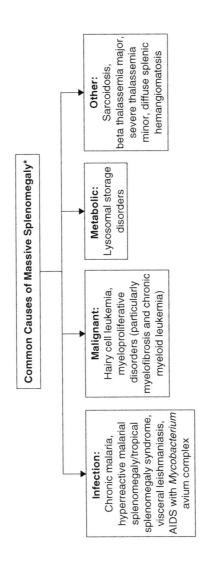

Figure 13.3 Differential for massive splenomegaly.

Table 13.5 Causes of Splenomegaly by Pathophysiology

I. Enlarging as it performs its normal functions

Clearance of microorganisms	Viral	Cytomegalovirus, HIV, hepatitis, infectious mononucleosis/Epstein–Barr virus
	Bacterial	Congenital syphilis, sepsis/subacute bacterial endocarditis, splenic abscess, tuberculosis, ehrlichiosis
	Parasitic	HMS (due to chronic inflammation, highest prevalence in Papua New Guinea), leishmaniasis, trypanosomiasis
	Fungal	Histoplasmosis
Clearance of defective erythrocytes	Immune destruction of RBCs	Paroxysmal nocturnal hemoglobinuria
	Hemoglobinopathies	Early Hgb SS, Hgb SC, HbS/β^+ thalassemia, beta thalassemia major
	Red cell membrane defects	Spherocytosis, ovalocytosis
	Other	Pernicious anemia
Synthesis of immunoglobulin	Immune cytopenias	Immune hemolytic anemias
	Rheumatoid arthritis	
	Systemic lupus erythematosus	
	Serum sickness	
Extramedullary hematopoiesis	Myelofibrosis	
	Marrow damage by toxins or radiation	
	Marrow infiltration by tumors	
	Leukemia	

II. Vascular congestion

    Portal hypertension, heart failure

    Splenic vein thrombosis

III. Infiltrative

Protein deposition	Collagen vascular diseases, amyloid
Granulomatous	Sarcoidosis, eosinophilic granulomas

(*continued*)

Table 13.5 Causes of Splenomegaly by Pathophysiology (*continued*)		
	Metabolic	Gaucher's disease causing lipid deposition and other lysosomal storage diseases (e.g., mucopolysaccharidoses)
	Tumor cells, malignant or benign	Angioimmunoblastic lymphadenopathy, splenic hemangioma/hamartoma/angiosarcoma, metastases
IV. Drug reactions		
Interleukin-2 therapy		
Granulocyte colony-stimulating factor given to healthy bone marrow donors for peripheral blood stem cell donation		
V. Fluid collections		
Splenic trauma with intracapsular hematoma formation		
Cysts		
HMS, hyperreactive malarial splenomegaly.		

associated with hyposplenism or asplenia. Spleens can be congenitally absent. Acquired asplenia has been described in patients with sickle cell disease, secondary to repeated infarctions, and in patients with splenic artery thrombosis. Hyposplenism or functional asplenia is associated with several other conditions including infiltrative diseases (e.g., sarcoidosis, amyloidosis), HIV infection, chronic graft-versus-host disease, autoimmune diseases, and celiac disease, among others. Patients with hyposplenism and asplenia are at increased risk of infections and should follow the same preventive measures and vaccinations as for patients who have undergone splenectomy.

Diagnosis

With no clear underlying etiology based on history and exam, clinicians may consider initial workup with routine CBC, peripheral smear, liver function tests, and HIV testing. Further, chest and abdomen/pelvis imaging (e.g., CT scans) may be considered to assess for LAD/malignancy, liver disease, or an underlying infection. An attempt to obtain a tissue diagnosis by biopsy may be considered according to clinical suspicion, for example, liver biopsy if liver disease is suspected and LN and/or bone marrow biopsies may be considered for infectious and hematologic disorders. Bone marrow aspirate, culture, and biopsy may have a diagnostic utility in evaluating an unexplained splenomegaly, which can aid in the diagnosis of not only hematologic neoplasms, but also mycobacterial/fungal infections, granulomatous disease, and even lipid storage diseases (such as Gaucher's disease). Splenic biopsies are of limited clinical utility and have been associated with increased risk of complications.

Key Diagnostic Dilemma

Unexplained splenomegaly remains a diagnostic challenge, and early referral to a hematologist may be considered. In one study of patients who underwent diagnostic splenectomy for unknown causes of splenomegaly or splenic masses (total of 122 patients), 57% of patients had leukemia/lymphoma. Less-common causes included metastatic sarcoma/carcinoma (11%), cyst/pseudocyst (9%), and benign/malignant vascular neoplasm (7%) (23).

Given that malignancy is the most common etiology for splenomegaly once liver disease has been excluded, clinicians may feel the pressure to obtain a diagnosis, even at the expense of splenectomy. A "watch and wait" strategy, however, may be appropriate for the young patient who is suspected to have an infection or the asymptomatic patient in whom diagnosis may not change management. For example, in the patient who may have a low-grade lymphoma with minimal symptoms and no or mild cytopenias, treatment is not always necessary. In such cases, a review of risks and benefits of obtaining a diagnosis can be discussed with the patient to determine the optimal management.

Management and Prognosis

Diagnostic or therapeutic splenectomy should be avoided for most patients with splenomegaly, given the relatively high morbidity and mortality rates associated with splenectomy. Splenectomy may be indicated for selected patients with steroid-refractory immune thrombocytopenia (ITP), symptomatic and refractory primary myelofibrosis, hereditary spherocytosis, and splenic trauma, among other much rarer common indications.

Patients with splenectomy are at increased long-term risk of infection, thrombosis, and malignancy. Given the significant increased risk of infections, the Centers for Disease Control and Prevention (CDC) recommends vaccination for splenectomized patients against encapsulated organisms as well as several viruses (Table 13.6). Although the risk of "overwhelming post-splenectomy infection" (OPSI) is rare, with an estimated incidence of 0.2% to 0.4% annually, the mortality of OPSI is up to 50% even with maximal treatment (24). The risk is highest in the first 2 years after splenectomy and higher in pediatric/younger patients compared to

Table 13.6 Vaccination Recommendations for Adults With Asplenia

Vaccine	Indication*	Dosing Schedule	Booster
HPV	Through age 21 for males, age 26 for females	Two or three doses	
Influenza	Universal	Every September/October	(Annual)
MMR	Not previously vaccinated (see CDC website for full details)	Two doses 4 to 8 weeks apart	Not recommended
Tetanus diphtheria pertussis	Universal	One dose of Tdap if not previously vaccinated	Td booster every 10 years
Varicella	No previous immunity, and age ≥50 years	Preferred: two doses of RZV administered 3 months apart (minimum 4 weeks apart) Alternative: one dose ZVL at age ≥60 years	Not recommended
HiB (ActHIB, Hiberix)	Universal	One dose	Not recommended
Meningococcal (both MenACWY/Menactra and MenB/Bexsero)	Universal	Menactra: Two doses, given 8 to 12 weeks apart MenB: Two doses for Bexsero, three doses for Trumenba	MenACWY: One dose every 5 years MenB: Not recommended
Pneumococcal (both Pneumovax/PPSV and Prevnar/PCV)	Universal	PCV first, followed by PPSV at least 8 weeks later	PPSV23: One dose 5 years after PPSV23

Notes: vaccination recommendations as of February 2018. **Bold** indicates encapsulated organisms.
*"Universal" refers to all patients with asplenia.
CDC, Centers for Disease Control and Prevention; HiB, *Haemophilus influenzae* B; HPV, human papillomavirus; MMR, measles, mumps, and rubella; RZV, recombinant zoster vaccine; ZVL, herpes zoster live-attenuated vaccine.

older patients. Many newer vaccines are protein subunit formulations, which are more effective in splenectomized patients due to their T-cell–inducing properties. *Streptococcus pneumoniae* is the most common causative organism, accounting for 50% to 80% of cases, and if splenectomy is elective and nonurgent, pneumococcal vaccination should occur at least 4 weeks prior to surgery.

LYMPHOCYTOSIS AND LYMPHOPENIA

Clinical Case 13.3

A 48-year-old male is referred to a hematologist for chronic leukocytosis over the past 2 years. He has a history of hypertension and hyperlipidemia. He has a 20-pack year tobacco history. His father died at age 69 from complications related to chronic lymphocytic leukemia (CLL). His 10-point review of systems is negative. His BMI is 30 kg/m². He has no adenopathy or hepatosplenomegaly on exam. Laboratory examination revealed a WBC count of 12,700 cells/mm³ (45% neutrophils, 45% lymphocytes, 9% monocytes, 1% eosinophils), hemoglobin 13.8 g/dL, MCV 89 fL, and platelets 262,000/μL. Flow cytometry of the peripheral blood is obtained and yields a 60% monoclonal B-cell population with expression of CD5, CD19, and CD23 and dim expression of CD20. CT scans of the chest, abdomen, and pelvis are negative for adenopathy or hepatosplenomegaly. The patient is reassured that he does not currently have a malignancy, but will require surveillance.

Introduction

There is no consensus definition of lymphocytosis, but it is generally defined as an absolute lymphocyte count (ALC) >4,000 cells/μL. Unless the patient is clinically unstable, a repeat CBC is always recommended before further evaluation is pursued.

Lymphopenia or lymphocytopenia is defined as an ALC <1,000/μL and is typically due to infection, systemic illness, drugs (e.g., chemotherapy or glucocorticoids) or rarely related to a congenital immunodeficiency disorder. Table 13.7 lists the common causes of lymphocytopenia.

Diagnosis

When an underlying monoclonal neoplastic condition is suspected, the gold standard test is flow cytometry of peripheral blood. With modern multicolor flow cytometry, sensitivity is high and capable of identifying one malignant cell in 10,000 or more normal cells. This sensitivity has led to high frequencies of monoclonal B-cell lymphocytosis (MBL), which is defined as a monoclonal population of B lymphocytes <5,000 cells/μL without any other identifiable cause or pathology in the general population. One study of

Table 13.7 Causes of Lymphopenia

Category	Cause	Examples
Iatrogenic	Antineoplastic therapy	Alemtuzumab, antilymphocyte globulin, cyclophosphamide
	Other drugs	Glucocorticoids, psoralen plus ultraviolet A treatment, Stevens–Johnson syndrome
	Other	ECMO (redistribution between peripheral blood and bone marrow, and tissue sequestration); extended field radiation therapy, for example, for Hodgkin lymphoma (not commonly used any longer)
Infections	Viral	HIV, West Nile, hepatitis, influenza, herpes simplex, HHV-6 and HHV-8, measles
	Bacterial/fungal	Sepsis, pneumonia, active tuberculosis
Nutritional	Ethanol abuse (most often in association with hypersplenism)	
	Deficiencies	Zinc deficiency, protein-losing enteropathy
Systemic illnesses	Bone marrow replacement	Aplastic anemia, myelofibrosis
	Autoimmune diseases	SLE, Sjögren syndrome, myasthenia gravis, vasculitis
	Acute physiologic stress	Myocardial infarction, pancreatitis, strenuous exercise, thermal injury, major surgery, trauma
	Malignancy	Hodgkin lymphoma
	Immunodeficiency syndromes	Wiskott–Aldrich and DiGeorge syndromes, ataxia telangiectasia, common variable immunodeficiency, idiopathic CD4+T lymphocytopenia
	Chronic illness	Sarcoidosis, congestive heart failure, uremia, celiac disease
	Other rare causes	Intestinal lymphangiectasia (increased lymphocyte loss)

ECMO, extracorporeal membrane oxygenation; HHV-6 and HHV-8, human herpes viruses types 6 and 8; SLE, systemic lupus erythematosus.

healthy adults in Spain reported an MBL prevalence of 12% among patients >40 years of age. Family history of CLL, age, and various infections, including hepatitis C, are the risk factors for acquiring MBL. Though MBL is a precursor state to CLL, progression to CLL requiring treatment occurs in ≤2% of patients with MBL annually (25).

As with other lymphoid disorders, the cornerstone for initial evaluation and subsequent testing of lymphopenia relies on the key findings from history and physical examination. Isolated lymphopenia without an associated diagnosis is rarely seen, and thus does not have a standard diagnostic approach. Diagnostic evaluation is often driven by associated symptoms or clinical findings.

Key Diagnostic Dilemma

The challenge for clinicians is to differentiate reactive (polyclonal) lymphocytosis from a monoclonal neoplastic disorder. Figures 13.4 and 13.5 outline the diagnostic approaches and list the probable causes of lymphocytosis.

In addition to history (e.g., constitutional symptoms) and physical examination (e.g., LAD, hepatosplenomegaly), the answers to three initial questions may guide subsequent evaluation:

1. **What is the patient's age and degree of lymphocytosis?** A patient <50 years of age with an ALC <5,000 is unlikely to have a monoclonal disorder, and observation is typically reasonable. ALC >5,000 should prompt a workup for malignancy. By combining age and ALC, one can predict the pretest probability of having an abnormal flow cytometry. Patients aged 50 to 67 years with ALC >6,700/µL or patients aged >67 years with ALC >4,000 cells/µL have a 95% sensitivity and 76% specificity for having a monoclonal B-cell disorder.

2. **Are there any other abnormal blood counts?** Lymphocytosis can be a sole abnormality, but is not infrequently associated with other cell count abnormalities. Reactive allergic, inflammatory, or infectious etiologies are commonly associated with elevated other WBCs such as eosinophils and/or neutrophils. Anemia and/or thrombocytopenia are relatively more common with other neoplastic conditions (e.g., CLL, other acute or chronic leukemias). Figure 13.4 outlines a diagnostic approach for lymphocytosis associated with other blood count abnormalities.

3. **What is the morphologic appearance of the lymphocytes on peripheral blood smear (PBS)?** Classic reactive lymphocytosis is often seen in infectious mononucleosis. The lymphocytes are pleomorphic, ranging from small/round to intermediate with abundant cytoplasm, even to immunoblasts.

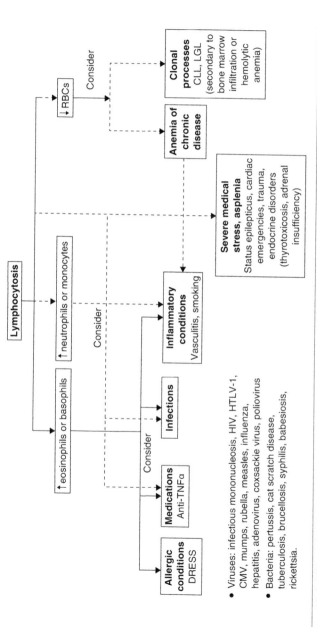

Figure 13.4 Differential diagnosis of lymphocytosis associated with other cell count abnormalities.

ALC, absolute lymphocyte count; CLL, chronic lymphocytic leukemia; CMV, cytomegalovirus; DRESS, drug reaction with eosinophilia and systemic symptoms; HTLV, human T-lymphotropic virus; LGL, large granular lymphocyte leukemia; RBC, red blood cell; TNFα, tumor necrosis factor alpha.

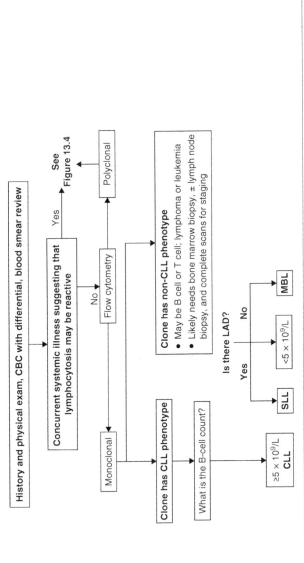

Figure 13.5 Approach to lymphocytosis, incorporating flow cytometry.

CBC, complete blood count; CLL, chronic lymphocytic leukemia; LAD, lymphadenopathy; MBL, monoclonal B-cell lymphocytosis; SLL, small lymphocytic lymphoma.

Source: Adapted from Strati P, Shanafelt TD. Monoclonal B-cell lymphocytosis and early-stage chronic lymphocytic leukemia: diagnosis, natural history, and risk stratification. *Blood.* 2015;126(4):454–462. doi:10.1182/blood-2015-02-585059

While monomorphic lymphocytes may suggest a lymphoproliferative disorder, important exceptions are *Bordetella pertussis* infection, polyclonal B lymphocytosis, and large granular lymphocytosis in response to viruses, malignancy, bone marrow transplantation, and chemotherapy.

Management and Prognosis

Treatment and prognosis of lymphocytosis or lymphopenia depend on the underlying etiology. Few retrospective reports identified lymphopenia as an independent risk factor for increased morbidity (mainly infections) and/or mortality (e.g., in patients with systemic lupus erythematosus [SLE], vasculitis, or for patients requiring intensive care unit admission). For patients who are otherwise healthy and with no significant identified treatable disease, no specific treatment intervention is warranted and patients may be followed conservatively.

Future Directions/Clinical Trials

The selected clinical trials are presented in Table 13.8.

Key Points

- A lymph node larger than 1 cm in diameter is considered abnormal. History and physical examination are the cornerstones for initial evaluation. Four percent of patients with unexplained LAD over the age of 40 will ultimately be diagnosed with malignancy.
- If a malignancy is suspected, an adequate biopsy is critical. Excisional biopsy is the gold standard, but fine needle cytology and core needle biopsies supplemented with ancillary tests such as flow cytometry and molecular analysis may substitute for an open biopsy under certain circumstances. Biopsy should also be considered for LAD persisting beyond 4 to 6 weeks.
- Approximately one third of patients with splenomegaly in the United States have underlying liver disease. Splenectomy should be avoided with a limited number of indications such as refractory ITP, splenic trauma, hereditary spherocytosis, and myelofibrosis. Splenectomized patients should be vaccinated for encapsulated organisms, in accordance with CDC guidelines, ideally prior to splenectomy when surgery is not urgent.
- Lymphocytosis is commonly related to benign conditions, but when a clonal neoplasm is suspected, a peripheral blood flow cytometry is the gold standard diagnostic test.

Table 13.8 Selected Clinical Trials Recruiting in the United States for Benign Idiopathic-Inflammatory Causes of Lymphadenopathy

Disease of Interest	Name of Trial	NCT Number	Phase	Last Update*
Castleman's disease, multicentric	Tocilizumab for KSHV-Associated Multicentric Castleman Disease	NCT 01441063	2	12/28/17
Castleman's disease, unicentric or multicentric	ACCELERATE (Advancing Castleman Care with an Electronic Longitudinal Registry, E-Repository, and Treatment/Effectiveness Research): An International Registry for Patients with Castleman Disease	NCT 02817997	Obs; cohort	7/17/17
IgG4-related disease	Study to Evaluate the Effect of XmAb®5871 on Disease Activity in Patients with IgG4-Related Disease (RD)	NCT 02725476	2	7/2/17
IgG4-related disease	Treatment of IgG4-Related Disease with Revlimid and Rituximab (TIGR2)	NCT 02705638	2	9/14/16
Inflammatory myofibroblastic tumor	Phase I Study of LDK378 in Pediatric, Malignancies with a Genetic Alteration in Anaplastic Lymphoma Kinase (ALK)	NCT 01742286	1	11/14/17
Posttransplant lymphoproliferative disorder	Biomarkers for Post-Transplant Lymphoproliferative Disorders in Children (CTOTC-06)	NCT 02182986	Obs; case control	11/20/17
Posttransplant lymphoproliferative disorder	Risk-stratified Sequential Treatment of Post-transplant Lymphoproliferative Disease (PTLD) With Rituximab SC [Hyaluronidase] and Immunochemotherapy (PTLD-2)	NCT 02042391	2	2/28/17
Rosai–Dorfman, multisystem	International Rare Histiocytic Disorders Registry (IRHDR)	NCT 02285582	Obs	4/27/16

*Recruiting as of this date (date of last update posted on ClinicalTrials.Gov).
NCT, National Clinical Trial; Obs, observational.

REFERENCES

1. Fijten GH, Blijham GH. Unexplained lymphadenopathy in family practice: an evaluation of the probability of malignant causes and the effectiveness of physicians' workup. *J Fam Pract*. 1988;27(4):373–376.
2. Gaddey HL, Riegel AM. Unexplained lymphadenopathy: evaluation and differential diagnosis. *Am Fam Phys*. 2016;94(11):896–903.
3. King D, Ramachandra J, Yeomanson D. Lymphadenopathy in children: refer or reassure? *Arch Dis Child*. 2014;99(3):101–110. doi:10.1136/archdischild-2013-304443
4. Misra UK, Kalita J, Rathore C. Phenytoin and carbamazepine cross reactivity: report of a case and review of literature. *Postgrad Med J*. 2003;79(938):703–704.
5. De Vriese AS, Philippe J, Van Renterghem DM, et al. Carbamazepine hypersensitivity syndrome: report of 4 cases and review of the literature. *Medicine*. 1995;74(3):144–151. doi:10.1097/00005792-199505000-00004
6. Simpson D. Epidemiology of castleman disease. *Hematol/Oncol Clin North Am*. 2018;32(1):1–10. doi:10.1016/j.hoc.2017.09.001
7. Fajgenbaum DC, Uldrick TS, Bagg A, et al. International, evidence-based consensus diagnostic criteria for HHV-8-negative/idiopathic multicentric Castleman disease. *Blood*. 2017;129(12):1646–1657. doi:10.1182/blood-2016-10-746933
8. Robinson D Jr, Reynolds M, Casper C, et al. Clinical epidemiology and treatment patterns of patients with multicentric Castleman disease: results from two US treatment centres. *Br J Haematol*. 2014;165(1):39–48. doi:10.1111/bjh.12717
9. Haap M, Wiefels J, Horger M, et al. Clinical, laboratory and imaging findings in Castleman's disease - The subtype decides. *Blood Rev*. 2018;32(3):225–234. doi:10.1016/j.blre.2017.11.005
10. Deshpande V, Zen Y, Chan JK, et al. Consensus statement on the pathology of IgG4-related disease. *Modern Pathology*. 2012;25(9):1181–1192. doi:10.1038/modpathol.2012.72
11. Sato Y, Yoshino T. IgG4-Related Lymphadenopathy. *Int J Rheumatol*. 2012;2012:572539. doi:10.1155/2012/572539
12. Stone JH, Zen Y, Deshpande V. IgG4-related disease. *N Engl J Med*. 2012;366(6):539–551. doi:10.1056/NEJMra1104650
13. Theilen TM, Soerensen J, Bochennek K, et al. Crizotinib in ALK(+) inflammatory myofibroblastic tumors—current experience and future perspectives. *Pediatr Blood Cancer*. 2018;65(4):e26920. doi:10.1002/pbc.26920

14. Jung IY, Ann HW, Kim JJ, et al. The incidence and clinical characteristics by gender differences in patients with Kikuchi-Fujimoto disease. *Medicine*. 2017;96(11):e6332. doi:10.1097/MD.0000000000006332

15. Iwai H, Nakae K, Ikeda K, et al. Kimura disease: diagnosis and prognostic factors. *Otolaryngol Head Neck Surg*. 2007;137(2):306–311. doi:10.1016/j.otohns.2007.03.027

16. Hicks J, Flaitz C. Progressive transformation of germinal centers: review of histopathologic and clinical features. *Int J Pediatr Otorhinolaryngol*. 2002;65(3):195–202. doi:10.1016/S0165-5876(02)00176-3

17. Emile J-F, Abla O, Fraitag S, et al. Revised classification of histiocytoses and neoplasms of the macrophage-dendritic cell lineages. *Blood*. 2016;127(22):2672–2681. doi:10.1182/blood-2016-01-690636

18. Louissaint A, Ferry J, Soupir CP, et al. Infectious mononucleosis mimicking lymphoma: distinguishing morphological and immunophenotypic features. *Modern Pathol*. 2012;25:1149–1159. doi:10.1038/modpathol.2012.70

19. Shah KK, Pritt BS, Alexander MP. Histopathologic review of granulomatous inflammation. *J Clin Tuberc Other Mycobact Dis*. 2017;7:1–12. doi:10.1016/j.jctube.2017.02.001

20. Schmitz N, de Leval L. How I manage peripheral T-cell lymphoma, not otherwise specified and angioimmunoblastic T-cell lymphoma: current practice and a glimpse into the future. *Br J Haematol*. 2017;176(6):851–866. doi:10.1111/bjh.14473

21. O'Reilly RA. Splenomegaly in 2,505 patients at a large university medical center from 1913 to 1995. 1963 to 1995: 449 patients. *West J Med*. 1998;169(2):88–97.

22. Isabel Fiel M, Reza Sima H, Desman G, et al. Increased thickness of abdominal subcutaneous adipose tissue occurs more frequently in steatohepatitis than in simple steatosis. *Arch Pathol Lab Med*. 2013;137(5):642–646. doi:10.5858/arpa.2012-0050-OA

23. Kraus MD, Fleming MD, Vonderheide RH. The spleen as a diagnostic specimen. *Cancer*. 2001;91(11):2001–2009. doi:10.1002/1097-0142(20010601)91:11<2001::AID-CNCR1225>3.0.CO;2-3

24. Morgan TL, Tomich EB. Overwhelming post-splenectomy infection (OPSI): a case report and review of the literature. *J Emerg Med*. 2012;43(4):758–763. doi:10.1016/j.jemermed.2011.10.029

25. Strati P, Shanafelt TD. Monoclonal B-cell lymphocytosis and early-stage chronic lymphocytic leukemia: diagnosis, natural history, and risk stratification. *Blood*. 2015;126(4):454–462. doi:10.1182/blood-2015-02-585059

14 Transfusion Medicine

Hatice Gur and Elizabeth A. Hartwell

Clinical Case 14.1

A 70-year-old man was being treated for anemia due to gastrointestinal bleeding. The patient reported no prior history of cardiac or respiratory disease. Following admission, his hemoglobin (Hgb) level was noted to be 7.5 g/dL and two units of red blood cells (RBCs) were ordered for transfusion. The patient had no history of previous transfusions and no history of allo- or autoantibodies. No alloantibodies were detected on testing the pretransfusion blood sample. Crossmatch-compatible RBCs were made available for transfusion. Following transfusion of approximately 50 mL of the first RBC (15 minutes into the transfusion), the patient developed tachycardia and dyspnea. The vital signs were as follows:

Vital Sign	Pretransfusion	Posttransfusion
BP (mmHg)	110/55	120/60
Pulse (bpm)	116	150
Respiratory rate (bpm)	21	36
Temperature (°F)	97.7	98.1
SaO$_2$	98% at room air	99% at room air
BP, blood pressure.		

The transfusion was discontinued, and the remaining blood product and a new patient blood sample were sent to the blood bank for a transfusion reaction investigation. The patient's tachycardia and dyspnea resolved following discontinuation of the transfusion. His vital signs and clinical status were stable in the following days.

INTRODUCTION

Blood transfusion is one of the most commonly used (and overused) medical interventions. Transfusion of any blood component must consider the balance between providing benefit to the recipient and avoiding the associated potential risks (Table 14.1) (1,2). In

Table 14.1 Estimated Relative Risk and Window Period for Transfusion-Transmitted Infections

Infectious Agent	Relative Residual Risk	Window Period (Days)
HIV	1:2.1 million	9.1
HBV	1:1.2 million	18.5 to 26.5
HCV	1:1.1 million	7.4
HTLV	1:2.7 million	51
West Nile virus	Rare	Unknown; low with testing
Trypanosoma cruzi (Chagas)	Rare	N/A

HBV, hepatitis B virus; HCV, hepatitis C virus; HTLV, human T-lymphotropic virus.

Source: From Fung MK, Eder AF, Spitalnik SL, et al (eds). *Technical Manual.* 19th ed. Bethesda, MD: AABB; 2017; Osterman JL, Arora S. Blood product transfusions and reactions. *Hematol Oncol Clin North Am.* 2017;31(6): 1159–1170. doi:10.1016/j.hoc.2017.08.014

an effort to improve judicious utilization of blood products, multiple guidelines for transfusion have been published. The majority of these focus on transfusion of RBCs, while guidelines for plasma and platelet transfusion continue to be developed.

PRETRANSFUSION TESTING

Pretransfusion testing includes ABO/Rh determination, screening for blood group antibodies with antibody identification, if needed, and compatibility testing (aka "the crossmatch"). Positive identification of the patient requires adherence to strict labeling guidelines, since patient and sample misidentification is the most common cause of acute hemolytic transfusion reactions. Both red cells and plasma/serum are required for testing. According to regulatory guidelines, if a patient has been pregnant or transfused within the past 3 months, the sample for pretransfusion testing in anticipation of transfusion of RBC-containing components must be collected within 3 days of the anticipated transfusion. Since this information is often not known or available, the majority of transfusion services simply require a new sample every 3 days, with the day of collection being Day 0 (1).

When requesting blood components for a patient, either a Type and Screen (T/S) or a Type and Cross (T/C or Crossmatch) is ordered. A T/S includes ABO and Rh typing and a screen of the patient's plasma or serum for the presence of unexpected blood group antibodies. A **T/S** is recommended when the likelihood of RBC transfusion is low, for instance, surgical procedures where blood loss is minimal, or when plasma-containing components only are needed. For transfusion of red cell–containing blood components (whole blood [WB] or RBCs), a **T/C** is required. A crossmatch is not required for transfusion of plasma, platelets, or cryoprecipitate.

ABO/RH TESTING

The **ABO system** is the most important blood group system in transfusion medicine. Failure to honor ABO compatibility in the transfusion of RBCs can result in immediate and life-threatening hemolytic reactions. The ABO system is composed of four phenotypes: O, A, B, and AB. If the ABO antigen is present on a patient's red cells, the corresponding ABO antibody is not produced. Rather, naturally occurring antibodies against the missing A and/or B antigens are produced. Table 14.2 summarizes the antigens and antibodies expected in an individual based on the ABO group.

Testing is designed to detect the presence or absence of A and B antigens on the RBCs ("forward typing") and the presence or absence of anti-A and anti-B in the serum ("reverse typing"). If a discrepancy occurs between the two tests, it must be resolved prior to transfusion. The most common typing discrepancy is the patient who is a weak subgroup of A and forms anti-A$_1$. In this case, the patient will have a forward type of "A" (A antigen only detected on the RBCs), but a reverse type of "O" (both the expected anti-B and the unexpected anti-A detected in the serum). The majority of group A individuals are group A$_1$ and forward and reverse type as expected. However, a small percentage of them have a subgroup of A (A$_2$) and may form anti-A$_1$. These individuals require transfusion with group A$_1$ RBCs. Typically, group O RBCs are used as these are easier to obtain.

Although the **Rh system** is composed of more than 50 different antigens, only the "D" antigen is considered important in routine testing. If the D antigen is detected, the individual is Rh Positive; if it is not detected, the individual is Rh Negative. Typing for the D antigen is part of the T/S procedure. Unlike the ABO system, anti-D is not a naturally occurring antibody in Rh-Negative individuals and it is only formed upon exposure to Rh-Positive RBCs due to prior pregnancy or transfusion. If present, the D antigen is detected by the antibody screening test as anti-D.

There are two uncommon variants of the D antigen: weak D and partial D. Individuals with fewer than average D antigenic sites

Table 14.2 ABO Compatibility* for Blood Components

Recipient ABO	Antigens Present	Antibodies Present	Whole Blood[†]	RBCs[†]	Plasma[‡]	Platelets[§]	Cryoprecipitate[‡]
O	None	Anti-A, Anti-B	O	O	O, A, B, AB	O, A, B, AB	All types okay
A	A	Anti-B	A	A, O	A, AB	A, AB, B, O	All types okay
B	B	Anti-A	B	B, O	B, AB	B, AB, A, O	All types okay
AB	A, B	None	AB	AB, A, B, O	AB	AB, A, B, O	All types okay
			Must be ABO identical to recipient	Must be ABO compatible with recipient's plasma	Must be ABO compatible with recipient's red cells	ABO identical preferred; otherwise, ABO compatible with recipient's red cells	All ABO groups and Rh types acceptable

*Listed in order of ABO group preference.

[†]Rh-Negative recipients should receive Rh-Negative whole blood or RBCs, if possible, especially females of childbearing potential. Rh-Positive recipients may receive either Rh-Positive or Rh-Negative whole blood or RBCs.

[‡]Can be transfused regardless of Rh type.

[§]If possible, Rh-Negative females of childbearing potential should receive Rh-Negative platelets.

RBC, red blood cell.

on their red cells are termed **"weak D"** ("D^u" in older literature). These individuals do not form anti-D antibodies since they possess the D antigen on their red cells. However, depending on the detection capabilities of the Rh testing assays used, these individuals may type as Rh Negative at one facility and Rh Positive at another. Extended Rh typing is, therefore, only required for blood donors who initially type as Rh Negative. If the blood donor is shown to have weak D, the unit is labeled as Rh Positive. Such extended typing is not required on patients, since transfusion of an Rh-Negative unit to a weak D individual is acceptable. Likewise, pregnant women should not be tested for weak D during pregnancy; they will be classified as Rh Negative. An exception occurs for Rh-Negative infants born to Rh-Negative women; these infants must be tested for weak D for purposes of determining maternal candidacy for Rh immune globulin.

The second D variant is **"partial D."** The D antigen is a mosaic structure composed of at least 30 epitopes. If some or many of the epitopes are missing, the individual has the potential of forming a D-like antibody to the missing epitopes. These individuals will type as Rh Positive, be transfused with Rh-Positive RBCs, and later found to have formed anti-D. The anti-D reagent antisera used today in Rh testing is designed to detect the majority of partial D phenotypes. An individual with a known partial D variant should be transfused only with Rh-Negative blood to avoid the formation of anti-D.

Detection of these variants is of particular importance in the obstetric patient. Rh-Negative women who carry an Rh-Positive fetus are at risk of Rh D alloimmunization. The availability and routine use of Rh D immune globulin (RhIG) has reduced the rate of alloimmunization significantly (3). Established protocols for administration of RhIG are available and provide evidence-based guidelines for management of women at risk for Rh D alloimmunization (Table 14.3).

ANTIBODY DETECTION/IDENTIFICATION

The test for blood group antibodies is termed an indirect antiglobulin test (IAT), indirect Coombs test, or antibody screen. The IAT is designed to detect alloantibodies (antibodies directed against blood group antigens that the recipient lacks) and, to a lesser degree, autoantibodies (those directed against "self"-antigens). Blood group antibodies are typically IgM or IgG; rarely, an antibody will be IgA. IgM antibodies are often naturally occurring (no previous exposure to the antigen), have an optimal reaction temperature of room temperature (20°C–24°C) and below, and can be potent complement binders. This is especially true for the

Table 14.3 Indications for Administration of Rh Immune Globulin in Unsensitized* Rh-Negative Women

Indication	
During pregnancy[†]	• At 28 weeks • Invasive diagnostic procedures (amniocentesis, chorionic villus sampling, cordocentesis) • Abdominal trauma • Antenatal hemorrhage in second or third trimester
Postpartum	• Within 72 hours following delivery of an Rh-Positive infant • Additional doses may be needed for fetal–maternal hemorrhage of >30 mL whole blood
Other	• External cephalic version • Molar pregnancy with uterine evacuation • Spontaneous miscarriage (especially if second or third trimester) • Pregnancy termination (medical or surgical) • Ectopic pregnancy • Fetal death in second or third trimester

*Unsensitized indicates that the woman has not already formed anti-D.

[†]It is assumed that the fetus is Rh Positive, unless the Rh status of the fetus is known with certainty.

Standard dose of RhIG is 300 mcg (covers exposure to 30 mL fetal WB or 15 mL fetal RBCs). Additional doses may be required for fetal maternal bleed for >30 mL.

RBC, red blood cell; RhIg, Rh D immune globulin.

Source: From Prevention of Rh D alloimmunization. ACOG Practice Bulletin, *Obstet Gynecol.* 2017;130:57–69.

ABO antibodies. In contrast, IgG antibodies are formed following exposure to the antigen via prior transfusion or pregnancy, typically react at body temperature (37°C), and, with the exception of IgM ABO antibodies, are considered more clinically significant than IgM antibodies. Therefore, a complete transfusion and pregnancy history is of utmost importance when a blood group antibody is identified.

The antibody screen is designed to detect clinically significant IgG antibodies and incorporates the use of anti-human globulin (AHG) reagent, typically anti-IgG. If the antibody screen is positive, the antibody(ies) are identified by using a panel of selected reagent RBCs. This process can be time-consuming, depending on the specificity of the antibody, the number of antibodies present, and whether the patient has an alloantibody, autoantibody, or both (Table 14.4). Good communication with the transfusion service will provide the clinician with an expected turnaround time. The most

Table 14.4 Special Techniques Used in Antibody Identification

Technique	Purpose
Panel	• Composed of 10 to 16 reagent red cells of known antigen composition • Used to determine specificity of blood group antibodies detected in antibody screening
Elution	• Used to dissociate IgG antibody from red cells • Panel performed on resulting solution (the eluate) to determine blood group specificity, if present
Adsorption	• Used to remove autoantibody from recipient's serum in order to determine presence or absence of underlying alloantibodies • Can be used with warm- and cold-reactive autoantibodies • Depending on the strength of autoantibody, multiple adsorptions may be required • If the recipient has not been recently transfused, recipient's own red cells are used for autoadsorption • If the recipient is recently transfused, reagent red cells are used, requiring additional time to perform the procedure
Titer	• Used to determine relative amount of antibody present • Serial twofold dilutions of patient serum performed; titer is expressed as reciprocal of highest dilution showing agglutination • Used commonly in prenatal studies where clinically significant IgG antibody is identified
Phenotype	• Used to determine blood group antigens present on individual's RBCs • Recipient should lack the blood group antigen(s) to which alloantibody(ies) is/are made • May not be valid in a recently transfused individual • Uses special antisera; may not be available for all blood group antigens
Genotype	• Used to determine the blood group alleles present on individual's RBCs • Can be used for a recently transfused individual • Increased time and expense to perform
Thermal amplitude	• Used to determine the highest reaction temperature (up to 37°C) of a cold-reactive autoantibody • Sample collection extremely important and can affect results • Cold-reactive autoantibodies associated with immune hemolysis often react at $\geq 30°C$

RBC, red blood cell.

Source: From Fung MK, Eder AF, Spitalnik SL, et al (eds). *Technical Manual.* 19th ed. Bethesda, MD: AABB; 2017.

commonly detected antibodies are those directed against antigens in the Rh, Kell, Duffy, and Kidd blood group systems; these are IgG in nature and, therefore, considered clinically significant for transfusion purposes (1).

CROSSMATCH

In a crossmatch, the patient's serum or plasma is tested against the donor RBCs using an in vitro system. A crossmatch is required prior to transfusion of WB, RBCs, and granulocytes. The RBCs selected for crossmatching must be ABO compatible with the recipient's serum/plasma. Rh-Positive individuals may receive either Rh-Positive or Rh-Negative RBCs. Since the D antigen is strongly immunogenic, Rh-Negative individuals should receive only Rh-Negative RBCs. Exceptions are during shortages of Rh-Negative RBCs, thereby reserving Rh-Negative RBCs for transfusion of Rh-Negative females of childbearing potential.

If the antibody screen is negative and there is not a historical record of clinically significant antibodies, the crossmatch can be abbreviated and completed within 10 to 15 minutes. However, if a clinically significant antibody is identified (or the patient has a history of one), RBCs that lack the corresponding antigen(s) must be located and crossmatched. Depending on the incidence of the antigen in the donor population, additional time for release of crossmatched units should be anticipated. For instance, if the patient has an anti-K, approximately 90% of donor units will lack the antigen and be compatible. However, if the patient has formed an anti-e, only 2% of donor units are expected to be compatible.

Plasma and cryoprecipitate do not contain red cells, therefore crossmatching is not required. Plasma components are transfused based on ABO compatibility only; the Rh type is not important. Since the cryoprecipitate contains such a small amount, neither ABO nor Rh compatibility is required. Platelet components also do not require a crossmatch; however, typically, units of the same ABO group are used, if possible, to avoid transfusion of incompatible ABO isoagglutinins. Rh-Negative platelets are preferred for transfusion of Rh-negative females of childbearing potential.

ABO compatibility of red cell- and plasma-containing components based on the recipient's ABO is shown in Table 14.2.

URGENT TRANSFUSION

If blood components, usually RBCs, are needed urgently before the completion of pretransfusion testing, uncrossmatched blood can be issued. If the patient's ABO/Rh has not been determined during the current admission, group O RBCs will be issued. When possible, Rh-Negative RBCs should be used for patients of childbearing potential or for children. If a current specimen from the patient has been tested for ABO/Rh, ABO/Rh-compatible units can be issued. In either circumstance, the ordering physician must acknowledge in writing that the clinical situation was of sufficient urgency to require release of blood components prior to completion of compatibility testing.

BLOOD COMPONENTS

Blood components are presented in Table 14.5.

A unit of WB contains approximately 500 mL of blood in an anticoagulant preservative solution. All anticoagulant solutions used for blood collection contain some formulation of citrate. The hematocrit of a WB unit is approximately 36% to 44% and the shelf life (time the unit can be stored before expiration) ranges from 21 to 35 days, depending on the anticoagulant preparation used. With storage, the levels of coagulation factors present in the plasma and platelet function are expected to decrease significantly after only 5 to 7 days of cold storage. The primary indication for use of WB is treatment of patients who are actively bleeding, typically in a trauma setting; therefore, this product is not routinely available for transfusion. Most often, donated units of WB are processed into individual blood components, including packed RBCs (PRBCs), plasma, platelets, and cryoprecipitate. This allows maximum use of the WB donation as well as providing a patient only with the specific blood component(s) needed.

Red Blood Cells

RBCs are prepared from WB by removal of the plasma. RBCs may also be collected through apheresis techniques. Various additive and preservative solutions can then be added to the RBCs to extend the shelf life of the product. The most common additive solutions allow storage of RBCs for up to 42 days; this product has a volume of approximately 300 to 350 mL with a hematocrit of 55% to 65%. Although approximately 30 mL of plasma remains in the RBC unit, there are no functional platelets or coagulation factors present. Each RBC unit contains approximately 200 to 250 mg of iron, primarily in the form of Hgb.

Transfusion guidelines for RBCs are controversial and vary among specialty societies (4–8). The Hgb threshold, or "transfusion trigger," has consistently been lowered over the past 10 years. For stable, asymptomatic patients, most current guidelines

Table 14.5 Blood and Blood Components

Blood Component	Storage Temperature	Storage Time/Expiration Date	Volume	Notes
Whole blood	1°C to 6°C	ACD/CPD/CP2D* - 21 days CPDA - 1 to 35 days	500 mL	• Hct approximately 40% • 1 unit raises Hgb by 1 g/dL (Hct by 3%)
Red blood cells (includes leukocyte reduced)	1°C to 6°C	CPD/CP2D - 21 days CPDA - 1 to 35 days Additive solution - 42 days	300 to 330 mL	• Hct approximately 50% to 55% • 1 unit raises Hgb by 1 g/dL (Hct by 3%)
Frozen red blood cells (thawed/deglycerolized)	1°C to 6°C	24 hours (open system) 14 days (closed system)	180 mL	• Must be thawed prior to use • Hct approximately 75% (open system) or 50% (closed system) • 1 unit raises Hgb by 1 g/dL (Hct by 3%)
Red blood cells, irradiated	1°C to 6°C	Original expiration date or 28 days from irradiation, whichever is sooner	300 to 330 mL	• Hct approximately 50% to 55% • 1 unit raises Hgb by 1 g/dL (Hct by 3%)
Red blood cells, washed	1°C to 6°C	24 hours	180 mL	• Hct approximately 75% • 1 unit raises Hgb by 1 g/dL (Hct by 3%)

(continued)

Table 14.5 Blood and Blood Components (*continued*)

Blood Component	Storage Temperature	Storage Time/Expiration Date	Volume	Notes
Plasma (thawed)	1°C to 6°C	24 hours; can be extended to 5 days	200 to 220 mL (whole blood derived) 300 to 600 mL (apheresis)	• Must be thawed prior to use • 1 unit of each coagulation factor + 2 to 4 mg fibrinogen/mL plasma • Typical dose is 2 to 3 units
Cryoprecipitate (thawed)	20°C to 24°C	6 hours (single units or closed-system pool) 4 hours (open-system pool)	15 mL	• Must be thawed prior to use • Usually pooled (5 units) for use • 200 to 250 mg fibrinogen/unit • 80 to 120 units factor VIII/unit
Platelets, apheresis (includes leukocyte reduced and irradiated)	20°C to 24°C	5 days 7 days if additional bacterial testing	300 mL	• Requires constant agitation during storage
Platelets, whole blood derived	20°C to 24°C	5 days	50 mL	• Usually pooled (5–6 units) for use • Must be infused within 4 hours of pooling

ACD, acid-citrate-dextrose; CPD, citrate-phosphate-dextrose; CP2D, citrate-phosphate-dextrose-dextrose; Hgb, hemoglobin; Hct, hematocrit.

Table 14.6 Indications for Red Blood Cell Transfusion*

Hgb	Indications
<7 g/dL	• Adult patient in an intensive care unit • Gastrointestinal bleeding in a hemodynamically stable patient
<8 g/dL	• Patient undergoing orthopedic or cardiac surgery • Postoperative surgical patients • Hemodynamically stable patient with pre-existing cardiovascular/coronary artery disease • Symptomatic anemia (chest pain, orthostatic hypotension/tachycardia unresponsive to fluid resuscitation, shortness of breath, or congestive heart failure)
Special situations	• Massive transfusion (>30% of blood volume) • Moderately severe bleeding (>15%–30% of blood volume) and unresponsive to fluid resuscitation • Red blood cell exchange
Studies not yet available to determine Hgb threshold	• Patients with acute coronary syndrome • Patients treated for hematological or oncological disorder

*Transfusion decisions should be influenced by symptoms as well as the Hgb concentration.

Hgb, hemoglobin.

Source: From Carson JL, Guyatt G, Heddle NM, et al. Clinical practice guidelines from the AABB: red blood cell transfusion thresholds and storage. *JAMA.* 2016;316(19):2025–2035. doi:10.1001/jama.2016.9185; Carson JL, Grossman BJ, Kleinman S, et al. Red blood cell transfusion: a clinical practice guideline from the AABB. *Ann Intern Med.* 2012;157:49–58. doi:10.7326/0003-4819-157-1-201206190-00429; Carson JL, Triulzi DJ, Ness PM. Indications for and adverse effects of red-cell transfusion. *NEJM.* 2017;377:1261–1272. doi:10.1056/NEJMra1612789; Goodnough LT, Panigrahi AK. Blood transfusion therapy. *Med Clin North Am.* 2017;101(2):431–447. doi:10.1016/j.mcna.2016.09.012; Rees DC, Robinson S, Howard J. How I manage red cell transfusion in patients with sickle cell disease. *Br J Hematol.* 2018;80:607–617. doi:10.1111/bjh.15115

advise use of a restrictive transfusion threshold of 7 to 8 g/dL. The criteria that determine asymptomatic versus symptomatic anemia can be controversial as well, particularly when considering patients with cardiovascular disease (Table 14.6). RBCs should be transfused on a unit-by-unit basis, except in severe bleeding, with Hgb level and clinical assessment performed after each unit.

Plasma

Like RBCs, plasma can be prepared either from a WB collection or obtained via apheresis technology. Once collected, plasma must be frozen at −18°C or colder within 24 hours; it is kept in the frozen state until needed for use. This storage prevents loss of significant amounts of factors V and VIII, the labile coagulation factors. The exception is liquid plasma, which is kept at 1°C to 6°C and never frozen. When needed, frozen plasma is thawed at 37°C and can then be stored at 1°C to 6°C for up to 5 days (depending on the particular plasma component and the preparation method). Most clinicians refer to all plasma products as fresh frozen plasma (FFP), since this was the only component available for a number of years. There are now several different plasma preparations, and most can be used interchangeably in terms of coagulation factors present. When an order for "plasma" is placed, typically, the Blood Bank will supply FFP, plasma frozen within 24 hours (PF24), or thawed plasma (Table 14.7, Box 14.1 [13], Box 14.2), depending on the blood supplier and availability.

Table 14.7 Plasma Product Types

Plasma Product	Specifications
FFP	• 200 to 250 mL or 400 to 600 mL (apheresis collection; also called "jumbo" plasma) • Normal levels of all coagulation factors, including FV and FVIII
PF24	• 200 to 250 mL or 400 to 600 mL (apheresis collection) • Slightly reduced levels of FVIII and protein C; however, still within hemostatic levels • Used interchangeably with FFP
Thawed plasma	• FFP or PF24 that has been thawed at 37°C and stored at 1°C to 6°C • Can be stored for up to 5 days post-thaw • Allows ready availability of plasma for transfusion without waiting for a 30-minute thaw period
Liquid plasma	• Never frozen plasma; stored at 1°C to 6°C for variable time periods • Coagulation factor profile variable • Contains viable lymphocytes (not indicated for patients at risk for TA-GVHD) • Used for massive transfusion and trauma management
S/D plasma	• Treated with agents that inactivate variety of viruses, bacteria, and parasites • Prepared from large pools of donor plasma units

Table 14.7 Plasma Product Types (*continued*)

Plasma Product	Specifications
Pathogen-inactivated plasma	• Same as S/D plasma, however using different inactivation system • Pooled plasma is not used; all units are from a single donor
Cryoprecipitate-reduced plasma	• Cryoprecipitate removed from FFP after thawing • Deficient in fibrinogen, FVIII, FXIII, high-molecular-weight multimers of vWF, and fibronectin • Used for plasmapheresis and/or transfusion of patients with TTP
Dried plasma	• Lyophilized or spray-dried plasma that must be reconstituted at the time of infusion • Stored at room temperature prior to reconstitution • Used by the military in France and Germany; undergoing trials in the United States

FV, factor V; FVIII, factor VIII; FXIII, factor XIII; FFP, fresh frozen plasma; PF24, plasma frozen within 24 hours; S/D, solvent/detergent; TA-GVHD, transfusion-associated graft-versus-host disease; TTP, thrombotic thrombocytopenic purpura; VWF, von Willebrand factor.

Plasma contains hemostatic levels of all coagulation factors, including fibrinogen. One milliliter of plasma contains approximately 1 unit of coagulation factor activity. The accepted dose is 10 to 20 mL/kg, equivalent to 3 to 6 units in an adult. This dose would be expected to increase the levels of clotting factors by 20% to 30%, which are the values considered sufficient for hemostasis.

Box 14.1 Indications for Plasma Transfusion

• Management of a bleeding patient who requires replacement of multiple coagulation factors (liver disease, DIC)

• Massive transfusion when clinically significant coagulation deficiencies exist

• Rapid reversal of warfarin effect in patient who is bleeding or requires an immediate invasive procedure, and time does not permit correction with vitamin K

• Therapeutic plasma exchange in selected patient populations (TTP, diffuse alveolar hemorrhage associated with Goodpasture's disease)

• Congenital factor deficiencies for which no specific coagulation concentrate is available (e.g., FV, FXI)

• Management of patients with selected plasma protein deficiencies (C1 esterase inhibitor), when recombinant products are not available

DIC, disseminated intravascular coagulation; FV, factor V; FXI, factor XI; TTP, thrombotic thrombocytopenic purpura.

Box 14.2 **Contraindications for Plasma Transfusion**

- Minimal elevation of INR in a non-bleeding patient or prophylaxis for invasive procedure (most current practice guidelines advocate an INR of ≤ 1.5 as acceptable for radiologically guided or surgical procedures)
- Providing intravascular volume expansion
- Protein source in nutritionally deficient patient
- Treatment to correct heparin therapy

INR, International Normalized Ratio.

Platelets (Tables 14.8, 14.9, and 14.10)

Table 14.8 Platelet Products

Component/Product	Platelet Concentration	Volume
Random donor platelet (whole blood–derived platelet, platelet concentrate)	$\geq 5.5 \times 10^{10}$/unit	50 mL
Apheresis platelet	$\geq 3 \times 10^{11}$/unit	300 mL
PAS platelet	Same as apheresis platelet; however, 65% of plasma replaced with sterile buffered solution	300 mL
Leukocyte-reduced apheresis platelet	$\geq 3 \times 10^{11}$/unit ($<5 \times 10^6$ WBCs/unit)	300 mL

PAS, platelet additive solution; WBC, white blood cell.

Source: From Fung MK, Eder AF, Spitalnik SL, et al (eds). *Technical Manual.* 19th ed. Bethesda, MD: AABB; 2017.

Table 14.9 Platelet Dosage

Patient Weight (kg)	Dose	Expected Increment
<35	5 to 10 mL/kg	30,000 to 60,000/mm³, when measured 10 to 60 minutes posttransfusion
≥ 35	One apheresis platelet or five to six whole blood–derived platelet pool	

Source: From Fung MK, Eder AF, Spitalnik SL, et al (eds). *Technical Manual.* 19th ed. Bethesda, MD: AABB; 2017.

Table 14.10 Indications for Platelet Transfusion

Platelet Count (per µL)	Indication
>100,000	• Patient on ECMO • Confirmed or suspected platelet dysfunction (cardiac bypass, uremia, medication related) • CNS or ophthalmic procedure/bleeding • Pulmonary hemorrhage

(*continued*)

Table 14.10 Indications for Platelet Transfusion (*continued*)

Platelet Count (per µL)	Indication
>50,000	• Planned surgical or invasive procedure • Active bleeding
>20,000	• Sepsis • DIC
≤20,000	• Bleeding prophylaxis in a stable patient

CNS, central nervous system; DIC, disseminated intravascular coagulation; ECMO, extracorporeal membrane oxygenation.

Source: From Fung MK, Eder AF, Spitalnik SL, et al (eds). *Technical Manual.* 19th ed. Bethesda, MD: AABB; 2017.

Platelet Transfusion: A Clinical Practice Guideline from the AABB (1,7,9)

- Transfusing hospitalized adult patients with a platelet count of <10 × 10^9 cells/L to reduce the risk for spontaneous bleeding is recommended.
- Transfusing patients having elective central venous catheter placement with a platelet count of <20 × 10^9 cells/L is recommended.
- Prophylactic platelet transfusion for patients having elective diagnostic lumbar puncture with a platelet count of <50 × 10^9 cells/L is recommended.

Platelet Refractoriness

Platelet refractoriness is defined as the repetitive failure to reach and sustain satisfactory platelet counts after platelet transfusions. A pragmatic approach is to define an inappropriate response to platelet transfusion as failure to obtain a posttransfusion platelet increment of >10, 000/µL one hour after transfusion. A failure to achieve this response on more than one occasion suggests alloimmune platelet refractoriness (Box 14.3). Refractoriness may be due to a variety of clinical factors, as listed in Table 14.11. In up to 20% of cases, the etiology is related to an immune-mediated mechanism.

Human leukocyte antigen (HLA) sensitization is the most common immune cause of refractoriness. Patient-generated alloantibodies against HLA Class I and human platelet antigens (HPAs) expressed by donor platelets cause platelet clearance after multiple transfusions. Alloantibodies against HLA-A and HLA-B antigens are more common than antibodies against HPA antigens, ranging from 7% to 55% versus 2% to 5%, respectively. Even if an immune-mediated cause is identified, a non-immune factor is often simultaneously present. Therefore, correcting the underlying non-immune causes is important for management of platelet refractoriness.

> **Box 14.3** Calculation of the Platelet Corrected Count Increment
>
> A posttransfusion platelet increment that is less than expected
>
> A CCI of $<5 \times 10^9$/L after two sequential transfusions:
> - Using ABO-compatible platelets
> - At least one of which had been stored for no more than 48 hours
> - Posttransfusion platelet count obtained within 1 hour after transfusion
>
> **CCI = [posttransfusion platelet count/L – pretransfusion platelet count/L] × BSA (m²)**
> **Platelets transfused**
> - Average adult BSA = 2.0 m²
> - Platelets transfused = 4×10^{11} platelets/apheresis unit or 0.7×10^{11} platelets/whole blood–derived platelet
>
> BSA, body surface area; CCI, correct counted increment.

Several management strategies are described in Box 14.4 (15), Figure 14.1, and Table 14.12 (3,9–11). Each approach has certain advantages and disadvantages. Relying on HLA-matched platelets requires a large pool of HLA-typed donors and does not necessarily lead to receiving HLA-identical or even well-matched platelets. In addition, it can lead to exclusion of donors whose HLA types are different from that of the recipient, but may still be suitable for transfusion.

Cryoprecipitate

Cryoprecipitate is prepared by thawing a unit of FFP at 1°C to 6°C, followed by centrifugation and removal of majority of the plasma supernatant. The remaining precipitate is resuspended in 10 to 15 mL plasma and the product refrozen until needed. For transfusion, the frozen cryoprecipitate is thawed at 37°C and should be transfused immediately. Cryoprecipitate is a concentrated form of fibrinogen, factor VIII (FVIII), factor XIII (FXIII), von Willebrand

Table 14.11 Etiology of Platelet Refractoriness

Non-Immune Mediated	Sepsis
	DIC
	GVHD
	Splenomegaly
	Medications
	Bleeding
Immune mediated	Alloimmunization (anti-HLA, anti-HPA-1a)

GVHD, graft-versus-host disease.

Box 14.4 Management of Platelet Refractoriness

Non-immune causes should be assessed and, if possible, corrected and controlled

ABO-matched and **freshest platelets** available should be used, when possible

If antibodies are identified, there are three possible strategies for identifying compatible platelet units:
- HLA matching (recipient's HLA type must be known)
- Crossmatching random platelet units
- Obtaining HPA-1a matched platelets (or antigen-matched platelets)

All three methods have similar results in terms of posttransfusion CCI counts.

CCI, correct counted increment; HLA, human leukocyte antigen; HPA, human platelet antigen.

---

factor (VWF), and fibronectin (Box 14.5); it is usually indicated for replacement of fibrinogen (Box 14.6). In an average adult, one unit of cryoprecipitate increases the fibrinogen level by 5 to 10 mg/dL; therefore, it is typically pooled into doses of five or 10 units for patient use.

BLOOD COMPONENT MODIFICATIONS

The blood component modifications are presented in Table 14.13.

TRANSFUSION REACTIONS

The blood supply is much safer today due to the data-driven improvements in transfusion practices. However, it is not without risk. The U.S. Biovigilance Network is a national collaboration among government and non-government organizations developing a hemovigilance surveillance system. This system is designed to collect and analyze information on the complications of transfusion. One of the main purposes of developing a hemovigilance program is to improve reporting of transfusion-related adverse events.

Many common clinical signs and symptoms are associated with more than one type of adverse reaction. Early recognition and prompt cessation of the transfusion are the key factors for improved outcomes.

Transfusion-related acute lung injury (TRALI), hemolytic transfusion reactions (HTRs), and transfusion-associated circulatory overload (TACO) are the three most commonly reported causes of

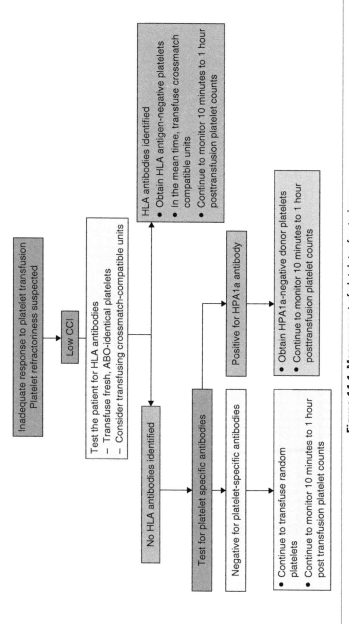

Figure 14.1 Management of platelet refractoriness.

CCI, correct counted increment; HLA, human leukocyte antigen.

Table 14.12 Different Management Strategies for Platelet Refractoriness

	HLa-Matched Platelets	Crossmatched Platelets	Antibody Specificity Selection
Methodology	• Both the patient and donor are HLA typed • HLA-matched donors are selected	• Donor platelets are incubated with patient serum; donor platelets that are crossmatch compatible are selected for transfusion	• Specific antibodies to platelet antigens are detected in the patient • Donor platelets lacking the corresponding antigen are selected
Advantage	• Prevents future alloimmunization, if fully matched	• HLA typing not required • Relatively rapid availability • Useful for both HLA and HPA antibodies	• HLA typing not required
Disadvantage	• Both patient and donor must be HLA typed • Must select HLA-matched platelets • Full HLA matching unlikely • Limited donor pool for rare HLA types	• Requires frequent crossmatching • Does not prevent future HLA alloimmunization • Difficult to find compatible donor in highly sensitized patient	• Difficult to find compatible donors • Does not prevent future HLA alloimmunization

HLA, human leukocyte antigen; HPA, human platelet antigen.

Source: Reproduced with permission from Juskewitch JE, Norgan AP, De Goey SR, et al. How do I manage the platelet transfusion-refractory patient? *Transfusion.* 2017;57(12):2828–2835.

> **Box 14.5** Composition of Cryoprecipitate (Per Unit)
>
> **Fibrinogen**: 150 to 250 mg
>
> **Factor VIII**: 80 to 150 international units
>
> **Factor XIII**: 50 to 75 international units
>
> **von Willebrand factor**: 100 to 150 international units

transfusion-related mortality. Therefore, each case should be investigated to rule out these three main adverse transfusion reactions. The most common transfusion reactions have been summarized in Table 14.14 and Figure 14.2, along with appropriate workup and treatment paradigms (14).

FUTURE DIRECTIONS

- Use of a **platelet additive solution** (PAS) in apheresis platelets results in removal of 60% to 70% of plasma and replacement with a sterile buffered solution. Reduction of the amount of plasma can reduce the incidence of allergic transfusion reactions. Not yet widely available.
- **Pathogen reduction technology** is being used to improve transfusion safety. Pathogen inactivation systems have been approved for use with plasma and apheresis platelets in the United States. Although this technology significantly reduces bacterial, viral, and parasitic pathogens in the blood component, it is not yet widely available. Phase 3 clinical trials are underway using this technology with RBCs. This technology also inactivates WBCs

text continues on page 461

> **Box 14.6** Indications for Cryoprecipitate Transfusion
>
> - Massive blood loss and low fibrinogen levels (usually <100 mg/dL)
> - Inherited disorders of fibrinogen and no fibrinogen concentrates available
> - Liver disease associated with bleeding or need for invasive/surgical procedure
> - Disseminated intravascular coagulation (DIC)
> - Uremic bleeding, unresponsive to desmopression (DDAVP)
> - Preparation of fibrin sealant (fibrin glue)
>
> DDAVP, 1-deamino-8-d-arginine vasopressin; DIC, disseminated intravascular coagulation.

Table 14.13 Blood Component Modifications

Modification	Description	Indications
Leukocyte reduction	• Removal of WBCs from a blood component, typically at the time of collection (pre-storage leukocyte reduction) • Final WBC count is <5 × 10^6/unit • Used for WB, RBCs, platelets • "Universal leukocyte reduction" is the standard of care in the majority of U.S. hospitals • Should not be used on granulocytes intended for transfusion	• Reduce incidence of febrile non-hemolytic transfusion reactions • Reduce HLA alloimmunization • Reduce HLA-mediated platelet refractoriness • Reduce the risk of transfusion-transmitted CMV infection (leukocyte-reduced components are considered "CMV safe" and can be used interchangeably with CMV-negative components)
Irradiation	• Gamma irradiation used to render T-lymphocytes inactive • Typically used for cellular components only (not plasma or cryoprecipitate) • Decreases the shelf life of RBC units due to damage to RBC membrane with resultant K$^+$ leakage into supernatant	• Prevention of TA-GVHD • Indicated for severely immunocompromised patients, recipients of IUT, units from donors who are blood relatives or HLA-matched, BMT, or PBSC recipients
Washed	• Remove the plasma proteins from RBCs or platelets • RBC expires 24 hours after washing; platelet expires 4 hours after washing	• History of recurrent severe allergic transfusion reactions • IgA-deficient patient with anti-IgA • Use of maternal platelets for neonatal/intra-uterine transfusion and maternal plasma has anti-HPA-1a

(continued)

Table 14.13 Blood Component Modifications (*continued*)

Modification	Description	Indications
CMV seronegative	• Testing for anti-CMV antibodies performed on donor unit as a method to detect possible CMV infectivity • Use of leukocyte-reduced RBCs and platelets is considered an acceptable alternative and provides equivalent safety profile • Not usually immediately available as routine inventory	• Organ transplant recipient, stem cell transplant recipient, low-birth-weight infant – who are already known to be CMV negative and severely immunocompromised
Volume reduction	• Removal of majority of plasma and anticoagulant solution from platelet products • Less commonly used for removal of anticoagulant/preservative solution from RBCs • Shelf life is reduced to 4 to 24 hours (depending on the system used) • Will result in some loss of platelets	• Decrease the volume of component transfused to patients at risk for circulatory overload • Reduce exposure to incompatible ABO isoagglutinins
Aliquoting	• Separation of a blood component into a smaller volume bag or syringe • Decreases the shelf life of the component	• Neonatal transfusion • Need for small volume transfusion
Pooling	• Provides clinically effective dose of a blood component • Decreases expiration date based on the system used	• Used for whole blood–derived platelets and cryoprecipitate • May be used for plasma for plasma exchange procedures

BMT, bone marrow transplant; CMV, cytomegalovirus; HLA, human leukocyte antigen; IUT, intrauterine transfusion; PBSC, peripheral blood stem cell; RBCs, red blood cells; TA-GVHD, transfusion-associated graft-versus-host disease; WB, whole blood; WBC, white blood cell.

Table 14.14 Common Transfusion Reactions

Type	Incidence	Etiology/Blood Product	Signs and Symptoms	Diagnosis	Prevention/Treatment	Notes
			Acute Transfusion Reactions (<24 hours)			
Urticarial allergic reaction	1% to 3%	Preformed antibodies in recipient against donor plasma allergens	Urticaria, flushing, pruritis, angioedema	R/O hemolytic reaction (negative DAT)	Premedicate with antihistamine (25–50 mg diphenhydramine), if not sufficient prednisone (20–50 mg oral) or methylprednisolone (125 mg IV) Routine prophylaxis for all recipients before transfusion is not indicated Is the only transfusion reaction in which the transfusion can be safely resumed if patient responds to prompt treatment	For patients whose reactions are severe and unresponsive to premedication: washed blood products (RBC or platelets), deglycerolized RBC or volume-reduced products may be considered Consult your blood bank
Anaphylaxis	1:20,000 to 1:50,000	Preformed antibodies in recipient against donor plasma allergens	Bronchospasm, respiratory distress, wheezing, hypotension, anxiety, urticaria	R/O hemolytic reaction (negative DAT) Check IgA levels; if low, test for anti-IgA	Trendelenburg position Epinephrine (0.2–0.5 mL of 1:1,000 solution SC or IM) Severe cases: 1:10,000 IV, initial rate 1 mcg/min Antihistamines, corticosteroids, beta2 agonists IgA-deficient patients should receive blood components from IgA-deficient donors (IgA <0.05 mg/dL)	

(continued)

Table 14.14 (continued)

Type	Incidence	Etiology/Blood Product	Signs and Symptoms	Diagnosis	Prevention/Treatment	Notes
FNHTR	0.1% to 1%	Accumulated cytokines in cellular components, particularly with platelet transfusion Recipient anti-HLA antibodies against donor leukocytes	Fever, rigors/chills, headache, vomiting	R/O hemolytic reaction (negative DAT) R/O infection/sepsis	Premedicate with antipyretics, for example, acetaminophen Meperidine for rigors, if there is no contraindication	Leukoreduced blood products
AHTR	1:40,000	RBC incompatibility	Chills, fever/rigors, hypotension, renal failure with oliguria, DIC, pain/oozing from IV lines, back pain, dark urine	Check the blood component (clerical error) Visual inspection for hemolysis Repeat patient's DAT ABO, pre- and posttransfusion sample Tests to detect hemolysis: LDH, bilirubin, haptoglobin, urine analysis for hemoglobinuria	Stop transfusion immediately Keep the urine output >1 mL/kg/hr with fluids and IV diuretics (furosemide) Analgesics (may need morphine) Pressors for hypotension (low-dose dopamine) Supportive treatment if DIC develops	Rapid hemolysis of as little as 10 mL of incompatible blood can produce symptoms of AHTR The most common presenting symptom is fever with or without accompanying chills/rigors

(continued)

Table 14.14 (*continued*)

Type	Incidence	Etiology/Blood Product	Signs and Symptoms	Diagnosis	Prevention/Treatment	Notes
TRALI	1:1,200 to 1:190,000	Antibodies to leukocyte antigens (HLA Class I, HLA Class II, and human neutrophil antigens); presence of biologic response modifiers	Hypoxia, hypotension, respiratory failure, fever, bilateral pulmonary edema	R/O hemolytic reaction (negative DAT) Chest x-ray Decreased BNP levels R/O cardiogenic pulmonary edema (TACO) R/O other causes of ALI WBC antibody screen in donor and recipient; if positive, antigen typing may be indicated WBC crossmatch	Supportive care until recovery of respiratory distress Usually resolves within 48 to 72 hours, but the mortality rate is 10% In most instances, no special requirements are necessary to manage further transfusions; however, if TRALI is due to recipient HLA antibodies, leukoreduced products are indicated	Suspected TRALI reactions should be reported to blood bank Implicated donors are deferred from blood donations; additional components from the same donor are quarantined or recalled Donor plasma is tested for HLA antibodies; if positive, the recipient is typed for cognate HLA antigens The donor of the implicated unit is often a multiparous woman; therefore, plasma products and whole blood collections are made from male donors, never pregnant female donors, or females who have been tested for HLA antibodies since their last pregnancy

(*continued*)

Table 14.14 (continued)

Type	Incidence	Etiology/Blood Product	Signs and Symptoms	Diagnosis	Prevention/Treatment	Notes
TACO	<1%	Volume overload Elderly and infants are at risk High flow rates are frequent cofactors	Dyspnea, orthopnea, cough, tachycardia, hypertension Elevated CVP, new ST and T wave changes on EKG Elevated serum troponin Elevated BNP Wide cardiothoracic ratio	Chest x-ray BNP R/O TRALI	Seated position, O_2 supplementation, IV diuretics	Slow transfusion rate (2–4 mL/min)
Transfusion-associated sepsis	Varies by blood product	Bacterial contamination of unit Platelets most commonly implicated	Fever, chills, hypotension	Gram stain/culture of patient and blood product R/O hemolysis	Broad-spectrum antibiotics until sensitivities are available	Most common bacterium in RBC transfusion is *Yersinia enterocolitica* Platelets are the main culprits in transfusion-associated sepsis, since they are stored at room temperature Most common bacteria after platelet transfusions are *Staphylococcus aureus*, *Escherichia coli*, *Bacillus* species, and *Salmonella* species

(continued)

Table 14.14 (*continued*)

Type	Incidence	Etiology/Blood Product	Signs and Symptoms	Diagnosis	Prevention/Treatment	Notes
Hypotension associated with ACE inhibitors	Varies by clinical condition		Flushing and hypotension	R/O hemolysis, DAT negative	Stop ACE inhibitor Avoid bedside leukocyte filtration	
Nonimmune hemolysis	Rare	Physical or chemical destruction of RBC	Hemoglobinemia and hemoglobinuria	R/O immune-mediated hemolysis, DAT negative		
Hypocalcemia, citrate toxicity	Varies by clinical setting	Rapid citrate infusions, massive transfusions of citrated blood, plasmapheresis	Perioral paresthesia, tetany, muscular spasms, arrhythmia, nausea, hyperventilation	Ionized Ca levels Prolonged QT interval	Slow Ca infusions while monitoring ionized Ca levels	Plasma, whole blood, and platelets contain citrate as anticoagulants. When large amounts are transfused rapidly, plasma citrate levels increase, binding calcium and causing hypocalcemia
Hypothermia	Varies by clinical setting	Rapid infusion of cold blood	Cardiac arrhythmia	Check body temperature	Use blood warmers	

(*continued*)

Table 14.14 (continued)

Type	Incidence	Etiology/Blood Product	Signs and Symptoms	Diagnosis	Prevention/Treatment	Notes
			Delayed transfusion reactions (>24 hours)			
DHTR due to RBC alloimmunization	1%	Immune response to foreign antigens on RBC, develops between 1 and 28 days Positive elution test with alloantibody present on the transfused RBCs OR Newly identified RBC alloantibody in recipient serum	Fever and anemia days to weeks after transfusion No increase in hemoglobin concentration following transfusion or rapid fall in hemoglobin back to pretransfusion levels	DAT, antibody screen	Avoid unnecessary transfusions Anemia is corrected by transfusing antigen-negative RBC as needed	Blood group antibodies associated with DHTRs include Kidd, Duffy, Kell, and MNS system, in order of decreasing frequency DSTR is the rapid development of alloantibody in the absence of laboratory evidence of hemolysis
Alloimmunization (HLA antigens)	10%	Immune response to WBCs and platelets	Platelet refractoriness, delayed hemolytic reaction	Platelet antibody screen HLA antibody screen	Avoid unnecessary transfusions Leukoreduced blood products	Refer to the section "Platelet Refractoriness"

(continued)

Table 14.14 (continued)

Type	Incidence	Etiology/Blood Product	Signs and Symptoms	Diagnosis	Prevention/Treatment	Notes
GVHD	Rare	Donor lymphocytes in transfused blood product attack the host tissue	Usually symptoms appear 8 to 10 days after transfusion Maculopapular rash, fever, enterocolitis with watery diarrhea, elevated liver functions, pancytopenia	Skin biopsy HLA typing Molecular analysis for chimerism	Corticosteroids and cytotoxic agents Irradiated blood components for patients at risk	**Well-documented indications:** Intrauterine transfusions Prematurity, low birth weight, erythroblastosis fetalis in newborns Congenital immunodeficiency Hematologic malignancy or solid tumors (neuroblastoma, sarcoma, Hodgkin disease) Peripheral blood stem cell/ marrow transplantation Components that are crossmatched, HLA matched or directed donations from family members Fludarabine therapy Granulocyte components **Potential indications:** Other malignancies, including those treated with cytotoxic agents Donor recipient pairs from genetically homogeneous populations **Usually not indicated:** Patients with HIV Full-term infants Non-immunosuppressed patients

(continued)

Table 14.14 (*continued*)

Type	Incidence	Etiology/Blood Product	Signs and Symptoms	Diagnosis	Prevention/Treatment	Notes
PTP	Rare	Recipient platelet antibodies destroy autologous platelets. Presence of platelet-specific alloantibodies in patients previously exposed to platelet antigens via pregnancy or transfusion	Profound thrombocytopenia (platelets <10,000/μL), wet purpura, bleeding 8 to 10 days after transfusion	Platelet antibody screen	IVIG. HPA-1a–negative platelets. Plasmapheresis	HPA-1a is the most common antibody (70% of PTP cases). HPA-1b alloantibodies and HLA antibodies are also implicated. Use of leukoreduced blood components may decrease the incidence of PTP. PTP usually does not recur; however, in patients with PTP history, efforts to obtain components from antigen-matched donors should be made

ACE, angiotensin converting enzyme; AHTR, acute hemolytic transfusion reaction; ALI, acute lung injury; BNP, brain natriuretic peptide; CVP, central venous pressure; DAT, direct antiglobulin test; DHTR, delayed hemolytic transfusion reaction; DIC, disseminated intravascular coagulation; DSTR, delayed serologic transfusion reaction; FNHTR, febrile non-hemolytic transfusion reaction; GVHD, graft-versus-host disease; HLA, human leukocyte antigen; IM, intramuscular; IV, intravenous; IVIG, intravenous immunoglobulin; LDH, lactate dehydrogenase; PTP, posttransfusion purpura; RBC, red blood cell; SC, subcutaneous; TACO, transfusion-associated circulatory overload; TRALI, transfusion-related acute lung injury.

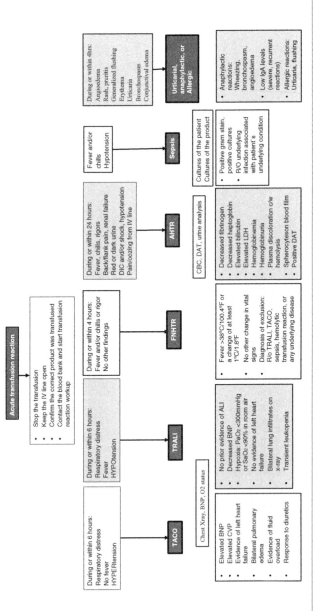

Figure 14.2 Recognition of common transfusion reactions.

AHTR, acute hemolytic transfusion reaction; CBC, complete blood count; DIC, disseminated intravascular coagulation; FNHTR, febrile non-hemolytic transfusion reaction; IV, intravenous; LDH, lactate dehydrogenase; TACO, transfusion-associated circulatory overload; TRALI, transfusion-related acute lung injury.

present in transfused blood components, thereby eliminating the requirement for irradiation to prevent graft-versus-host disease (GVHD) in susceptible patient populations.

- **Patient blood management (PBM)** programs are designed to reduce the need for RBC transfusion in the perioperative period (12). This is accomplished through preoperative screening for and treatment of anemia in patients scheduled for surgical procedures, as well as identifying those patients at increased risk for bleeding. Treatment strategies may include oral or IV iron supplementation, adjustment of antiplatelet and anticoagulant medications, and intraoperative and postoperative red cell salvage techniques.
- Correction of the effects of **antiplatelet medications** and **factor Xa inhibitors** in patients who require acute interventions where bleeding likely represents challenges in blood transfusion. Standard dosage of platelet and/or plasma transfusions may not be effective, and potential benefit versus harm should be assessed (9). Specific reversal agents are undergoing clinical trials.
- **Transfusion of WB** is becoming more common in trauma settings. Several studies have shown that group O WB with low titers of anti-A and anti-B can be safely transfused to actively bleeding patients regardless of the individual's ABO blood group.

KEY POINTS

- Blood transfusion is not without risk. Appropriate informed consent should be obtained.
- Avoid ordering "multiples" of blood products ("Why give two, when one will do") in a hemodynamically stable patient. Assess the need for continued transfusion with monitoring of laboratory values and patient symptoms.
- RBC transfusion guidelines have been published by several specialty societies. They distinguish between use of a restrictive (Hgb 7–8 g/dL) versus a liberal (Hgb 8–10 g/dL) transfusion threshold based on Hgb levels.
- Assessment of posttransfusion Hgb level can be performed as early as 15 minutes following completion of the transfusion.
- Plasma should not be transfused solely to correct a minimally elevated International Normalized Ratio (INR) in a patient who is not bleeding and/or scheduled for an immediate invasive procedure.

- Diagnosis of platelet refractoriness requires checking the platelet count 10 to 60 minutes after completion of the platelet transfusion. To qualify as platelet refractoriness, the CCI should be <5 × 10^9/L after two sequential platelet transfusions.
- Many common clinical signs/symptoms occurring during or immediately after transfusion can be associated with more than one type of reaction. Early recognition and prompt cessation of the transfusion are the key factors for improved outcome.
- The most commonly reported causes of transfusion-related mortality are hemolytic transfusion reactions, TRALI, and transfusion-associated circulatory overload (TACO).
- Acute HTRs are often due to sample or patient misidentification. Accurate patient identification is mandatory in all processes associated with transfusion.
- HLA-matched platelets are more likely to cause transfusion-associated GVHD; therefore, HLA-matched platelets should be irradiated.
- Cryoprecipitate is ineffective in reversing the anticoagulant effects of warfarin or other vitamin K antagonists.
- Allergic reactions range from mild urticarial to severe anaphylactic reactions. Patients experiencing severe reactions should be checked for IgA deficiency. Patients with absolute IgA deficiency (IgA <0.05 mg/dL) should receive plasma from IgA-deficient donors. Other cellular components (RBC, platelets) can be depleted of plasma by washing.

REFERENCES

1. Fung MK, Eder AF, Spitalnik SL, et al., eds. *Technical Manual.* 19th ed. Bethesda, MD: AABB; 2017.
2. Osterman JL, Arora S. Blood product transfusions and reactions. *Hematol Oncol Clin North Am.* 2017;31(6):1159–1170. doi:10.1016/j.hoc.2017.08.014
3. Prevention of Rh D alloimmunization. ACOG Practice Bulletin. *Obstet Gynecol.* 2017;130(2):57–69.
4. Carson JL, Guyatt G, Heddle NM, et al. Clinical practice guidelines from the AABB: red blood cell transfusion thresholds and storage. *JAMA.* 2016;316(19):2025–2035. doi:10.1001/jama.2016.9185
5. Carson JL, Grossman BJ, Kleinman S, et al. Red blood cell transfusion: a clinical practice guideline from the AABB. *Ann Intern Med.* 2012;157:49–58. doi:10.7326/0003-4819-157-1-201206190-00429

6. Carson JL, Triulzi DJ, Ness PM. Indications for and adverse effects of red-cell transfusion. *NEJM.* 2017;377:1261–1272. doi:10.1056/NEJMra1612789

7. Goodnough LT, Panigrahi AK. Blood transfusion therapy. *Med Clin North Am.* 2017;101(2):431–447. doi:10.1016/j.mcna.2016.09.012

8. Rees DC, Robinson S, Howard J. How I manage red cell transfusion in patients with sickle cell disease. *Br J Hematol.* 2018;80:607–617. doi:10.1111/bjh.15115

9. Gremmel T, Panzer S. Oral platelet therapy: impact for transfusion medicine. *Vox Sanguinis.* 2017;112:511–517. doi:10.1111/vox.12537

10. Juskewitch JE, Norgan AP, De Goey SR, et al. How do I manage the platelet transfusion-refractory patient? *Transfusion.* 2017;57(12):2828–2835. doi:10.1111/trf.14316

11. Pine AB, Lee E-J, Sekeres M, et al. Wide variations in blood product transfusion practices among providers who care for patients with acute leukemia in the United States. *Transfusion.* 2017;57:289–295.

12. Yazer MH, Waters JH. What in the world of transfusion medicine isn't patient blood management? *Transfus Med.* 2018;28(2):89–91. doi:10.1111/tme.12522

13. Alcorn K, Ramsey G, Souers R, et al. Appropriateness of plasma transfusion. *Arch Pathol Lab Med.* 2017;141:396–401. doi:10.5858/ARPA.2016-0047-CP

14. Delaney M, Wendel S, Bercovitz RS, et al. Transfusion reactions: prevention, diagnosis, and treatment. *Lancet.* 2016;388:2825–2836. doi:10.1016/S0140-6736(15)01313-6

15. Wang J, Xia W, Deng J, et al. Analysis of platelet-reactive allo-antibodies and evaluation of cross-match-compatible platelets for the management of patients with transfusion refractoriness. *Transfus Med.* 2018;28(1):40–46. doi:10.1111/tme.12423

15 Pharmacology

Anthony Wiseman and Rosetta Lee

Clinical Case 15.1

A 46-year-old female with history of HIV diagnosed 6 months ago is taking emtricitabine, tenofovir alafenamide, and raltegravir. She also receives rifampin, isoniazid, pyrazinamide, and ethambutol for pulmonary tuberculosis. Her last viral load was undetectable, with a CD4 count of 460 cells/mm³. She has a history of unprovoked right lower extremity deep vein thrombosis (DVT) 5 years earlier and was treated with therapeutic enoxaparin for 3 years followed by aspirin 325 mg/d. She had recurrence of right lower extremity DVT with pulmonary embolism and has since been treated with warfarin. She presents to hematology clinic to discuss alternative oral anticoagulant therapy. She has had labile International Normalized Ratios (INRs) and is within therapeutic range only 50% of the time. The patient dislikes the dietary restrictions and frequent INR checks associated with warfarin use. She refuses to self-administer subcutaneous low-molecular-weight heparin (LMWH).

VITAMIN K ANTAGONISTS

Vitamin K antagonists (VKAs) have a long-standing history of use in the treatment of venous thromboembolism (VTE) and in stroke prevention secondary to atrial fibrillation (AF). Warfarin is the most commonly prescribed anticoagulant despite the inception of the direct acting oral anticoagulants (DOACs).

Pharmacology

Normal clotting requires carboxylation of factors II, VII, IX, and X; this carboxylation process is regulated by vitamin K epoxide reductase, the enzyme which converts the oxidized form of vitamin K to the active reduced form. Warfarin inhibits vitamin K epoxide reductase, decreasing the concentrations of reduced vitamin K required for the vitamin K-dependent carboxylase, ultimately inhibiting the conversion of factors II, VII, IX, and X into their active forms (1). Of note, when warfarin therapy is initiated, it takes a number of days before the previously active vitamin K-dependent clotting factors

Table 15.1 Approximate Half-Life Values of Endogenous Coagulation Factors II, VII, IX, X, Protein C, and Protein S

Coagulation Factor	Half-Life (hours)
Factor II	50
Factor VII	6
Factor IX	24
Factor X	36
Protein C	8
Protein S	24

are cleared. Initially, warfarin exerts a procoagulant effect because it inhibits the naturally occurring anticoagulants, protein C, and protein S, due to their very short half-lives (Table 15.1).

Pharmacokinetics

Warfarin is 100% bioavailable and is completely absorbed with its maximum concentration occurring between 2 and 6 hours. The volume of distribution is 0.14 L/kg; it is 98% to 99% bound to albumin in the plasma, indicating that only a small amount of warfarin is pharmacologically active once absorbed (2,3). Once metabolized, warfarin is eliminated through the urine unchanged.

Two enzymes associated with variant genetic polymorphisms contribute to the interpatient variability observed in the dose–response relationship of warfarin: CYP2C9 and vitamin K epoxide reductase complex 1 (VKORC1). While wild-type CYP2C9 (*1/*1 alleles) confers normal warfarin metabolism, studies have shown that the *2 and *3 alleles are associated with decreased metabolism and may lead to overanticoagulation, requiring dose reductions, especially when initiating therapy (1). Genetic variants of VKORC1 are associated with single missense polymorphisms and are known to influence warfarin dosing (4,5). A summary of CYP2C9 and VKORC1 polymorphisms and their effect on warfarin metabolism can be found in Table 15.2. While there is evidence to support the use of genotype-based warfarin dosing, the availability, time, and cost of testing prohibit its utilization.

Initiation and Management of Warfarin

There is significant debate surrounding the most appropriate dose for warfarin initiation (5). The use of genotyping to arrive at the optimal starting dose is not currently recommended due to cost. Consequently, most practitioners initiate warfarin therapy at a starting dose of 5 mg once daily, but it may be individualized based on clinical factors such as age, comorbidities, and organ dysfunction.

Table 15.2 Common CYP2C9 and Vitamin K Epoxide Reductase Complex 1 Polymorphisms and Their Effects on Warfarin Dosing

Polymorphism	Warfarin Metabolism Alterations
CYP2C9 *2/*2	Decrease
CYP2C9 *2/*3	Decrease
CYP2C9 *3/*3	Decrease
VKORC1A: G3673A (−1639G > A)	Increase
VKORC1A: G9041A (−3730G > A)	Decrease

VKORC1, vitamin K epoxide reductase complex 1.

The American College of CHEST Physicians guidelines suggest a starting dose of less than 5 mg for patients >60 years of age, malnourishment, congestive heart failure, and liver dysfunction.

Warfarin does not exert its full anticoagulant effect immediately. Prothrombin, the end target of warfarin therapy for anticoagulation, has the longest half-life, approximately 60 to 100 hours (Table 15.1), and hence, the recommendation for bridging therapy with a shorter-acting anticoagulant such as unfractionated heparin (UFH) or an LMWH (e.g., enoxaparin) for at least 5 days.

Chronic warfarin management requires diligent and ongoing therapeutic monitoring. Previously, prothrombin time (PT) was used to measure warfarin's anticoagulation effects. But due to the variability of thromboplastin used to obtain PT results, the INR was developed to provide a more standardized result and is now the most recognized approach in warfarin monitoring. Doses should be titrated based on the target INR, depending on the indication for use (Table 15.3). Due to its narrow therapeutic window, subtherapeutic INR increases the risk of clotting, while supratherapeutic INR increases the risk of bleeding. If alterations are warranted, modifications should be based on calculations of the total weekly dose of warfarin and should be either increased or decreased by 5% to 25%. Furthermore, dose adjustments should only be made after waiting for a minimum of 3 days, since changes in INR occur slowly based on the aforementioned half-lives of the vitamin K coagulation factors.

Interactions

One of the most significant challenges of warfarin therapy is the myriad of food and drug interactions that may alter the INR and result in deleterious clinical outcomes (Tables 15.4, 15.5). Patients

Table 15.3 Target International Normalized Ratio (INR) Levels Based on Indication

Indication	Target INR
VTE treatment	2 to 3
Stroke prophylaxis in atrial fibrillation	2 to 3
Hypercoagulable states (e.g., antiphospholipid syndrome)	2 to 3
Prosthetic heart valves	2.5 to 3.5
VTE, venous thromboembolism.	

should be advised to maintain a consistent level of vitamin K-rich foods on a daily basis as fluctuations in vitamin K concentrations may disrupt the INR goal. It is important that clinicians conduct a thorough investigation and educate patients on these interactions, including prescription and nonprescription medications, to make appropriate adjustments based on INR levels. Patients should be advised to communicate with their providers if any changes occur with their medications and to discuss any inconsistencies with their diet, so that appropriate modifications can be made after subsequent INR testing (1,6).

Table 15.4 Vitamin K-Rich Foods and Their Vitamin K Content per One Cup Serving Size

Food Name	Vitamin K Content (mcg)
Kale, boiled	1,062
Parsley, raw	984
Spinach, boiled	888
Collards, boiled	836
Swish chard, boiled	574
Turnip greens, boiled	530
Mustard greens, boiled	210
Broccoli, cooked	220
Brussel sprouts, cooked	219
Endive, raw	116

Source: Adapted from https://www.cc.nih.gov/ccc/patient_education/drug_nutrient/coumadin1.pdf

Table 15.5 List of Drug Interactions and Their Relevant Cytochrome P450 Enzyme Effects on Warfarin

Drug/Supplement	INR Effect	Mechanism
Amiodarone	Increase	CYP1A2, 2C9, 3A4 inhibitor
Bitter orange	Increase	CYP3A4 inhibitor
Carbamazepine	Decrease	CYP1A2, 2C9, 2C19, 3A4 inducer
Cimetidine	Increase	CYP1A2 inhibitor
Ciprofloxacin	Increase	CYP1A2 inhibitor
Clarithromycin	Increase	CYP3A4 inhibitor
Cranberry	Increase	CYP2C9 inhibitor
Diltiazem	Increase	CYP3A4 inhibitor
Echinacea	Increase	CYP3A4 inhibitor
Erythromycin	Increase	CYP3A4 inhibitor
Eucalyptus	Increase	CYP1A2, 2C9, 2C19, 3A4 inhibitor
Fluconazole	Increase	CYP2C9, 3A4 inhibitor
Fluvoxamine	Increase	CYP2C19 inhibitor
Garlic	Increase	CYP 2C9, 2C19, 3A4 inhibitor
Ginseng	Decrease	CYP inducer
Goldenseal	Increase	CYP3A4 inhibitor
Grapefruit juice	Increase	CYP1A2, 3A4 inhibitor
Itraconazole	Increase	CYP3A4 inhibitor
Isoniazid	Increase	CYP2C19 inhibitor
Kava Kava	Increase	CYP1A2, 2C9, 2C19, 3A4 inhibitor
Ketoconazole	Increase	CYP3A4 inhibitor
Metronidazole	Increase	CYP2C9 inhibitor
Milk thistle	Increase	CYP2C9, 3A4 inhibitor
Phenobarbital	Decrease	CYP1A2, 2C9, 3A4 inducer
Phenytoin	Decrease	CYP2C9, 2C19, 3A4 inducer
Rifampin	Decrease	CYP1A2, 2C9, 2C19, 3A4 inducer
Ritonavir	Increase	CYP2C9, 2C19, 3A4 inhibitor
St. John's wort	Decrease	CYP3A4 inducer
Telithromycin	Increase	CYP3A4 inhibitor
Tobacco (smoking)	Decrease	CYP1A2 inducer

(*continued*)

Table 15.5 List of Drug Interactions and Their Relevant Cytochrome P450 Enzyme Effects on Warfarin (*continued*)

Drug/Supplement	INR Effect	Mechanism
Trimethoprim/ sulfamethoxazole	Increase	CYP2C9 inhibitor
Valerian root	Increase	CYP3A4 inhibitor
Verapamil	Increase	CYP3A4 inhibitor
Wild cherry	Increase	CYP3A4 inhibitor

CYP3A4, cytochrome P450 3A4.

VKA Reversal

For patients who are receiving VKA therapy and require immediate reversal, especially in the setting of a life-threatening hemorrhage, the pretreatment INR guides dosing (please see the section "Prothrombin Complex Concentrate" for additional information). Patients should also receive an intravenous (IV) infusion of 5 to 10 mg vitamin K over 1 hour.

Key Points

1. Warfarin is a highly effective anticoagulant that alters the vitamin K-dependent coagulation process.

2. Warfarin is associated with significant challenges in its management, given its narrow therapeutic index, its need for continuous monitoring, and the burden it presents to patients and clinicians due to its numerous amounts of food and drug interactions.

DIRECT ORAL ANTICOAGULANTS

Direct oral anticoagulants (DOACs) are a newer class of agents that do not require the lifestyle changes or frequent therapeutic monitoring that VKAs mandate. Meta-analyses show that DOACs have safer bleeding profiles and, in some circumstances, are more efficacious than VKAs.

Currently, five DOACs are approved by the Food and Drug Administration (FDA) across a number of indications (Box 15.1). Dabigatran is the only oral direct thrombin (factor IIa) inhibitor, while rivaroxaban, apixaban, edoxaban, and betrixaban are all factor Xa inhibitors. All DOACs are reversible, competitive, and selective inhibitors for their respective targets. Unlike heparins, the DOACs do not require antithrombin activity to function. Once bound to the prothrombinase complex, activated factor X or factor

---

Box 15.1 Indications for Direct Oral Anticoagulant Use

Stroke prevention in nonvalvular atrial fibrillation

Acute VTE

Maintenance therapy for VTE

Risk reduction and prevention of recurrent VTE

Prevention of VTE in postoperative knee and hip arthroplasty

VTE, venous thromboembolism.

II retains potent activity in converting prothrombin into thrombin. Whereas heparins only bind free activated serine proteases, DOACs have activity against both free and bound serine proteases (7). DOACs inhibit platelet aggregation indirectly by blocking thrombin formation, and thus thrombin-mediated platelet aggregation.

Betrixaban is the only approved DOAC for VTE prophylaxis for hospitalized patients in the acute setting (8). There are no direct head-to-head trials comparing the DOACs to one another, so it is imperative that clinicians be familiar with the subtle differences between each agent in order to choose the most appropriate therapy for the individual patient. DOACs are contraindicated in the setting of active pathologic hemorrhage, hemodynamically unstable VTE, patients with valvular heart disease (e.g., rheumatic mitral disease, history of mitral valve repair, prosthetic/mechanical heart valves), pregnant and breastfeeding mothers, and neuroaxial spinal anesthesia (9).

Pharmacokinetics and Special Populations

In general, patients are more likely to experience bleeding complications on DOACs when they are older (age >75 years), have low body weight (<60 kg), and exhibit renal dysfunction (creatinine clearance by Cockcroft–Gault formula [CrCl]: <30–50 mL/min). The risk of bleeding further increases with concomitant use of drugs that either modulate metabolic enzyme activity (e.g., P-glycoprotein [P-gp] or cytochrome P450 [CYP]) or further increase the risk of bleeding independent of the DOAC (e.g., nonsteroidal anti-inflammatory agents, antiplatelets, aspirin, possibly selective serotonin reuptake inhibitors/serotonin and norepinephrine reuptake inhibitors [SSRI/SSNIs]). Thus, review of potential drug–drug interactions and pharmacology, especially the pharmacokinetics (PK), of the DOACs is imperative when considering their use (Tables 15.6–15.9).

Extra caution is recommended when considering DOAC therapy in the following: women of childbearing age without "proper contraceptive measures"; pregnant or nursing mothers; HIV patients (with or without use of protease inhibitors); when there is concomitant use of strong cytochrome P450 3A4 (CYP3A4) inducers or

text continues on page 477

Table 15.6 Dosing Guidelines of Direct Oral Anticoagulants in Nonvalvular Atrial Fibrillation

	Dabigatran	Rivaroxaban	Apixaban	Edoxaban
Normal dose	150 mg PO BID	20 mg PO daily (with evening meal)	5 mg PO BID	60 mg PO daily if CrCl ≤95 mL/min
Important trials	RE-LY	ROCKET-AF	ARISTOTLE, AVERROES	ENGAGE AFTIMI 48
Dose reduced	75 mg PO BID	15 mg PO daily (with evening meal)	2.5 mg PO BID	30 mg daily
Indications for dose reduction	CrCl 15 to 30 mL/min (from PK data) CrCl 30 to 50 mL/min and P-gp inhibitor	CrCl 15 to 50 mL/min (15–30 mL/min from PK data)	If more than one factor present: Age ≥80 years Wt ≤60 kg Cr ≥1.5 mg/dL	CrCl 15 to 50 mL/min
	Dronedarone and systemic ketoconazole		Strong combined P-gp and CYP3A4 inhibitors (2.5 mg PO BID)	
Avoid use/ contraindications	CrCl <30 mL/min and using P-gp inhibitors in general	Combined P-gp and strong CYP3A4 inhibitors/inducers	Severe hepatic impairment	If CrCl >95 mL/min
			Strong combined P-gp + CYP3A4 inducers	Moderate-to-severe hepatic impairment
	"Mechanical heart valves"	"Prosthetic heart valves"	"Prosthetic heart valves"	Mechanical heart valves
				Moderate-to-severe mitral stenosis

(continued)

Table 15.6 Dosing Guidelines of Direct Oral Anticoagulants in Nonvalvular Atrial Fibrillation (*continued*)

	Dabigatran	Rivaroxaban	Apixaban	Edoxaban
No dosing recommendation available or other notes	CrCl <15 mL/min Trials excluded LFT elevation >2× ULN	Any hepatic impairment	Moderate hepatic impairment	Any hepatic impairment

BID, twice daily; CrCl, creatinine clearance by Cockcroft and Gault formula; CYP3A4, cytochrome P450 3A4; DOACs, direct oral anticoagulants; P-gp, P-glycoprotein; PK, pharmacokinetics; PO, per os; ULN, upper limit of normal.

Table 15.7 Direct Oral Anticoagulant Dosing Guidelines in Acute Venous Thromboembolism, Recurrence, or Prophylaxis

Acute VTE, Recurrence, Prophylaxis	Dabigatran	Rivaroxaban	Apixaban	Edoxaban
Important trials	RE-COVER I, II RE-MEDY RE-SONATE	EINSTEIN PE EINSTEIN CHOICE	AMPLIFY, AMPLIFY-EXT	Hokusai VTE Hokusai VTE cancer
Acute VTE dose	After 5 to 10 days of parenteral anticoagulation, start 150 mg BID	15 mg BID with meals for 21 days, then 20 mg with evening meals daily	10 mg BID for 7 days, then 5 mg BID	After 5 to 10 days of parenteral anticoagulation, start 60 mg daily (Note: no CrCl upper limit compared to A.fib.)
Prevention of VTE recurrence dose	150 mg BID	20 mg q evening meal 10 mg q evening meal	After ≥6 months of therapy, 2.5 mg BID	Data noninferior, but not approved
Post-op prophylaxis THA	Not indicated	10 mg for 35 days	2.5 mg BID for 35 days	Not indicated
TKA	Not indicated	10 mg for 12 days	2.5 mg BID for 12 days No adjustment for low CrCl (trials excluded ESRD, CrCl <15)	Not indicated

(continued)

Table 15.7 Direct Oral Anticoagulant Dosing Guidelines in Acute Venous Thromboembolism, Recurrence, or Prophylaxis (*continued*)

Acute VTE, Recurrence, Prophylaxis	Dabigatran	Rivaroxaban	Apixaban	Edoxaban
Indications for dose reduction	No recommendation available	No recommendation available	Decrease dose by 50% if more than one factor present: Age ≥80 years Wt ≤60 kg Cr ≥1.5 mg/dL Or Strong combined P-gp and CYP3A4 inhibitors	30 mg daily if: CrCl 15 to 50 mL/min, weight ≤60 kg, use of certain P-gp inhibitors (such as verapamil, quinidine, dronedarone; trial excluded patients taking ritonavir, nelfinavir, indinavir, saquinivar, cyclosporine)
Avoid use or contraindications	Hepatic impairment*	Moderate-to-severe hepatic impairment	Severe hepatic impairment	Moderate-to-severe hepatic impairment
	CrCl <50 mL/min and using P-gp inhibitors	CrCl ≤30 mL/min	Indications for 2.5 mg dose and taking strong combined P-gp and CYP3A4 inhibitors	Mechanical heart valves or moderate-to-severe mitral stenosis
				Rifampin use
No dosing recommendation available	CrCl ≤30 mL/min	Use combined P-gp and strong CYP3A4 inhibitors/inducers	Moderate hepatic impairment	

Note: Synonymous terms in cirrhosis for mild, moderate, and severe hepatic impairment are Child–Pugh A, B, and C, respectively.

*See the section "Dabigatran."

A, fib, atrial fibrillation; BID, twice daily; CrCl, creatinine clearance by Cockcroft and Gault formula; CYP3A4, cytochrome P450 3A4; DOACs, direct oral anticoagulants; ESRD, end stage renal disease; P-gp, P-glycoprotein; PO, per os (by mouth); THA, total hip arthroplasty; TKA, total knee arthroplasty; VTE, venous thromboembolism.

Table 15.8 Pharmacokinetic Parameters of Direct Oral Anticoagulants

	Dabigatran	Rivaroxaban	Apixaban	Edoxaban	Betrixaban
Target of inhibition	IIa	Xa	Xa	Xa	Xa
Prodrug	Yes, four active metabolites	No	No	No	No
Bioavailability, oral	3% to 7% (Increases by 75% without capsule shell. AUC not affected by food. Absorption may be decreased by PPIs)	80% to 100% (66% without food)	50% (Not affected by food or if crushed)	62% (Not affected by food)	34% (C_{max} and AUC with food reduced by 61%–70%)
Time to C_{max} (hours)	1 to 3	2 to 4	3 to 4	1 to 2	3 to 4
Half-life (hours)	12 to 17	5 to 13*	9 to 14	10 to 14	19 to 27
Renal clearance (%)	80	33	25	50	11
Liver metabolism	Minimal	Yes	Yes	Minimal	Minimal[†]
Metabolism and routes of drug interactions	P-gp	P-gp CYP3A4	P-gp CYP3A4	P-gp	P-gp

*Rivaroxaban's half-life is 5 to 9 hours in young healthy volunteers aged between 20 and 45 years and 11 to 13 hours in elderly patients.

[†]Betrixaban is not recommended for use in patients "with hepatic impairment."

AUC, area under the curve; CYP3A4, cytochrome P450 3A4; P-gp, P-glycoprotein; PPIs, proton pump inhibitors.

Table 15.9 Potential Drug–Drug Interactions With Direct Oral Anticoagulants When Used in Combination

Inhibitors: strong combined P-gp and CYP3A4	Azoles: itraconazole, posaconazole, ketoconazole (high dose)
	Macrolide antibiotics: erythromycin, clarithromycin, azithromycin
	HIV protease Inhibitors: ritonavir (Norvir), ritonavir + lopinavir (Kaletra), indinavir (Crixivan)
	Quinidine
Inhibitors: strong P-gp and weak-to-moderate CYP3A4	Antiarrhythmics (Class III): dronedarone, amiodarone
	Calcium channel blockers, non-dihydropyridine: diltiazem, verapamil
	Azoles: fluconazole, voriconazole, ketoconazole (low dose)
Other notable CYP3A4 inhibitors with possible interactions	Anastrazole, tamoxifen, exemestane, letrozole Busulfan, cyclophosphamide, ifosfamide, cytarabine, docetaxel, doxorubicin, etoposide, irinotecan, vinblastine, vincristine, vinorelbine Erlotinib, gefitinib, imatinib Corticosteroids, tretinoin
Inducers: strong combined P-gp and CYP3A4	Rifampin
	Antiepileptics: phenytoin, carbamazepine
	Herbal supplements: St. John's wort

CYP3A4, cytochrome P450 3A4; DOACs, direct oral anticoagulants; P-gp, P-glycoprotein.

Source: Adapted from Scripture CD, Figg WD. Drug interactions in cancer therapy. *Nat Rev Cancer.* 2006;6(7):546–558.

inhibitors (cardiac medications, macrolides, antifungals, rifampin, antiepileptics) (see Table 15.10); patients taking additional anticoagulants other than low-dose aspirin; dual antiplatelet therapy; chronic nonsteroidal anti-inflammatory drug (NSAID) use; uncontrolled hypertension (with blood pressures, in general, greater than 170/100 mmHg); and pre-existing coagulopathy including thrombocytopenia. Even though patients who were very overweight or underweight were not excluded from DOAC trial enrollment, concern remains that patients at the extremes of body weight are at an increased risk of DOAC treatment failure. For patients with a body mass index (BMI) >40 kg/m^2 or an actual body weight >120 kg, the pharmacokinetic and pharmacodynamic data suggest that these

Table 15.10 Clinical Pearls Quick Reference

	Dabigatran	Rivaroxaban	Apixaban	Edoxaban
Taken with food	No	Yes (10 mg dose indications can be taken without food)	No	No
Administration	Keep in bottle, do not put in pill box DO NOT remove from capsule shell	May crush tablet, mix apple sauce, or suspend and take with food. Use caution if used through J tube (distal to stomach)	May be crushed, suspended in D5W, and given through gastric feeding tubes (stable for up to 4 hours)	No data available regarding the bioavailability of edoxaban tablets upon crushing and/or mixing into food, liquids, or administration through feeding tubes
Kidney dysfunction dose adjustments	Yes	Yes	Yes	Yes
Hemodialysis clearance	Yes	No	No	Minimal
Avoid in hepatic impairment	No recommendations available*	Moderate to severe	Severe	Moderate to severe
Potential drug interactions	Minimal CYP3A4 P-gp	CYP3A4 P-gp	CYP3A4 P-gp	Minimal CYP3A4 P-gp
Use in acute DVT/PE requires parenteral bridge	Yes	No	No	Yes

(continued)

Table 15.10 Clinical Pearls Quick Reference (*continued*)

	Dabigatran	Rivaroxaban	Apixaban	Edoxaban
Conversion between anticoagulants (see Table 15.12)	When transitioning off dabigatran to another agent may need to be overlapped, duration based on kidney function	No overlap generally required	No overlap generally required	When transitioning off edoxaban to VKA, requires overlap period with 50% of the planned edoxaban dose
Miscellaneous	Side effects gastritis/dyspepsia (from tartaric acid), but inconsistently observed across trials	May contain lactose	May contain lactose	Avoid in nonvalvular AF if CrCl is >95 mL/min

*Studies with MODERATE showed inconsistent and large interpatient variability; therefore, no dose reduction recommendations can be made. But LFT elevations >2× ULN excluded from most trials.

AF, atrial fibrillation; CrCl, creatinine clearance by Cockcroft and Gault formula; CYP3A4, cytochrome P450 3A4; D5W, 5% dextrose solution; DVT, deep vein thrombosis; PE, pulmonary embolism; P-gp, P-glycoprotein; ULN, upper limit of normal; VKA, vitamin K antagonist; VTE, venous thromboembolism.

patients experience decreased drug exposures, reduced peak concentrations, and have shorter drug half-lives (i.e., faster clearance). There are not enough clinical data available to demonstrate that the current approved DOAC dosages are safe and efficacious in patients >120 kg, and VKA therapy is instead recommended (10).

DOAC Metabolism, Drug–Drug Interactions, and Clinical Implications

Dabigatran

Dabigatran etexilate (Pradaxa) is a prodrug with low bioavailability that is hydrolyzed to the active dabigatran by carboxylesterases without relying on CYP metabolism (11). Interactions with P-gp inhibitors and inducers affect the absorption of dabigatran, altering its efficacy, especially in the setting of renal dysfunction. It is recommended to decrease the dose of dabigatran to 75 mg twice daily (BID) in patients with a calculated CrCl between 30 and 50 mL/min. Concomitant use of strong P-gp inhibitors and inducers should generally be avoided.

Rivaroxaban

Rivaroxaban (Xarelto) also utilizes the P-gp transport mechanism, but unlike dabigatran, undergoes hepatic metabolism via the CYP3A4 pathway. Combined use of rivaroxaban with strong P-gp and strong CYP3A4 inhibitors can cause an increase in rivaroxaban exposure, and clinicians are advised to use caution when considering the use of concomitant P-gp and/or CYP3A4 modulators with rivaroxaban (Table 15.10).

Apixaban

Apixaban (Eliquis) utilizes similar mechanisms of metabolism as rivaroxaban. The major hepatic mechanism of apixaban metabolism is the CYP3A4 pathway, while minor pathways include CYP1A2, 2J2, 2C8, 2C9, and 2C19. Additionally, apixaban is also a P-gp substrate. Standard doses of apixaban should be reduced by 50% when used with combined strong CYP3A4 and P-gp inhibitors, while use is not recommended in the setting of CYP3A4 and P-gp inducers (i.e., rifampin, phenytoin, carbamazepine; Table 15.10)

Edoxaban

Edoxaban (Savaysa) is eliminated by nonmetabolic pathways, via urinary and biliary excretion (12). Hepatic metabolism via the cytochrome pathway accounts for approximately 10% of edoxaban's elimination, and theoretically, is minimally altered by drugs that modulate CYP enzymes. However, edoxaban is a substrate of P-gp and its pharmacokinetics are affected by P-gp inhibitors and inducers. The use with P-gp inhibitors and inducers is not recommended while on edoxaban (Table 15.10). Interestingly, the ENGAGE AF-TIME 48 trial observed an increased number of ischemic strokes in patients with CrCl higher than 95 mL/min. Pharmacokinetic studies showed that these patients experienced approximately 40% lower edoxaban blood levels compared to patients with poorer kidney function.

Betrixaban

The betrixaban (Bevyxxa) molecule is the predominant active form and, like dabigatran, does not undergo significant CYP-mediated metabolism and is a substrate for the P-gp transporter. Despite this, to date betrixaban has not been studied in hepatic impairment and the package label recommends against its use in such patients. Dose adjustments for severe renal impairment (CrCl 15–29 mL/min) are recommended. For the indications of VTE prophylaxis post–total hip arthroplasty (THA) or total knee arthroplasty (TKA), betrixaban must be taken with food for its absorption, and may be a challenge if patients have not resumed oral intake postoperatively. Betrixaban is the only DOAC shown to prolong the QT interval.

Drug Interactions and DOACs, in Summary

Each of the DOACs has a number of drug interactions with medications that are metabolized by CYP3A4 or transported via P-gp, and their concomitant use with medications that inhibit or induce CYP3A4 must be taken into consideration in addition to medications that inhibit P-gp. Clinicians should be familiar with the potential for interactions and carefully consider dose reductions, utilizing alternative medications, or discontinuing the offending agent if possible. Please see Table 15.9 for summary.

Future Directions

While DOAC pharmacokinetic studies have been performed in patients with advanced kidney disease and formal dosing recommendations have been made in patients with reduced kidney function, more evidence is needed in other special populations, such as patients with liver dysfunction, regarding efficacy and safety. Advanced or active liver disease has been excluded in most DOAC trials, especially those with Child–Pugh class B cirrhosis or higher (e.g., moderate-to-severe hepatic impairment), in addition to earlier-stage cirrhosis associated with concomitant coagulopathy. Even though dabigatran has the least hepatic metabolism, patients with mild transaminitis were excluded from clinical trials. Thus, caution is advised when using DOACs in either kidney or liver dysfunction patient populations. For more details about specific DOAC dose reduction recommendations, see Tables 15.6 to 15.8.

For years, the standard of care for cancer-associated VTE has been the use of LMWH over VKA (8). Results from the Hokusai VTE cancer study demonstrated that edoxaban was noninferior to dalteparin (LMWH) for treatment of acute cancer-associated VTE. When compared to dalteparin, edoxaban had less-recurrent VTE (not statistically significant), but more statistically significant upper gastrointestinal (GI) bleeding, driven mostly by GI cancers (8). Likewise, rivaroxaban use in cancer-associated VTE has recently been published in the acute VTE setting compared to LMWH (SELECT-D) and for thromboprophylaxis in high-risk patients (CASSINI) (Table 15.11). Additionally, apixaban is currently being investigated for cancer-associated VTE in the CARAVAGGIO and ADAM-VTE trials (Table 15.11).

Conversions Between DOACs and Anticoagulants

Conversions between anticoagulants are driven by the half-life of each agent. Transitioning from warfarin to DOAC is dependent on the INR level. Prescribing information for each DOAC has specific recommendations for starting therapy based on the INR level, which is summarized in Table 15.12. Generally, a new agent can be initiated at the time of the dose that the previous agent would be due. Specific recommendations can be found in Table 15.12 (13).

Key Points

1. Currently, five FDA-approved DOACs are used for a wide array of indication and offer a variety of advantages over VKA therapy including no therapeutic drug monitoring and less food and drug interactions.

2. To date, there are no head-to-head trials comparing DOACs; therefore, clinicians need to be familiar with the subtle and unique differences between the DOACs in regard to pharmacokinetics (Table 15.8) and administration with or without food (Table 15.10).

3. In addition to clinical factors such as dose adjustment factors (age, weight, kidney dysfunction) (Tables 15.6, 15.7), clinicians must consider scenarios where CYP-mediated drug–drug interactions might have clinically significant effects on the efficacy and safety (Table 15.9).

DOAC ANTICOAGULATION REVERSAL

Clinical Case 15.2

A 67-year-old female with history of hypertension, diabetes, chronic kidney disease (CKD) stage III (CrCl 45 mL/min) presented to the emergency

text continues on page 488

Table 15.11 Direct Acting Oral Anticoagulant Use in Treatment of Cancer-Associated Venous Thromboembolism

Trial	Size (n)	Design	Drug	Comparator	Primary Outcome	Follow-Up Duration	Results
SELECTeD	530	Randomized open label superiority	Rivaroxaban	Dalteparin	VTE recurrence Major bleeding Safety and efficacy of continued therapy if RVT at 5 months Compliance, QOL, cost	12 months	Rivaroxaban had lower VTE recurrence (4% vs. 11%), comparable major bleeding (6% vs. 4%), and higher clinically relevant nonmajor bleeding (13% vs. 4%). Most bleeding events were gastrointestinal or urologic
CARAVAGGIO	1,126	Randomized, open label, blinded endpoint; noninferiority	Apixaban	Dalteparin	VTE recurrence Major bleeding	6 months	Ongoing, no preliminary data available yet
ADAM-VTE	300	Randomized, open label, superiority	Apixaban	Dalteparin	Major bleeding	6 months	Apixaban was associated with rates of bleeding (0% vs. 2.1%) and significantly lower VTE recurrence (3.4% vs. 14.1%) with superior QOL outcome measures compared to parenteral dalteparin in the treatment of cancer-associated VTE

(continued)

Table 15.11 Direct Acting Oral Anticoagulant Use in Treatment of Cancer-Associated Venous Thromboembolism (*continued*)

Trial	Size (n)	Design	Drug	Comparator	Primary Outcome	Follow-Up Duration	Results
CASSINI	700	Randomized; 6-month, double-blind treatment period; prophylactic	Rivaroxaban	Placebo	Time to symptomatic VTE	180 days treatment 30 days follow-up	In high-risk ambulatory patients with cancer, treatment with rivaroxaban did not significantly lower the incidence of VTE or VTE-associated death in 180-day period. (6% vs. 8.8%, $p = .10$) During the intervention period, rivaroxaban lowered the incidence of VTE (2.6% vs. 6.4%), with a low incidence of major bleeding (2.0% vs. 1.0%)
AVERT	563	Randomized, placebo controlled, double blind; prophylactic	Apixaban	Placebo	Objectively documented VTE	180 days	Apixaban significantly lowered the rate among intermediate-to-high risk ambulatory patients with cancer starting chemotherapy (4.2% vs. 10.2%). The rate of major bleeding episodes was higher with apixaban than with placebo (3.5% vs. 1.8%).

QOL, quality of life; RVT, recurrent venous thromboembolism; VTE, venous thromboembolism.

Table 15.12 Conversion to and From Anticoagulants

Anticoagulant	DBG	RVX	APX	EDX	UFH*	LMWH*	VKA
VKA	Stop VKA INR <2	Stop VKA INR <3	Stop VKA INR <2	Stop VKA INR ≤2.5	Stop VKA Initiate infusion when INR <2	Stop VKA Initiate agent when INR <2	
LMWH (enoxaparin, dalteparin, fondaparinux)	Stop LMWH Start DOAC prior to the time of next scheduled LMWH dose	Stop VKA Start DOAC ≤2 hours prior to the time of next scheduled LMWH infusion	Stop LMWH Start DOAC at time of next scheduled LMWH dose		Stop LMWH agent Start heparin infusion at a time when the next dose of LMWH is due		Begin when clinically indicated. Will need to overlap therapy a minimum of 5 days to achieve INR goal
UFH	Stop UFH Start DOAC at the time of stopping UFH infusion			Stop UFH Start EDX 4 hours after stopping UFH		Stop UFH Start agent 30 minutes to 2 hours after UFH stopped	Begin when clinically indicated Will need to overlap therapy a minimum of 5 days to achieve INR goal

(continued)

Table 15.12 Conversion To and From Anticoagulants (*continued*)

Anticoagulant	DBG	RVX	APX	EDX	UFH*	LMWH*	VKA
DBG		Stop DBG Initiate RVX <2 hours prior to the next regularly scheduled DBG	Stop DBG Initiate DOAC at the time of next regularly scheduled DBG		INSERT SAYS: If CrCl ≥30, wait for 12 hours before start IV. If <30, wait for 24 hours	INSERT SAYS: If CrCl ≥30, wait for 12 hours before start IV. If <30, wait for 24 hours	CrCl >50 mL/min, start VKA 3 days before stopping DBG; CrCl >30 to 49 mL/min, start VKA 2 days before stopping DBG; CrCl 15 to 29 mL/min, start VKA 1 day before stopping DBG; CrCl <15 mL/min, not recommended. Start INR monitoring 2 days after stopping DBG (sooner INR levels may be falsely elevated)
RVX	Stop RVX Begin DOAC at a time when the next RVX is due		Stop RVX Begin DOAC at a time when the next RVX is due		Stop RVX Begin infusion when the next RVX dose is due		Stop RVX Start VKA and consider starting bridging agent at a time when the next RVX is due. Begin INR monitoring 2 days after stopping RVX. Stop bridging agent once INR goal is achieved

Table 15.12 Conversion To and From Anticoagulants (*continued*)

Anticoagulant	DBG	RVX	APX	EDX	UFH*	LMWH*	VKA
APX	Stop APX Begin DOAC when the next dose of APX is due			Stop APX Begin EDX when the next dose of APX is due	Stop APX Begin infusion when the next RVX dose is due		Stop APX Start VKA and consider bridging agent when APX is next due Start INR monitoring 2 days after stopping APX (sooner INR levels may be falsely elevated) Stop bridge when INR is at goal
EDX	Stop EDX Begin DOAC at a time when the next dose of EDX is due				Stop EDX Begin infusion when the next RVX dose is due		If taking 60 mg: reduce dose to 30 mg daily and begin VKA concomitantly. Discontinue when INR is at goal If taking 30 mg daily: reduce dose to 15 mg daily and begin VKA concomitantly. Stop when INR is at goal OR Begin parenteral anticoagulant and VKA at a time the next dose of EDX is due. Stop parenteral drug when INR is at goal

*CrCl are all listed in mL/min.

APX, apixaban; CrCl, creatinine clearance by Cockcroft and Gault formula; DOAC, direct acting oral anticoagulant; DBG, dabigatran; EDX, edoxaban; INR, International Normalized Ratio; IV, intravenous; LMWH, low-molecular-weight heparin; RVX, rivaroxaban; VKA, vitamin K antagonist.

Source: Adapted from Table 5 of Kovacs RJ, Flaker GC, Saxonhouse SJ, et al. Practical management of anticoagulation in patients with atrial fibrillation. *J Am Coll Cardiol.* 2015;65(13):1340–1360. doi:10.1016/j.jacc.2015.01.049

department for 1 day of dyspnea, lightheadedness, and palpitations. She was taking lisinopril and metformin. Her pulse was irregularly irregular and rapid, and EKG showed atrial fibrillation with rapid ventricular response. Chest x-ray was unremarkable. Serum troponin measurements were negative three times. Heart rate was controlled with IV metoprolol and subsequent oral equivalents. Complete blood count (CBC) and prothrombin time (PT)/ activated partial thromboplastin time (aPTT) were within normal limits. Therapeutic LMWH w/ enoxaparin at 1 mg/kg every 12 hours for 5 days was initiated. On hospital day 6, dabigatran 150 mg BID was started in the morning and she continued to receive therapeutic enoxaparin. On hospital day 6, 2 hours after receiving enoxaparin, dabigatran, and night time administration of subcutaneous insulin, the patient became confused and had a mechanical fall with trauma to the head that was witnessed by a hospital staff. Blood sugar was found to be low and she was given dextrose 50% solution with correction of glucose to 253 mg/dL, but she remained impaired. Stat head CT without contrast noted right-sided epidural hematoma with associated underlying temporal skull fracture. Neurosurgical and Hematology consultations were placed, and urgent surgical intervention was planned.

An advantage of DOAC therapy is the lack of therapeutic drug monitoring. That being said, there is no standardized or FDA-approved validated assay that can be used to predict therapeutic and/or bleeding risk. This is a major disadvantage of DOAC therapy when it is important to determine if the drug and its anticoagulant effect are still present. Although one would expect factor II and X inhibitors to affect routine coagulation assays (PT, partial thromboplastin time [PTT], and thrombin time [TT]), elevations in these clotting time assays are not sensitive to the presence of the drug and its effects. Studies show wide variability in the dose–response relationship using traditional coagulation assays due to reagent sensitivities, calibration studies, and patient factors. Altogether, the clinical approach to a patient on DOAC therapy who has indications for urgent anticoagulant reversal remains a challenge.

Up to 4% to 6% of patients taking oral anticoagulant therapy will experience a major bleeding event or have an indication for urgent invasive intervention (14). Large meta-analyses of the clinical trials comparing DOACs and VKAs have shown that DOACs have safer bleeding profiles, prevent more strokes/systemic thromboembolism, and have less all-cause mortality (15–17). Despite these encouraging data, the paucity of prospectively demonstrated safe and effective reversal agents for the DOACs remains a large hurdle for expanding their implementation. Whereas the INR in VKA therapy is a well-established and standardized therapeutic drug monitoring strategy indicative of how much anticoagulation remains in the system, this is not the case for DOACs. As of May 2018, the FDA approved the first anti-Xa reversal agent, andexanet alfa,

Table 15.13 Perioperative Management of Warfarin

Pre-op INR	Pre-op Plan	Post-op Plan
2.0 to 3.0	Stop 5 days before	Resume within 24 hours or the next day if hemostasis is achieved and the surgeon agrees
3.0 to 4.5	Stop 6 days before	
>4.5	Stop 6 to 7 days before, consider recheck 2 to 3 days later Consider vitamin K if indicated	

INR, International Normalized Ratio.

Source: Adapted from https://www.uwhealth.org/files/uwhealth/docs/anticoagulation/Periprocedural_Anticoagulation_Guideline.pdf

which joins the dabigatran-specific reversal agent, idarucizumab (approved in October 2015). Our field's experience with DOAC reversal agents is still in its infancy.

The management of nonurgent perioperative anticoagulant is beyond the scope of this section, but general guidelines can be found summarized in Tables 15.13 to 15.17.

Idarucizumab

Idarucizumab (Praxbind™) is an FDA-approved reversal agent for only dabigatran and does not have activity against the other

Table 15.14 Perioperative Management of Direct Acting Oral Anticoagulants

Drug	Minor Surgery or Normal Bleeding Risk	Major Surgery or High Bleeding Risk
Dabigatran	Stop 1 to 2 days before	Stop 2 to 4 days before
Rivaroxaban	Stop 24 hours before	Stop 48 hours before
Apixaban	Stop 24 hours before	Stop 48 hours before
Edoxaban	Stop 24 hours before	Stop 48 hours before

In the setting of kidney dysfunction, consider stopping an additional 24 hours earlier than the above recommendation if CrCl ≤30 mL/min (rivaroxaban), creatinine ≥1.5 mg/dL (apixaban), CrCl <50 mL/min (edoxaban); 3 to 5 days before minor surgery or ≥5 days for major or high-risk surgery if CrCl (dabigatran) CrCl <50 mL/min.

Postoperative anticoagulation may be resumed, if in agreement with the surgeon, within 24 hours after minor or normal bleeding risk surgery or within 72 hours after major or high bleeding risk surgery.

CrCl, creatinine clearance (Cockcroft–Gault formula); DOACs, direct oral anticoagulants.

Source: Adapted from https://www.uwhealth.org/files/uwhealth/docs/anticoagulation/Periprocedural_Anticoagulation_Guideline.pdf

Table 15.15 Perioperative Management of Parenteral Anticoagulation

Drug	Preprocedure Factor	Pre-op Plan (all Bleeding Risks)	Resume Post-op in Minor Surgery or Normal Bleeding Risk*	Resume Post-op in Major Surgery or High Bleeding Risk*
UFH	Prophylactic dose	Ok to give morning of procedure	Within 12 hours	Within 24 hours
	Therapeutic dose	Stop 4 to 6 hours before		
Enoxaparin	Prophylactic dose	Stop 12 hours before	Within 24 hours	Within 72 hours
	Therapeutic dose	Stop 24 hours before		
Fondaparinux	CrCl ≥50 mL/min	Stop 3 days before	Within 24 hours	Within 72 hours
	CrCl <50 mL/min	Stop 5 days before		
Argatroban	Normal hepatic function	Stop 3 hours before	Within 12 hours	Within 24 hours
	Child–Pugh >6	Stop 9 hours before		
Bivalirudin	CrCl ≥30 mL/min	Stop 1.5 hours before	Within 12 hours	Within 24 hours
	CrCl <30 mL/min	Stop 3 hours before		

*Restarting anticoagulation postoperatively should be done in conjunction with the surgeon.

CrCl, creatinine clearance (Cockcroft–Gault formula); UFH, unfractionated heparin.

Source: Adapted from https://www.uwhealth.org/files/uwhealth/docs/anticoagulation/Periprocedural_Anticoagulation_Guideline.pdf

DOACs. Idarucizumab is a humanized IgG monoclonal antibody that selectively binds and neutralizes both free and bound dabigatran by binding the drug with 350 times more affinity than thrombin. While it has structural similarities to thrombin, it lacks enzymatic activity and does not affect coagulation (18). Preclinical studies with dabigatran and prothrombin complex concentrate (PCC) failed to demonstrate in vitro correction of coagulation assays when compared to placebo (19). The recommended dose of

Table 15.16 Perioperative Management of Antiplatelet Agents

Drug	Pre-op Plan	Post-op Plan, to Resume ___*
Aspirin • Low risk for CV event • High risk for CV event	Stop 7 to 10 days before May continue	Within 24 hours
Clopidogrel	Stop 5 days before	Within 24 to 48 hours
Prasugrel	Stop 5 to 7 days before	Within 24 to 48 hours
Ticagrelor	Stop 5 days before	Within 24 to 48 hours
Cilostazol	Stop 1 to 2 days before	Within 24 hours
Dipyridamole	Stop 1 to 2 days before	Within 24 hours

*Restarting anticoagulation postoperatively should be done in conjunction with the surgeon.

CV, cardiovascular.

Source: Adapted from https://www.uwhealth.org/files/uwhealth/docs/anticoagulation/Periprocedural_Anticoagulation_Guideline.pdf

Table 15.17 Classification of Surgery and Bleeding Risks

Minor surgery or procedures with low bleeding risk	• Cataracts • Laparoscopic cholecystectomy • Endoscopy or colonoscopy including planned biopsy • Coronary angiography • Majority of cutaneous surgeries • Dental procedures: hygiene, simple extractions, restoration, endodontics, prosthetics
Minor surgery or procedures with moderate bleeding risk	• Major intra-abdominal or intrathoracic surgery • Biopsy of prostate, kidney • Colon polypectomy • Pacemaker implantation • Invasive dental or ophthalmic procedures

(*continued*)

Table 15.17 Classification of Surgery and Bleeding Risks (*continued*)

Major surgery or procedures with high bleeding risk	• Neurosurgery: intracranial, spinal, epidural interventions
	• Cardiovascular surgery: heart valve or aneurysm repair, coronary or peripheral artery bypass
	• Bowel polypectomy
	• Genitourinary surgery: bladder, prostate
	• Orthopedic surgery: knee and hip replacements
	• Reconstructive plastic surgery
	• Any major cancer surgery

Source: Data from https://www.uwhealth.org/files/uwhealth/docs/anticoagulation/Periprocedural_Anticoagulation_Guideline.pdf

idarucizumab is 5 g given as two separate 2.5-g infusions within 15 minutes of each other. The onset of action for idarucizumab is rapid and occurs immediately after administration. Prior to initiation of idarucizumab, a baseline PTT should be obtained, as intermittent PTT monitoring starting a few hours after initial dosing serves as a surrogate marker for the effects of idarucizumab (18). Incomplete reversals have been described and can be observed by a rising PTT despite initial correction; this has been attributed to the pharmacokinetic properties of dabigatran. Because dabigatran is highly protein bound, once it has been removed by idarucizumab, active drug will redistribute into the blood, increasing its plasma concentration. In the event of an incomplete reversal or clinically significant hemorrhage after the first dose, a second dose of idarucizumab at 5 g can be considered. Toxicities from idarucizumab include hypersensitivity reactions and thromboembolic sequelae (both arterial and venous). It is recommended to resume anticoagulant therapy based on the clinical situation. If dabigatran is to be resumed, it can be restarted 24 hours after the administration of idarucizumab as per the drug labeling.

In the absence of idarucizumab availability and an indication for urgent dabigatran reversal, alternatives such as PCC (Kcentra™), activated PCC (FEIBA™), and activated recombinant FVII (NovoSeven™) can be considered, although there are only experimental healthy volunteer data to support their use (14). Dabigatran can be removed by dialysis, though the efficacy of urgent hemodialysis for the treatment of dabigatran-associated hemorrhagic complications has not been established. Activated charcoal reduces oral absorption and can be considered if oral ingestion was recent.

Andexanet Alfa

Andexanet alfa (Andexxa) is a genetically modified protein that mimics a catalytically inactive form of factor Xa that acts as a "decoy" to bind and sequester factor Xa inhibitors, as well as LMWH and activated antithrombin. The FDA-approved label states that andexanet is limited to the reversal of apixaban and rivaroxaban. Preclinical data show that andexanet may be active in edoxaban and betrixaban reversal as well. There are two dosing schedules available for use, with both schedules requiring a bolus followed by an IV infusion for 2 hours (Table 15.18). Depending on the dose of the factor Xa inhibitor, and the time of its last administered dose, a low-dose versus high-dose schedule is recommended for andexanet use (Table 15.19). Repeat doses for incomplete reversal have not been studied. The half-life of andexanet is approximately 1 hour, and at a steady state, it was able to provide a rapid and dose-dependent reversal of factor Xa inhibitors.

Prothrombin Complex Concentrate

The most frequently used factor concentrates for reversal of drug-induced coagulopathy are three-factor concentrates and four-factor concentrates (4F-PCC), also known as PCC. These formulations comprise vitamin K–dependent factors (II, VII, IX, X), with

Table 15.18 Andexanet Alfa Food and Drug Administration–Approved Dosing Schedules

	Initial IV Bolus	IV Infusion
Low dose	400 mg at a target rate of 30 mg/min	4 mg/min for up to 120 minutes
High dose	800 mg at a target rate of 30 mg/min	8 mg/min for up to 120 minutes

IV, intravenous.

Table 15.19 Recommended Dosing Schedule for Andexanet Alfa

FXa inhibitor	FXA inhibitor last dose	Time since last dose <8 hours or unknown	Time since last dose ≥8 hours
Rivaroxaban	≤10 mg	Low dose	Low dose
	>10 mg/ unknown	High dose	
Apixaban	≤5 mg	Low dose	
	>5 mg/unknown	High dose	

FXa, factor Xa.

the major difference between three-factor and 4F-PCC being the latter's higher factor VII content. Another important nomenclature difference is "activated" PCC has activated FVII, whereas inactivated PCC contains mostly inactive factors. These agents were originally developed to treat hemorrhagic complications in patients with hemophilia and factor inhibitors. Their use was subsequently expanded to treat VKA-associated hemorrhagic complications. There are no prospective randomized clinical data demonstrating similar safety and efficacy of factor concentrates in patients with significant hemorrhage on DOACs (19). Coagulation assay abnormalities induced by DOACs have been shown to correct with PCC in vitro, and data from animal models and healthy volunteers suggest correction of assays. Still, PCCs are not FDA approved for DOACs and clinical efficacy in patients remains mostly anecdotal. In addition, meta-analysis from VKA reversal with PCC clinical data demonstrates the rates of arterial and/or VTE with the use of three-factor PCC as 0.7%, 4F-PCC as 1.8%, and an overall mortality rate of 10.6% (20). Thus, PCC product labels carry black box warnings for their use in patient populations not included in original studies, including disseminated intravascular coagulation (DIC), myocardial infarction, unstable angina, transient ischemic attack/cerebrovascular accident, other systemic thromboembolic event, or severe peripheral artery disease within the past 3 months. Due to the uncertainty about the safety and efficacy in addition to possible devastating side effects, off-label use of PCC is not recommended outside of emergent situations, such as intracranial hemorrhage or massive hemorrhage with hemodynamic instability.

Kcentra is a 4F-PCC product that is available in the United States. Data from healthy volunteers suggest that the 4F-PCC off-label use for anticoagulation reversal from non-VKAs should be given as one-time dose of 50 units/kg (not to exceed 5,000 units) (21). If another dose is felt to be necessary, an additional dose of 25 units/kg can be administered. For those who receive VKA therapy and require immediate reversal, pretreatment INR guides dosing of 4F-PCC (Table 15.20). When given for VKA therapy reversal, patients should also receive an IV infusion of 5 to 10 mg vitamin K over 4 hour.

Table 15.20 Kcentra Dosing for Vitamin K Antagonist Reversal

INR Value	Recommended Kcentra Dose
<4	25 units/kg (max dose: 2,500 units)
4 to 6	30 units/kg (max dose: 3,500 units)
>6	50 units/kg (max dose: 5,000 units)

INR, International Normalized Ratio.

Alternative Removal Agents or Procedures

Fresh frozen plasma (FFP) has not been studied in the setting of DOAC hemorrhage and its efficacy and safety are unknown. The onset of action of FFP is slow compared to PCC, and the volumes of product required put patients at risk for fluid overload, transfusion reactions, and transmission of infection.

Activated charcoal can decrease oral absorption if the last dose was within approximately 2 hours, and it typically works best with prodrugs like dabigatran. Of note, oral absorption of rivaroxaban saturates and becomes limited after doses greater than 50 mg.

Anti-Xa DOACs are highly protein bound (rivaroxaban 92%–95%, apixaban 87%, edoxaban 55% in vitro) and they are minimally cleared through hemodialysis. Edoxaban is expected to have only 7% clearance after 4 hours of hemodialysis. Dabigatran is the DOAC that is most amenable to removal through dialysis.

Future Directions DOAC Reversal Agents

There are other DOAC reversal agents in development including ciraparantag, which is a small, positively charged molecule that binds to and neutralizes factor Xa inhibitors through noncovalent interactions.

Key Points

1. Relatively new agents are available for the reversal of DOAC effects, such as the dabigatran-specific idarucizumab and andexanet alfa for anti-Xa inhibitors.

2. Concentrated factor preparations such as PCC have been used in emergency situations to reverse DOAC effects in the absence of access to idarucizumab or andexanet alfa, but factor concentrates have limited safety and efficacy data outside the scenarios of bleeding due to VKA or factor inhibitor and should be used with caution due to the possibility of thrombosis.

3. There are limited roles for FFP, hemodialysis, and activated charcoal for DOAC reversal.

HEPARINOIDS

Heparin for commercial use is isolated from porcine intestinal mucosa or beef lung. UFH is composed of sulfated glycosaminoglycan saccharide chains of variable lengths between 3 and 30 kDa (mean 15 kDa). UFH exerts its antithrombotic activity through its pentasaccharide active site sequence that specifically binds with antithrombin and then goes on to form a tripeptide complex that inhibits the propagation of thrombosis, while endogenous fibrinolytic pathways work to resorb the clot. The UFH–antithrombin complex not only interacts with prothrombin, but also with factors Xa, IX and, XII.

The pharmacokinetic and pharmacodynamics parameters of UFH display significant interpatient variability. These differences are, in part, due to additional protein and non-protein binding sites for heparin that must be saturated before UFH reaches a therapeutic steady state. Subcutaneous or intravenous UFH has dose-dependent half-lives. At low doses (i.e., prophylaxis), UFH clearance is dependent on heparinases and desulfatases, along with interactions within the reticuloendothelial system (half-life typically 30–90 minutes). At high doses of UFH (i.e., such as those used in cardiac surgery), renal clearance plays a more significant role and the half-life can become longer than 150 minutes (2). Despite this, there is no evidence to guide renal dose adjustments for large doses of UFH; thus, UFH remains a mainstay for the acute treatment of thrombosis in patients with severe renal insufficiency.

Mechanism of Action

LMWH lengths are less variable owing to depolymerization isolation methods leading to mean sizes of 4.2 kDa (enoxaparin) and 6.0 kDa (dalteparin). Fondaparinux, a synthetic pentasaccharide, is composed of only a five-sugar pentasaccharide molecular sequence that makes up the active site for all the heparinoids. Of importance, the varying lengths of the heparins correlate with the risk of causing heparin-induced thrombocytopenia and thrombosis (HITT) (covered in Chapter 10, "Platelet Disorders"). The pentasaccharide sequence binds to the active site of antithrombin, undergoes a conformational change, then goes on to bind and inhibit activated tissue factors in a ternary protein complex, including thrombin and factor Xa, thus inhibiting the coagulation cascade and thrombogenesis. The LMWHs more selectively bind the ternary complex formed with factor Xa over thrombin due to their shorter length. The degree of factor inhibition is variable depending on the heparin being used, with inhibition of thrombin:factor Xa by UFH occurring at a ratio of about 1:1 and LMWH at a ratio of 3 to 4:1 (dalteparin 2.7:1, enoxaparin 3.8:1) (2). Fondaparinux, which has the shortest length among the heparinoids (1.7 kDa), is not long enough to form any ternary complexes with thrombin, and therefore, it is 100% specific for factor Xa binding and inhibition. UFH ultimately inhibits the formation of fibrin clot through inhibition of factor Xa and its role in the conversion of inactivated factor II to thrombin. When there is active and ongoing thrombosis, larger doses of heparin inactivate thrombin and prevent ongoing conversion of fibrinogen to fibrin and inhibit the activation of fibrin-stabilizing factors, thus destabilizing current clots and making them more susceptible to endogenous fibrinolytics; however, heparinoids do not possess fibrinolytic activity.

The dosages for UFH and the LMWH dalteparin are prepared according to standardized in vitro anticoagulant activity and labeled in units that correlate with the expected anticoagulant effect in vivo at the dose provided.

Metabolism and Drug Monitoring

The two major LMWHs in clinical use today are enoxaparin (Lovenox) and dalteparin (Fragmin). The LMWHs are primarily metabolized in the liver via two routes, desulfation and by degradation of the polymers into lower-molecular-weight heparins that have less-potent anticoagulant properties. Renal excretion of active compound is observed. Exposure to LMWHs increases with the level of kidney dysfunction, and as such, dose adjustments for patients with severe renal impairment are necessary. Patients with severe renal impairment (CrCl <30 mL/min) on enoxaparin were observed to have 65% exposure to enoxaparin at repeated prophylactic subcutaneous doses of 40 mg daily and those on dalteparin experienced dose accumulations after a week of prophylactic doses of 5,000 U/d. In renal insufficiency, enoxaparin has been better characterized than dalteparin; therefore, the package label for enoxaparin has recommendations for dose adjustments in CrCl <30 mL/min. Current recommendations state that in renal insufficiency, dalteparin needs to be dose adjusted based on a target anti-Xa level of 0.5 to 1.5 IU/mL. Target anti-Xa level for enoxaparin 4 hours post-dose is 0.6 to 1.0 U/mL for BID dosing and 1.0 to 2.0 U/mL for daily dosing. Routine therapeutic drug monitoring is not necessary for patients on an LMWH. In patients with severe renal dysfunction or at an increased risk of hemorrhage, dose adjustment based on anti-Xa levels is reasonable. The effects of hepatic impairment on enoxaparin and dalteparin exposure have not been studied and their use in this patient population is cautioned. LMWHs are not dialyzable and should be avoided in patients on dialysis.

Fondaparinux (Arixtra™) is eliminated unchanged predominantly through urine. Patients with renal dysfunction (CrCl <30 mL/min) have been observed to have a decrease in clearance up to 55%, and thus, fondaparinux use is contraindicated in patients with severe renal dysfunction. Fondaparinux clearance decreases in underweight individuals (<50 kg body weight) and is contraindicated in this patient population. Pharmacokinetics of fondaparinux has not been studied in patients with hepatic impairment. Elimination is lower in patients over 75 years of age. See Table 15.21 for more details.

Table 15.21 Heparinoid Half-Lives and Metabolism

Heparinoid	Half-Life (in Hours)	Bioavailability	Clearance
UFH, IV	0.5 to 1.5 (25 to 100 U/kg)	100%	RES
UFH, IV	2.5 (≥400 U/kg)	100%	RES + renal*
UFH, SC	2.0 to 4.0	30% to 70%†	RES
Enoxaparin, SC	4.5 to 7.5	100%	Renal + RES
Dalteparin, SC	3.0 to 5.0	PI: 87%	Renal + RES
Fondaparinux	17 to 21	100%	Renal 77%

*Clinical relevance of renal clearance is unclear; current level of evidence recommends no dose adjustments.

†Low doses of subcutaneous heparin have lower bioavailability compared to higher doses.

IV, intravenous; RES, reticuloendothelial system; SC, subcutaneous; UFH, unfractionated heparin.

Sources: Data from Dipiro JT, Talbert RL, Yee GC, et al. *Pharmacotherapy: a pathophysiologic approach.* 7th ed. China: McGraw-Hill Companies, 2008; ASH 2011 Clinical Practice Guide on Anticoagulant Dosing and Management of Anticoagulant Associated Bleeding Complications in Adults. Mary Cushman, Wendy Lim, Neil A Zakai. Presented by the American Society of Hematology, adapted in part from the: American College of Chest Physicians Evidence-Based Clinical Practice Guideline on Antithrombotic and Thrombolytic Therapy (8th Edition); Olsson P, Lagergren H, Ek S. The elimination from plasma of intravenous heparin: an experimental study on dogs and humans. *Acta Med Scand.* 1963;173:619–630.

Heparinoid Reversal

For heparin neutralization, protamine sulfate is an immediate reversal agent with onset of action within 5 minutes; yet, a number of factors limit its practical clinical use. When IV heparin is used at doses up to 25 units/kg, it has a half-life of about 30 minutes; therefore, discontinuation of IV infusion is enough to eliminate it from the circulation and for the PTT to normalize after 2 to 2.5 hours without a reversal agent. Protamine sulfate has endogenous anticoagulant properties that may cause hemorrhage if used at doses higher than required to neutralize the expected blood levels of heparin. If the decision to use it is made, the calculated dose of protamine sulfate must account for the total heparinoid dose received within the past 2 to 3 hours for UFH and the past 8 hours for LMWHs. Depending on the source of heparin, either beef lung or porcine products, protamine sulfate neutralizes approximately 100 units of heparin per 1 mg of protamine sulfate. Protamine is administered by a slow injection over 10 minutes with a maximum

Table 15.22 Ratios for Neutralization of Protamine Sulfate:Heparinoid Dose

Protamine Sulfate	Heparinoid
1 mg	Per 100 U UFH received in the past 2 to 3 hours
1 mg	Per 1 mg enoxaparin received within the past 8 hours
1 mg	Per 100 IU dalteparin received within the past 8 hours

IU, international units of anti-Xa activity; U, units.

Dose addition protamine sulfate, as clinically indicated, with 0.5 mg per amount stated in the table and frequently monitor PTT (UFH) or anti-Xa level (LMWH).

Protamine sulfate is not expected to have a reversal effect on fondaparinux.

injection dose of 50 mg and no more than 100 mg over a short interval of time. If the injection solution needs to be diluted for use as a continuous infusion, such as with neutralization of subcutaneous heparin or LMWHs, then protamine sulfate can be diluted in normal saline or 5% dextrose. After protamine sulfate administration, either PTT or anti-Xa levels specific to the heparinoid can be monitored and additional protamine titrated to give the desired effect. See Table 15.22 for more details.

Severe and fatal hypotension and anaphylaxis have been described with protamine sulfate administration. Bedside treatments of anaphylaxis should be available during its use. Severe hypersensitivity reactions include pulmonary edema and pulmonary hypertension. Risk factors for severe reactions include history of prior protamine exposure through medications (most common being NPH insulin), fish allergies, "severe left ventricular dysfunction, abnormal pulmonary hemodynamics," or vasectomy. Protamine is incompatible with penicillins and cephalosporins.

Heparinoids are poorly dialyzed. FFP and recombinant tissue factor concentrate(s) do not reverse the activity of heparinoids.

Key Points

1. Chain length determines important differences between the heparinoid products, including half-life, onset of action, pharmacodynamic targets (inhibition of factor II and factor Xa), and renal clearance.
2. Protamine sulfate can reverse heparinoid anticoagulant effects. Dose of protamine is critically dependent on the type of heparinoid (not for fondaparinux), total dose of heparinoid received, and time of administration.

ANTIPLATELET THERAPY

Clinical Case 15.3

An 83-year-old male with hypertension, multivessel coronary artery disease, and non-ST segment elevation myocardial infarction (NSTEMI) 11 weeks ago with placement of single drug-eluting stent takes aspirin, ticagrelor, atorvastatin, and carvedilol. He presents to the emergency department for altered mental status. Family members report onset of headache 2 weeks earlier, which had become progressively worse. Imaging demonstrates a large acute chronic right subdural hematoma with midline shift. Hematology is consulted for recommendations on antiplatelet reversal prior to urgent operative management.

Upon vascular and endothelial injury, platelet activation is initiated through a variety of G-coupled protein interactions. Thromboxane A2, adenosine diphosphate (ADP), thrombin, and epinephrine are ligands that bind to their respective receptors, thereby leading to increased intracellular calcium levels and decreased cyclic adenosine monophosphate (cAMP) concentrations. Ultimately, platelet glycoprotein IIb/IIIa (GPIIb/IIIa) is activated and binds to fibrinogen, leading to platelet aggregation and stabilization (22).

Aspirin

Thromboxane A2 is synthesized from arachidonic acid via a pathway mediated by cyclooxygenase (COX). Aspirin is a COX-1 inhibitor that irreversibly inactivates the production of thromboxane A2 when dosed daily. Aspirin is rapidly absorbed and has a 45% to 50% oral bioavailability, which is significantly reduced with enteric coated formulations (2). Peak plasma concentrations are achieved 30 minutes after ingestion. Platelet function is restored 7 to 10 days after aspirin is discontinued.

ADP Receptor (P2Y12) Antagonists

ADP plays a central role in activating platelets. Platelets express two types of adenosine receptors, P2Y1 and P2Y12, which stimulate platelet aggregation when activated. While P2Y1 is a G-coupled seven-membrane protein that activates the phospholipase C and phosphatidylinositol pathway, P2Y12 is an inhibitory G-protein receptor that decreases adenylyl cyclase and subsequently decreases intracellular cAMP levels. This ultimately leads to increased cytosolic calcium, which triggers dimerization of GPIIb to GPIIIa, allowing it to bind to fibrinogen and promote platelet aggregation (23). The P2Y12 receptor has a more prominent role in platelet aggregation than P2Y1, and thus has been the preferred drug target. There are five different P2Y12 antagonists approved by the FDA in two general classes: thienopyridine and non-thienopyridine antagonists.

Thienopyridines undergo hepatic transformation by the CYP system into active metabolites that confer irreversible antiplatelet activity. Ticlopidine is a first-generation thienopyridine with dose-dependent inhibition of platelet activity. Ticlopidine inhibits platelet-derived growth factor (PDGF) and disrupts the interaction between von-Willebrand factor and GPIIb/IIIa (24,25). With chronic dosing, ticlopidine has a prolonged half -life between 20 and 50 hours, conferring maximum antiplatelet activity in 5 to 10 days. The most common adverse events include diarrhea, dyspepsia, and rash, while more serious toxicities include neutropenia, aplastic anemia, and thrombotic thrombocytopenic purpura.

Ticlopidine has fallen out of favor due to toxicity and has been replaced by clopidogrel (Plavix), a second-generation thienopyridine prodrug. Approximately 85% of clopidogrel is hydrolyzed to an inactive carboxylic acid derivative. The remaining 15% of clopidogrel is transformed by CYP enzymes into an active thiol metabolite that irreversibly binds to the ADP P2Y12 receptor (26). A loading dose of 300 mg allows the drug to reach steady-state concentrations rapidly and is followed by a maintenance dose of 75 mg once daily. Post-marketing data have shown significant interpatient variability in terms of response. Numerous factors contribute to altered response, including drug interactions and genetic polymorphisms, which have been studied extensively.

Proton pump inhibitors (PPIs) decrease the bioactivation of clopidogrel. While some studies suggest an increased risk of poor cardiovascular outcomes when the PPIs are used with clopidogrel, other studies suggest the risk is independent of clopidogrel use. Omeprazole and esomeprazole are more likely to interact with clopidogrel than pantoprazole, dexlansoprazole, and lansoprazole (27). Other drug interactions that have been implicated include statins and calcium channel blockers, but these have not been confirmed in larger studies. At high doses, clopidogrel can inhibit CYP2C9; therefore, caution is advised with concomitant warfarin therapy. Genetic polymorphisms in *CYP2C19* play an important role in clopidogrel metabolism (28).

Prasugrel (Effient), a third-generation thienopyridine, confers more potent activity and offers several advantages over clopidogrel. Prasugrel is rapidly absorbed and hydrolyzed to a thiolactone intermediate. The intermediate is then converted to the active form by CYP enzymes, in a single step process, which offers a more rapid onset of action and more efficient antiplatelet activity. Drug interactions with PPIs do not significantly alter the antiplatelet activity of prasugrel (29,30). Because prasugrel requires activation by CYP3A4, there appears to be a clinically significant drug interaction with ritonavir, such that it inhibits the activation of prasugrel, and therefore, this combination should be avoided.

Currently, prasugrel is only indicated for the reduction of cardiovascular events after percutaneous coronary intervention (PCI) for patients with unstable angina, non-ST elevation myocardial infarction (non-STEMI), or STEMI. In contrast to clopidogrel, prasugrel is associated with increased risk of major and minor bleeding. Risk factors include age greater than 75 years, patients undergoing coronary artery bypass surgery, body weight <60 kg, propensity to bleed, and use of medications that also cause increased risk of bleeding (including warfarin, NSAIDs, heparins). Prasugrel is contraindicated for patients with active bleeding or a prior history of stroke or transient ischemic attack.

An alternative to thienopyridines, non-thienopyridines such as ticagrelor (Brilinta) and cangrelor (Kengreal) block the adenosine P2Y12 receptor by mimicking adenosine triphosphate (ATP), the endogenous antagonist of P2Y12 (31).

Ticagrelor is an allosteric inhibitor that reaches a peak effect 2 hours after oral administration. It is metabolized by CYP3A4 and -3A5 to form a less-potent active metabolite. Ticagrelor is predominantly eliminated by hepatic metabolism, while the active metabolite is most likely excreted through biliary secretion. Renal elimination is not a primary method of ticagrelor excretion (31).

Cangrelor has a short half-life of 3 to 5 minutes and is administered as a continuous infusion following a loading dose. Once it is discontinued, platelet function is restored within 60 minutes as the drug is rapidly dephosphorylated by plasma enzymes (32). Because of its short activity, the loading dose (30 mcg/kg) of cangrelor should be initiated prior to the start of PCI and the maintenance dose (4 mcg/kg/min) should be continued for at least 2 hours or for the duration of the PCI procedure, whichever is longer. Patients should be transitioned to an oral P2Y12 inhibitor after PCI. Oral P2Y12 inhibitors should not be given during cangrelor infusion as they are rendered inactive, since cangrelor occupies the active site (33). Specific recommendations are made for when to start each P2Y12 antagonist (Table 15.23). Additional comparisons of ticagrelor and cangrelor can be found in Table 15.24. Given that cangrelor does not require hepatic transformation and is inactivated by phosphorylase enzymes, there are currently no known CYP450-mediated drug–drug interactions. Approximately 50% of cangrelor is recovered in the urine and 35% is excreted in the feces.

Aside from bleeding, the most common side effects of ticagrelor and cangrelor are dyspnea and bradyarrhythmias caused by delayed adenosine metabolism and increased plasma adenosine concentration due to inhibition of the erythrocyte equilibrium nucleoside transporter (ENT)-1 (34).

Table 15.23 Transitioning Patients From Cangrelor to Oral P2Y12 Antagonist

P2Y12 Antagonist	Transition Instructions
Clopidogrel	Give 600 mg immediately after discontinuation of cangrelor
Prasugrel	Give 60 mg immediately after discontinuation of cangrelor
Ticagrelor	Give 180 mg immediately after discontinuation of cangrelor

Glycoprotein IIb/IIIa Inhibitors

GPIIb/IIIa is the most common receptor on the platelet surface and is composed of two heterodimers, IIb and IIIa, which bind to fibrinogen when activated. Ultimately, this cross-linkage between platelets leads to aggregation.

Currently, there are three GPIIb/IIIa inhibitors available for use. All three agents are administered IV. While several oral GPIIb/IIIa antagonists have been developed, they have not been approved due to increased toxicity and mortality in phase 3 trials.

Abciximab (ReoPro) is a reversible chimeric human/murine monoclonal antibody that has high affinity for the GPIIb/IIIa receptor.

Table 15.24 Pharmacokinetic Comparison Between Ticagrelor and Cangrelor

	Ticagrelor	Cangrelor
Bioavailability	36%*	100% (IV)
Volume of distribution	88 L	3.9 L
Protein bound	>99%	97% to 99%
Metabolism	Predominantly hepatic (CYP3A4)	Enzymatic dephosphorylation
Half-life	7 hours (parent drug) 9 hours (active metabolite)	3 to 6 minutes
Elimination	58% feces 26% urine	58% urine 35% feces

*When taken with a high-fat meal, ticagrelor's AUC decreased by 21%, but C_{max} remained the same; ticagrelor may be taken with or without regards to food.

AUC, area under the curve; IV, intravenous.

The Fc portion of the molecule was removed to decrease the risk of hypersensitivity. Abciximab confers its activity by providing steric bulk to block the active site of the receptor. Alternatively, eptifibatide (Integrilin) and tirofiban (Aggrastat) are synthetic GPIIb/IIIa inhibitors that take advantage of the peptide sequence arg–gly–asp (RGD), which inhibits ligand binding and competitively blocks the active site on GPIIb/IIIa (35). Eptifibatide is a cyclic heptapeptide incorporating a lysine–glycine–aspartate (KGD) sequence, while tirofiban is a non-peptide tyrosine analog that mimics the structure of the RGD sequence. These agents are reversible antagonists of GPIIb/IIIa and inhibit platelet aggregation. The GPIIb/IIIa inhibitors are associated with major and minor bleeding, as well as thrombocytopenia. Pharmacokinetic differences and cost of therapy are important considerations when choosing the most appropriate therapy (Table 15.25).

Urgent Reversal Strategies on Antiplatelet Agents

In the setting of severe hemorrhage, discontinuation of the antiplatelet agent or agents is the first step. The intravenous antiplatelet

Table 15.25 Comparative Pharmacokinetics Among Glycoprotein IIb/IIIa Inhibitors

	Abciximab	**Eptifibatide**	**Tirofiban**
Bioavailability	100% (IV)	100% (IV)	100% (IV)
Volume of distribution	1.44 L/kg	0.2 L/kg	21 to 87 L
Protein bound	See below*	25%	64%
Metabolism	Enzymatic degradation	Enzymatic deamination	Enzymatic degradation
Half-life	10 minutes (first phase) 30 minutes (second phase)	2.5 hours	1 to 1.5 hours
Elimination	—	50% Urine	65% Urine 25% Feces

*Abciximab is continually redistributed among circulating platelets and there is no drug-free platelet population.

IV, intravenous.

Sources: Data from Kondo K, Umemura K. Clinical pharmacokinetics of tirofiban, a nonpeptide glycoprotein IIb/IIIa receptor antagonist. *Clin Pharmacokinet.* 2002;41(3):187–195; Curran MP, Keating GM. Eptifibatide: a review of its use in patients with acute coronary syndromes and/or undergoing percutaneous coronary intervention. *Drugs.* 2005;65(14):2009–2035.

agents, including the monoclonal antibody abciximab, have short half-lives (1–2.5 hours) that are amenable to simply withholding further therapy. Unlike the anticoagulants reviewed in Case 1 and their antidotes in Case 2, there are no specific antiplatelet antidotes. Platelet transfusions can be considered for both reversible and irreversible (i.e., aspirin) platelet inhibitors, and repeat transfusions may be considered for agents with longer half-lives. Patients receiving antiplatelet agents are often medically complex and may have had a recent cardiovascular event for which the antiplatelet agent is currently indicated (e.g., NSTEMI, placement of drug-eluting coronary artery stent), requiring consultation with the appropriate subspecialty services. Any underlying coagulopathy, even if unrelated to antiplatelet therapy, should be investigated and reversed.

Key Points

1. Antiplatelet therapies are an essential tool to reduce the risk of atherothrombotic disease and are the mainstay in therapy for patients with cardiovascular, cerebrovascular, and/or peripheral artery disease.
2. Aspirin, P2Y12 antagonists, and GPIIb/IIIa inhibitors utilize different platelet targets to inhibit platelet aggregation.
3. Ticagrelor and cangrelor are the most recently FDA-approved antiplatelet agents, for which bleeding, dyspnea, and bradyarrhythmias are the most common side effects.
4. Antiplatelet reversal requires discontinuation of the offending agent, transfusion of platelets as needed, and should be a shared medical decision-making process (when available) with appropriate subspecialty colleagues.

GROWTH FACTORS

Clinical Case 15.4

A 62-year-old male with hypertension and end-stage renal disease has been on hemodialysis for 2 years. He receives darbopoetin alfa weekly, but still requires occasional blood transfusions with outpatient dialysis. He is being considered for kidney transplant and is referred to hematology clinic for consideration of preoperative growth factors for persistent neutropenia and thrombocytopenia. Absolute neutrophil count is 900 cells/mm³ and platelet count is 46,000 cells/ mm³. Review of outside records shows the neutropenia and thrombocytopenia have been worsening over the past 3 years.

Granulocyte Colony-Stimulating Growth Factors

There are multiple formulations available in the United States for granulocyte colony-stimulating factor (G-CSF) agents, including filgrastim (Neupogen™), tbo-filgrastim (Granix™), and sndz-fil-grastim (Zarxio™). Their administration is identical. Filgrastim is a 175-amino acid recombinant human G-CSF protein that stimulates production of granulocytes by binding to receptors on hemato-poietic progenitors to stimulate proliferation, differentiation, and enhance neutrophil functions such as phagocytic activity, respira-tory burst, antibody-dependent killing, and the expression of cell surface antigens.

Filgrastim and its biosimilar products exhibit complicated phar-macokinetics with multiple absorption and elimination pathways. The drugs are metabolized by neutrophil uptake, and thus, metab-olism depends on absolute neutrophil counts (36,37). Hepatic and renal elimination is negligible, and currently there are no indica-tions for dose adjustments in either setting.

Most dose indications for G-CSF use range between 5 and 10 mcg/kg/day. Of note, international dosing units may vary, and 1 mg is equivalent to 100,000 units. Filgrastim is available in 300 and 480 mcg doses and can be given IV or subcutaneously with similar half-lives (231 vs. 210 minutes, respectively). Subcutaneous bioavail-ability is 60% to 70%. Peak neutrophil counts occur at around 10 to 12 hours with IV administration and 20 to 24 hours when given subcutaneously (36). After discontinuation, the neutrophil counts can be expected to fall 50% within the first 2 days and will decrease back to baseline levels within 7 days. Filgrastim's effect to increase white blood cell count is dose dependent; but these dose-depen-dent effects diminish at or above 10 mcg/kg/day. Of note, the pack-age label reports that the increase in WBC count due to filgrastim has been observed to exceed 100,000 cells/mm^3.

Filgrastim should not be administered 24 hours before or after chemotherapy has begun, due to concerns of exposing rapidly dividing granulocyte hematopoietic precursors to cytotoxic che-motherapy. As per the package labeling, filgrastim may cause splenic rupture, sickle cell crisis, severe acute lung injury/acute respiratory distress syndrome (ARDS), anaphylaxis, alveolar hem-orrhage, capillary leak syndrome, thrombocytopenia, glomerulo-nephritis, cutaneous vasculitis, and Sweet's syndrome (i.e., acute febrile neutrophilic dermatosis). Use should be avoided if there is a history of anaphylaxis from filgrastim use. Its use should also be avoided if ARDS is present, and its use with bleomycin is contro-versial and warrants considerations of risk versus benefit due to theoretical lung toxicity (e.g., Hodgkin lymphoma, testicular can-cer) (38,39). G-CSF receptors have been found on tumor cell lines, and concerns about filgrastim's safety in myeloid malignancies and myelodysplasia are unresolved. Filgrastim also causes bone marrow enhancement on MRI and increased positron emission tomography (PET) avidity. Filgrastim has been described to cross the placenta and is a Pregnancy Category C drug, and its safety in breastfeeding is unclear.

Pegfilgrastim (Neulasta®) is the same recombinant filgrastim that is covalently bound to monomethoxypolyethylene glycol, which significantly increases the half-life of its conventional dosage form. Currently, it is only indicated for use in chemotherapy-induced myelosuppression with significant risk for febrile neutropenia and for acute exposure to myelosuppressive radiation. Pegfilgrastim does not have an indication for nonmalignancy-related neutropenia. The drug is administered as a single subcutaneous dose of 6 mg once per chemotherapy cycle (40); half-life is variable and ranges between 15 and 80 hours. Warnings and precautions for pegfilgrastim are similar to those for filgrastim, including avoidance if anaphylaxis occurs with either drug. Patients with acrylic allergies should avoid pegfilgrastim use. Additional common but milder side effects include arthralgias/bone pains, which may respond to second-generation antihistamine. Efficacy may decrease if left at room temperature or exposed to excess amounts of heat; therefore, G-CSFs should be refrigerated until the time for administration.

Key Points

1. G-CSFs come in a variety of biosimilar and bioequivalent preparations that have a wide array of approved indications. Clinicians should be familiar with doses and timing or administration depending on the clinical context.
2. Products need to remain refrigerated.
3. Clinicians should be familiar with critical timing considerations (such as timing before and after myelosuppressive chemotherapy) and side effects.

ERYTHROPOIETIN-STIMULATING AGENTS

The two major indications for erythropoietin stimulating agents (ESAs) are (a) anemia associated with CKD and (b) anemia due to myelosuppressive chemotherapy with at least 2 months of planned, non–curative-intent chemotherapy. The goal of therapy is to minimize blood transfusion burden in patients with baseline hemoglobin <10 g/dL. It is important to note that ESAs have not been demonstrated to improve patient's quality of life, fatigue, or well-being.

There are currently four FDA-approved ESAs available in the United States: epoetin alfa (manufactured as two different products: Procrit, Epogen), darbepoetin alfa (Aranesp), and epoetin beta (Mircera). ESAs are recombinant polypeptides that have the same underlying protein structure as endogenous erythropoietin, a 165-amino acid polypeptide chain, and function by binding to and stimulating erythroid progenitors. Glycosylation of erythropoietin leads to varying structural properties and pharmacokinetics that affect the stability and solubility among the ESAs (41). Darbepoetin alfa has higher sialic acid-carbohydrate content than epoetin alfa, which accounts for its longer half-life.

Prior to starting an ESA, patients should be evaluated for erythropoiesis substrate deficiencies, including iron stores (transferrin saturation <20% and/or ferritin <100 ng/mL), folate, and vitamin B12 levels. Nutritional deficiencies can result in ESA treatment failure, and therefore should be corrected prior to its initiation. Treatment response is not immediate; the reticulocyte count increases within a week of initiation, followed by an increase in hemoglobin in 2 to 6 weeks. The hemoglobin should increase by at least 1 g/dL after 4 weeks of therapy; patients not meeting the expected response after 4 weeks of therapy should have the dose increased by 25%. Weekly monitoring of hemoglobin at the start of therapy is recommended, as rapid increases in hemoglobin (such as ≥1 g/dL every 2 weeks) may occur. Dose adjustments for ESAs should not occur more frequently than once every 4 weeks to avoid rapid increases in hemoglobin associated with adverse events (see the following sections "Epoetin Alfa" and "Darbepoetin Alfa"). In patients not experiencing an expected rise in hemoglobin, clinicians should address patient compliance, administration techniques, and proper storage and handling (ESAs should be refrigerated to minimize instability). Patients whose hemoglobin fails to respond after 3 months of ESA dose escalation are unlikely to respond to further increases in dose, and so, ESA should be discontinued. As with any ESA, the lowest dose required to achieve the target hemoglobin should be used. Iron stores should be monitored throughout therapy to determine if adjunctive iron replacement is needed.

Epoetin Alfa

Epoetin alfa is marketed under two different trade names, Epogen and Procrit. Although they are manufactured by different companies, their indications and dosing schedules are the same. Epoetin alfa products are indicated for anemia in HIV patients on zidovudine treatment with EPO levels <500 mUnits/mL as well as for anemia in the perioperative setting for noncardiac, nonvascular elective surgeries to reduce the number of blood transfusions (limited to patients with hemoglobin levels between 11 and 13 g/dL).

Dosing schedules for epoetin alfa can be found in Table 15.26. Generally, higher doses are required for cancer patients and surgical patients in contrast to patients with CKD or HIV.

Darbepoetin Alfa

Darbepoetin alfa (Aranesp) is dosed less frequently than epoetin alfa. The half-life of darbepoetin is three times longer than that of epoetin (approximately 24 vs. 8.5 hours) and clearance of darbepoetin is four times slower (42). Recommended starting doses for darbepoetin alfa are 0.45 mcg/kg weekly or 0.75 mcg/kg every 2 weeks. Dosing can be IV or subcutaneous, but IV is preferred in dialysis patients because subcutaneous bioavailability is variable. Dialysis increases the clearance of darbepoetin alfa, therefore patients with CKD not on dialysis

Table 15.26 Epoetin Alfa Dosing Schedules as per Indication

Indication	Initial Dosing Schedule	Dose Modifications
Chronic kidney disease (dialysis)	50 to 100 units/kg IV or SC* three times weekly	• Titrate once in every 4 weeks as necessary • If Hgb increases >1 g/dL in 2-week period, decrease by at least 25%
Chronic kidney disease (non-dialysis)	50 to 100 units/kg IV or SC three times weekly	• If Hgb does not increase 1 g/dL in 4 weeks, increase dose by 25%
Zidovudine-induced anemia in HIV	100 units/kg IV or SC three times weekly	• Increase dose by 50 to 100 units/kg at 4- to 8-week intervals if inadequate response • If Hgb >12 g/dL, hold dose until Hgb <11 g/dL and reduce dose by 25% • Do NOT exceed 300 units/kg (if adequate response is NOT achieved within 8 weeks at this dose, discontinue treatment)
Cancer-related anemia	150 units/kg SC three times weekly **OR** 40,000 units SC once weekly until completion of chemotherapy course	• If Hgb increases >1 g/dL in a 2-week period or target Hgb level is met to avoid transfusion, decrease by 25% • If Hgb does not increase 1 g/dL in 4 weeks AND Hgb level remains <10 g/dL, increase to 300 units/kg SC three times weekly OR 60,000 units SC once weekly • Discontinue after 8 weeks if no response or transfusion requirements do not decrease

(*continued*)

Table 15.26 Epoetin Alfa Dosing Schedules as per Indication (*continued*)

Indication	Initial Dosing Schedule	Dose Modifications
Prevention of perioperative anemia[†]	300 units/kg SC for 15 days, starting 10 days prior to surgery **OR** 600 units/kg SC for four doses given 21, 14, and 7 days before surgery and once on the day of surgery	None

*IV route is the preferred route of administration in hemodialysis patients.

[†]Given high risk of DVT, prophylaxis is recommended for this indication.

DVT, deep vein thrombosis; Hgb, hemoglobin; IV, intravenous; SC, subcutaneous.

should start at 0.45 mcg/kg every 4 weeks (either IV or subcutaneous). Dose adjustments may be needed in non-dialysis patients on stable doses of darbepoetin alfa once dialysis is initiated. Higher doses are required for cancer patients on chemotherapy, and the manufacturer recommends either 500 mcg subcutaneously every 3 weeks or 2.25 mcg/kg subcutaneously weekly.

ESAs, like darbopoetin alfa, are routinely used off-label with the best example being use in myelodysplastic syndrome (MDS) to reduce transfusion burden in symptomatic anemia in patients with serum EPO levels <500 mU/mL (see NCCN guidelines for Myelodysplastic Syndrome, version 2.2019). Recommended subcutaneous darbopoetin alfa doses in MDS start at 150 to 300 mcg every other week.

ESAs have been associated with a number of adverse events including increases in blood pressure, and uncontrolled hypertension is a contraindication to the use of ESAs. Up to 40% of CKD patients on ESAs require interventions to optimize their antihypertensive regimens after ESA therapy begins. ESAs may need to be withheld until hypertension can be adequately controlled. ESAs have been associated with severe allergic reactions and pure red cell aplasia, and the occurrence of either side effect should prompt immediate discontinuation. The use of ESAs to target hemoglobin levels over 11 g/dL has been associated with increased mortality and cardiovascular events (e.g., myocardial infarction, congestive heart failure, stroke, and thromboembolism including DVT and hemodialysis access thrombosis). Use of ESAs in patients with a history of these events is cautioned, but not contraindicated. ESAs increase the risk of seizures due to hypertensive encephalopathy. In the setting of cancer, the use of ESAs has been associated with increased mortality and increased cancer-specific adverse outcomes, including an increase in locoregional recurrence, disease progression, and a decrease in overall survival. These adverse events have been observed in cancer patients receiving ESAs in the setting of chemotherapy or radiation therapy, including: cervical cancer; early-stage, that is, curable breast cancer;metastatic breast cancer; lymphoproliferative disorders; head and neck cancers;and non-small cell lung cancer (package insert). ESAs should only be used in the setting of chemotherapy-induced anemia for which the treatment goals are not curative, and ESAs should be discontinued once chemotherapy treatment is completed. Specifically, ESAs are not recommended for use in cancer-related anemia when patients are neither receiving active treatment nor receiving non-myelosuppressive chemotherapy (43). The FDA has lifted the Risk Evaluation and Mitigation Strategy (REMS) program restriction after concluding that prescribers demonstrated acceptable knowledge of the potential risks of ESA use in the setting of cancer and were appropriately prescribing ESAs (44).

ESAs carry a designation of Pregnancy Category C for single-use vials of Procrit, and multidose vials are contraindicated in pregnancy and breastfeeding due to the presence of benzoyl alcohol.

Key Points

1. Before starting an ESA, iron and vitamin B12 deficiencies should be corrected.
2. ESA therapy should be monitored to avoid an elevated hemoglobin level associated with increased risk for venous and arterial thrombotic events. The minimum dose needed to achieve therapeutic goals should be used.
3. ESAs should be avoided in cancer patients receiving therapy with curative intent.

THROMBOPOIESIS AGENTS

Thrombopoietin (TPO) is synthesized predominantly in the liver and is the major driver of megakaryocyte and platelet production. TPO is a 353-amino acid glycosylated polypeptide with two different domains. The receptor-binding domain resembles that of

EPO and a second highly glycosylated domain promotes protein stability and secretion. TPO binds to its receptor (also known as c-mpl) and induces receptor homodimerization and activates signal transduction primarily via the Janus kinase/signal transducers and activators of transcription (JAK/STAT) pathway to promote differentiation and production of platelets. TPO has minimal effect on the later stages of megakaryocyte development and platelet shedding (42).

Two recombinant TPO products were developed and underwent clinical trials, but never gained FDA approval as they were associated with the development of antibodies against both endogenous and recombinant TPO, paradoxically causing thrombocytopenia (45). Subsequently, the peptide and non-peptide/small-molecule TPO receptor agonists were developed and tested. These agents are FDA approved for chronic immune thrombocytopenia purpura (ITP) with persistent thrombocytopenia refractory to corticosteroids, IV immunoglobulin, or splenectomy that poses an increased risk for hemorrhage.

Romiplostim (Nplate™) is a recombinant "peptibody" composed of two domains. The receptor-binding domain is composed of four repeating amino acid peptides that share no sequence homology with endogenous TPO; this domain is bound to a human IgG Fc domain to prolong its pharmacological half-life. Romiplostim acts as a TPO mimetic and increases TPO receptor activity leading to increased platelet production. The recommended starting dose of romiplostim is 1 mcg/kg given as a subcutaneous injection once weekly. The thrombopoietic effect is dose dependent and often delayed by several days. Romiplostim requires careful monitoring and titration on a weekly basis to maintain a platelet count between 50 and 400×10^9 cells/L (with a maximum dose of 10 mcg/kg/week) (Table 15.27). The goal of therapy is not to normalize platelet levels, but rather to decrease bleeding risk related to the degree of thrombocytopenia. Concomitant ITP therapy may be utilized in combination with romiplostim if necessary (e.g., corticosteroids, immunoglobulins, but not eltrombopag), especially if the platelet goal of >50,000 cells/L has not been achieved, and therapy should be titrated accordingly. Romiplostim is generally well tolerated and thought to be associated with mild-to-moderate adverse effects that include headache, contusion, epistaxis, and nasopharyngitis. Thrombotic complications are rare and, in fact, pooled analyses of clinical trials show that these adverse events occurred at the same rate as that of patients treated with placebo or standard of care (46). Additionally, patients not on therapy tended to have higher risk of bleeding complications than those receiving therapy However, phase 1/2 clinical trials reported a potential risk for

Table 15.27 U.S. Recommendations for Romiplostim Titration

Platelet Count	Titration Recommendation
<50,000 cells/mcL	Increase dose by 1 mcg/kg
>200,000 cells/mcL for 2 consecutive weeks	Decrease dose by 1 mcg/kg
>400,000 cells/mcL	Hold dose, recheck platelet counts weekly Once the platelet count is <200,000 cells/mcL, decrease the dose by 1 mcg/kg from the previous dose

Discontinue romiplostim if platelet counts do not increase sufficiently after 4 weeks of therapy at a maximum dose of 10 mcg/kg

developing acute myeloid leukemia (AML) for MDS patients being treated with romiplostim (currently an off-label use), which led to study discontinuation. However, recent long-term follow-up results showed that there was, in fact, no increase in AML and no detrimental effect on overall survival for patients receiving romiplostim (46). Discontinuation of romiplostim may result in rebound thrombocytopenia to lower-than-pretreatment baseline platelet levels, and platelet counts should be monitored closely.

Thrombopoietic Receptor Agonists

Eltrombopag is a first-generation oral non-peptide thrombopoietic receptor agonist that is composed of three regions: an acidic region, a lipophilic region, and a metal chelating region (47,48). Eltrombopag does not occupy the same receptor-binding site, but interacts further downstream, possibly in the transmembrane region at histidine 499. Eltrombopag works in conjunction with TPO in an additive manner and causes direct activation of the JAK/STAT signaling pathway (48). Interestingly, binding of eltrombopag at this region is species specific for humans and chimpanzees, while other species (rat, mouse, cynomolgus monkey) express a leucine residue and eltrombopag is inactive in these species (48).

Pharmacokinetic studies indicate that the bioavailability of eltrombopag is significantly reduced when given with a high-fat meal. The recommended starting dose varies based on indication and is titrated accordingly (Tables 15.28–15.31). Patients of East Asian descent have increased sensitivity to eltrombopag and should be dose reduced accordingly. Eltrombopag is metabolized by the CYP450 system, and therefore, drug interactions must be taken into consideration (Table 15.32). Because eltrombopag can

Table 15.28 Initial Eltrombopag Dosing Regimens Based on Patient Populations

	Initial Dosing Regimen	East Asian Decent/ Hepatic Dysfunction
Adult patients with ITP (including pediatric patients >6 years of age)	50 mg once daily	25 mg once daily
Chronic hepatitis C–associated thrombocytopenia	25 mg once daily	—
Severe aplastic anemia	50 mg once daily	25 mg once daily

*Patients of non-East Asian decent or those who do not have hepatic dysfunction should be dosed based on the initial dosing regimen.

ITP, immune thrombocytopenia purpura.

act as a metal chelator, it is important to space out or eliminate concomitant use with antacids containing polyvalent cations. Additionally, hepatic impairment significantly increases plasma levels of eltrombopag by at least 40% and in severe impairment, doubles the half-life of the drug; hence, doses should be adjusted according to the patient's degree of hepatic impairment, that is, Child–Pugh score.

Patients receiving eltrombopag have an increased risk for thromboembolism (venous and arterial) compared to placebo, and

Table 15.29 Titration Recommendations for Eltrombopag in Immune Thrombocytopenia Purpura

Platelet Count	Titration Recommendation
<50,000 cells/mcL for at least 2 weeks	Increase daily dose by 25 mg (max: 75 mg daily)
>200,000 cells/mcL for 2 consecutive weeks	Decrease daily dose by 25 mg and observe response for 2 weeks (if taking 25 mg, reduce to 12.5 mg daily)
>400,000 cells/mcL	Hold therapy, increase platelet monitoring to twice weekly When platelet <150,000 cells/mcL, decrease daily dose by 25 mg (if taking 25 mg, reduce to 12.5 mg daily)
>400,000 cells/mcL for 2 weeks at the lowest dose	Discontinue eltrombopag

Table 15.30 Titration Recommendations for Eltrombopag in Hepatitis C Thrombocytopenia

Platelet Count	Titration Recommendation
<50,000 cells/mcL for at least 2 weeks	Increase daily dose by 25 mg (max: 100 mg daily)
>200,000 cells/mcL for 2 consecutive weeks	Decrease daily dose by 25 mg and observe response for 2 weeks (if taking 25 mg, reduce to 12.5 mg daily)
>400,000 cells/mcL	Hold therapy, increase platelet monitoring to twice weekly When platelet <150,000 cells/mcL, decrease daily dose by 25 mg (if taking 25 mg, reduce to 12.5 mg daily)
>400,000 cells/mcL for 2 weeks at the lowest dose	Discontinue eltrombopag

thrombosis was observed even at low-to-normal platelet counts. Patients should not exceed the lowest dose of eltrombopag necessary to meet their platelet goal targets, and the goal should not be to normalize the patient's platelet count. Caution is advised for use in those with history of thrombosis or with an inherited thrombotic diathesis. Eltrombopag can cause or worsen cataracts, thus patients should have a baseline eye exam prior to initiation of therapy.

Table 15.31 Titration Recommendations for Eltrombopag in Severe Aplastic Anemia

Platelet Count	Titration Recommendation
<50,000 cells/mcL for at least 2 weeks	Increase daily dose by 50 mg (max: 150 mg daily) Patients on 25 mg daily should be increased to 50 mg before titrating by 50 mg increments
>200,000 cells/mcL for 2 consecutive weeks	Decrease daily dose by 50 mg and observe response for 2 weeks
>400,000 cells/mcL	Hold therapy for 1 week, increase platelet monitoring to twice weekly When platelet <150,000 cells/mcL, decrease daily dose by 50 mg
>400,000 cells/mcL for 2 weeks at the lowest dose	Discontinue eltrombopag

Table 15.32 Pharmacokinetics of Eltrombopag

Pharmacokinetic Parameters	Eltrombopag
C_{max}	7.3 mcg/mL
T_{max}	2 to 6 hours
Absorption	52% (tablet) 77% (suspension) High-fat meal decreases absorption
Half-life	26 to 35 hours
Metabolism	UGT1A1, UGT1A3, CYP1A2, CYP2C8
Excretion	59% (feces) 31% (urine)

Avatrombopag (Doptelet) is a recently approved small-molecule TPO receptor agonist that is currently only indicated in the setting of secondary thrombocytopenia due to chronic liver disease prior to planned invasive procedure.

Combination therapy among TPO mimetics like romiplostim and eltrombopag has not been studied and the safety profile is unknown. Safe transitioning from eltrombopag to romiplostim and vice versa has been reported (46).

Spleen Tyrosine Kinase (Syk) Inhibition

Fostamatinib (Tavalisse) is a first-in-class agent that is approved for ITP that has not responded to previous treatment. This approval was based on two parallel double-blind, placebo-controlled trials, FIT-1 and FIT-2, for which the primary endpoint, stable platelet response, is defined as a platelet level $\geq$50,000 cells/mm^3 by week 24. Collectively, a total of 150 patients were included and patients were randomized to receive up to 150 mg of fostamatinib orally BID versus placebo. In both clinical trials, 18% versus 16% of patients achieved stable disease, respectively. When data were combined, statistically significant stable responses were seen in 17% of patients versus 2% on placebo. Common toxicities observed included diarrhea, hypertension, nausea, and elevations in liver transaminases. Currently, the approved dose is 100 mg orally BID, but if platelet counts have not increased to at least 50,000 cells/mm^3 within 4 weeks of treatment, fostamatinib can be increased to 150 mg orally BID.

Fostamatinib is formulated as a disodium hexahydrate prodrug that is metabolized by alkaline phosphatase to its active metabolite. Pharmacokinetic studies show that food decreases its absorption, but the overall exposure of the active component did not differ between fasting and fed states, and therefore, patients can take fostamatinib without regard to food (49). The half-life of fostamatinib is approximately 15 hours, and 80% of the drug is excreted by fecal route. Because fostamatinib is metabolized by liver enzymes, including CYP enzymes, drug interactions are a concern. Strong CYP3A4 inhibitors increase exposure of the active metabolite and may increase the risk for toxicity. Concomitant use of strong CYP3A4 inducers, which may increase the risk of treatment failure, is not recommended.

Key Points

1. TPO mimetics have unique structures and mechanisms of action as compared to G-CSF and ESA agents.
2. Eltrombopag considerations include: taking on an empty stomach and avoiding administration with antacids. Dose reductions are recommended in patients of East Asian descent due to inherited CYP450 factors and the risk of hepatotoxicity.
3. Monitoring is required during initiation and uptitration of TPO mimetics. Thrombotic events have been observed even with low platelet counts; the minimum dose needed to achieve therapeutic goals should be used.

REFERENCES

1. Schwarz UI, Ritchie MD, Bradford Y, et al. Genetic determinants of response to warfarin during initial anticoagulation. *N Engl J Med.* 2008;358(10):999–1008. doi:10.1056/NEJMoa0708078
2. Dipiro J, Talbert R, Yee G, et al. *Pharmacotherapy: A pathophysiologic approach.* 7th ed. China: McGraw-Hill Companies; 2008.
3. Wittkowsky AK. Warfarin. In: Murphy JE, ed. *Clincal Pharmacokinetics.* 6th ed. Bethesda, MD: American Society of Health-System Pharmacists; 2012.
4. Owen RP, Gong L, Sagreiya H, et al. VKORC1 pharmacogenomics summary. *Pharmacogenet Genomics.* 2010;20(10):642–644. doi:10.1097/FPC.0b013e32833433b6
5. Mahtani KR, Heneghan CJ, Nunan D, et al. Optimal loading dose of warfarin for the initiation of oral anticoagulation. *Cochrane Database Syst Rev.* 2012;12:CD008685. doi:10.1002/14651858.CD008685.pub2
6. Lynch T, Price A. The effect of cytochrome P450 metabolism on drug response, interactions, and adverse effects. *Am Fam Physician.* 2007;76(3):391–396.
7. Adcock DM, Gosselin R. Directoral anticoagulants (DOACs) in the laboratory: 2015 review. *Thromb Res.* 2015;136(1):7–12. doi:10.1016/j.thromres.2015.05.001

8. Kraaijpoel N, Carrier M. How I treat cancer-associated venous thromboembolism. *Blood*. 2019;133(4):291–298. doi:10.1182/blood-2018-08-835595

9. Horlocker TT, Vandermeuelen E, Kopp SL, et al. Regional anesthesia in the patient receiving antithrombotic or thrombolytic therapy: American Society of Regional Anesthesia and Pain Medicine evidence-based guidelines (fourth edition). *Reg Anesth Pain Med*. 2018;43(3):263–309. doi:10.1097/AAP.0000000000000763

10. Martin K, Beyer-Westendorf J, Davidson BL, et al. Use of the direct oral anticoagulants in obese patients: guidance from the SSC of the ISTH. *J Thromb Haemost*. 2016;14(6):1308–1313. doi:10.1111/jth.13323

11. Blommel ML, Blommel AL. Dabigatran etexilate: a novel oral direct thrombin inhibitor. *Am J Health Syst Pharm*. 2011;68(16):1506–1519. doi:10.2146/ajhp100348

12. Parasrampuria DA, Truitt KE. Pharmacokinetics and pharmacodynamics of edoxaban, a non-vitamin K antagonist oral anticoagulant that inhibits clotting factor xa. *Clin Pharmacokinet*. 2016;55(6):641–655. doi:10.1007/s40262-015-0342-7

13. Kovacs RJ, Flaker GC, Saxonhouse SJ, et al. Practical management of anticoagulation in patients with atrial fibrillation. *J Am Coll Cardiol*. 2015;65(13):1340–1360. doi:10.1016/j.jacc.2015.01.049

14. Tornkvist M, Smith JG, Labaf A. Current evidence of oral anticoagulant reversal: a systematic review. *Thromb Res*. 2018;162:22–31. doi:10.1016/j.thromres.2017.12.003

15. Lopez-Lopez JA, Sterne JAC, Thom HHZ, et al. Oral anticoagulants for prevention of stroke in atrial fibrillation: Systematic review, network meta-analysis, and cost effectiveness analysis. *BMJ*. 2017;359:j5058. doi:10.1136/bmj.j5058

16. Chai-Adisaksopha C, Hillis C, Isayama T, et al. Mortality outcomes in patients receiving direct oral anticoagulants: A systematic review and meta-analysis of randomized controlled trials. *J Thromb Haemost*. 2015;13(11):2012–2020. doi:10.1111/jth.13139

17. Makam RCP, Hoaglin DC, McManus DD, et al. Efficacy and safety of direct oral anticoagulants approved for cardiovascular indications: systematic review and meta-analysis. *PLoS One*. 2018;13(5):e0197583. doi:10.1371/journal.pone.0197583

18. Shaw JR, Siegal DM. Pharmacological reversal of the direct oral anticoagulants—a comprehensive review of the literature. *Res Pract Thromb Haemost*. 2018;2(2):251–265. doi:10.1002/rth2.12089

19. Eerenberg ES, Kamphuisen PW, Sijpkens MK, et al. Reversal of rivaroxaban and dabigatran by prothrombin complex concentrate: a randomized, placebo-controlled, crossover study in healthy subjects. *Circulation.* 2011;124(14):1573–1579. doi:10.1161/CIRCULATIONAHA.111.029017

20. Dentali F, Marchesi C, Giorgi Pierfranceschi M, et al. Safety of prothrombin complex concentrates for rapid anticoagulation reversal of vitamin K antagonists. A meta-analysis. *Thromb Haemost.* 2011;106(3):429–438. doi:10.1160/TH11-01-0052

21. Christos S, Naples R. Anticoagulation reversal and treatment strategies in major bleeding: update 2016. *West J Emerg Med.* 2016;17(3):264–270. doi:10.5811/westjem.2016.3.29294

22. Davi G, Patrono C. Platelet activation and atherothrombosis. *N Engl J Med.* 2007;357(24):2482–2494. doi:10.1056/NEJMra071014

23. Wallentin L. P2Y12 inhibitors: Differences in properties and mechanisms of action and potential consequences for clinical use. *European Heart Journal.* 2009;30(16):1964–1977. doi:10.1093/eurheartj/ehp296

24. Desager JP. Clinical pharmacokinetics of ticlopidine. *Clin Pharmacokinet.* 1994;26(5):347–355. doi:10.2165/00003088-199426050-00003

25. Flores-Runk P, Raasch RH. Ticlopidine and antiplatelet therapy. *Ann Pharmacother.* 1993;27(9):1090–1098. doi:10.1177/106002809302700915

26. Pelliccia F, Rollini F, Marazzi G, et al. Drug-drug interactions between clopidogrel and novel cardiovascular drugs. *Eur J Pharmacol.* 2015;765:332–336. doi:10.1016/j.ejphar.2015.08.059

27. Przespolewski ER, Westphal ES, Rainka M, et al. Evaluating the effect of six proton pump inhibitors on the antiplatelet effects of clopidogrel. *J Stroke Cerebrovasc Dis.* 2018;27(6):1582–1589. doi:10.1016/j.jstrokecerebrovasdis.2018.01.011

28. Trenk D, Hochholzer W. Genetics of platelet inhibitor treatment. *Br J Clin Pharmacol.* 2014;77(4):642–653. doi:10.1111/bcp.12230

29. Jackson LR, Peterson ED, McCoy LA, et al. Impact of proton pump inhibitor use on the comparative effectiveness and safety of prasugrel versus clopidogrel: Insights from the treatment with adenosine diphosphate receptor inhibitors: Longitudinal assessment of treatment patterns and events after acute coronary syndrome (TRANSLATE-ACS) study. *J Am Heart Assoc.* 2016;5(10): e003824. doi:10.1161/JAHA.116.003824

30. Siller-Matula J, Trenk D, Krähenbühl S, et al. Clinical implications of drug–drug interactions with P2Y12 receptor inhibitors. *J Thromb Haemost.* 2014;12(1):2–13. doi:10.1111/jth.12445

31. Dobesh PP, Oestreich JH. Ticagrelor: Pharmacokinetics, pharmacodynamics, clinical efficacy, and safety. *Pharmacotherapy.* 2014;34(10):1077–1090. doi:10.1002/phar.1477

32. Bhatt DL, Lincoff AM, Gibson CM, et al. Intravenous platelet blockade with cangrelor during PCI. *N Engl J Med.* 2009;361(24):2330–2341. doi:10.1056/NEJMoa0908629

33. Storey RF. Pharmacology and clinical trials of reversibly-binding P2Y12 inhibitors. *Thromb Haemost.* 2011;105(Suppl 1):S75–881. doi:10.1160/THS10-12-0769

34. Armstrong D, Summers C, Ewart L, et al. Characterization of the adenosine pharmacology of ticagrelor reveals therapeutically relevant inhibition of equilibrative nucleoside transporter 1. *J Cardiovasc Pharmacol Ther.* 2014;19(2):209–219. doi:10.1177/1074248413511693

35. Bledzka K, Smyth SS, Plow EF. Integrin $\alpha IIb\beta 3$: From discovery to efficacious therapeutic target. *Circ Res.* 2013;112(8):1189–1200. doi:10.1161/CIRCRESAHA.112.300570

36. Wang B, Ludden TM, Cheung EN, et al. Population pharmacokinetic-pharmacodynamic modeling of filgrastim (r-metHuG-CSF) in healthy volunteers. *J Pharmacokinet Pharmacodyn.* 2001;28(4):321–342. doi:10.1023/A:1011534529622

37. Wiczling P, Lowe P, Pigeolet E, et al. Population pharmacokinetic modelling of filgrastim in healthy adults following intravenous and subcutaneous administrations. *Clin Pharmacokinet.* 2009;48(12):817–826. doi:10.2165/11318090-000000000-00000

38. Yao D, Janakiram M, O'Brien TE. Pegfilgrastim use and risk of bleomycin induced pulmonary toxicity in hodgkin lymphoma. *Blood.* 2016;128(22):5350.

39. Martin WG, Ristow KM, Habermann TM, et al. Bleomycin pulmonary toxicity has a negative impact on the outcome of patients with hodgkin's lymphoma. *J Clin Oncol.* 2005;23(30):7614–7620. doi:10.1200/JCO.2005.02.7243

40. Lyman GH, Allcott K, Garcia J, et al. The effectiveness and safety of same-day versus next-day administration of long-acting granulocyte colony-stimulating factors for the prophylaxis of chemotherapy-induced neutropenia: a systematic review. *Support Care Cancer.* 2017;25(8):2619–2629. doi:10.1007/s00520-017-3703-y

41. Egrie JC, Browne JK. Development and characterization of novel erythropoiesis stimulating protein (NESP). *Nephrol Dial Transplant.* 2001;16(Suppl 3):3–13. doi:10.1093/ndt/16.suppl_3.3

42. Allon M, Kleinman K, Walczyk M, et al. Pharmacokinetics and pharmacodynamics of darbepoetin alfa and epoetin in patients undergoing dialysis. *Clin Pharmacol Ther*. 2002;72(5):546–555. doi:10.1067/mcp.2002.128374

43. National Comprehensive Cancer Network. Cancer- and chemotherapy-induced anemia. 2018. https://www.nccn.org/profes sionals/physician_gls/pdf/anemia.pdf

44. United States Food and Drug Administration. Information on erythropoiesis-stimulating agents (ESA) epoetin alfa (marketed as Procrit, Epogen), darbepoetin alfa (marketed as Aranesp). 2018. https://www.fda.gov/Drugs/DrugSafety/ucm109375.htm

45. Li J, Yang C, Xia Y, et al. Thrombocytopenia caused by the development of antibodies to thrombopoietin. *Blood*. 2001;98(12):3241–3248. doi:10.1182/blood.v98.12.3241

46. Al-Samkari H, Kuter DJ. Optimal use of thrombopoietin receptor agonists in immune thrombocytopenia. *Ther Adv Hematol*. 2019;10:2040620719841735. doi:10.1177/2040620719841735

47. Lam MS. Review article: Second-generation thrombopoietin agents for treatment of chronic idiopathic thrombocytopenic purpura in adults. *J Oncol Pharm Pract*. 2010;16(2):89–103. doi:10.1177/1078155209337668

48. Vlachodimitropoulou E, Chen YL, Garbowski M, et al. Eltrombopag: a powerful chelator of cellular or extracellular iron(III) alone or combined with a second chelator. *Blood*. 2017;130(17):1923–1933. doi:10.1182/blood-2016-10-740241

49. Baluom M, Grossbard EB, Mant T, Lau DT. Pharmacokinetics of fostamatinib, a spleen tyrosine kinase (SYK) inhibitor, in healthy human subjects following single and multiple oral dosing in three phase I studies. *Br J Clin Pharmacol*. 2013;76(1):78–88. doi:10.1111/bcp.12048

Index